DORLAND'S

Immunology/ Endocrinology

WORD BOOK

for Medical

Transcriptionists

DORLAND'S

Immunology/ Endocrinology WORD BOOK

for Medical Transcriptionists

Series
Editor: SHARON B. RHODES, CMT, RHIT

Edited &
Reviewed by: SUSAN PIERCE, CMT, RHIT

W.B. SAUNDERS COMPANY
A Harcourt Health Sciences Company

Philadelphia London New York St. Louis Sydney Toronto

W.B. Saunders Company
A Harcourt Health Sciences Company

The Curtis Center
Independence Square West
Philadelphia, Pennsylvania 19106

Library of Congress Cataloging-in-Publication Data

Dorland's immunology/endocrinology word book for medical transcriptionists /
Sharon B. Rhodes, editor; edited & reviewed by Susan Pierce.

p. cm.

ISBN 0-7216-9392-X

1. Immunology—Terminology. 2. Endocrinology—Terminology. 3. Medical
   transcription. I. Rhodes, Sharon B. II. Pierce, Susan K.

QR180.4.D67 2002

616.07′9′014—dc21   2001034184

Dorland's Immunology and Endocrinology Word Book for
Medical Transcriptionists   ISBN 0-7216-9392-X

I am proud to present the *Dorland's Immunology/Endocrinology Word Book for Medical Transcriptionists*—one of the ongoing series of word books being compiled for the professional medical transcriptionist. For over one hundred years, W.B. Saunders has published the *Dorland's Illustrated Medical Dictionary*. With the advent of medical transcription, it became the dictionary of choice for medical transcriptionists.

When I was approached in the fall of 1999 to help develop a new series of word books for W.B. Saunders, I have to admit the thought absolutely overwhelmed me. The *Dorland's Illustrated Medical Dictionary* was one of my first book purchases when I began my transcription career over thirty years ago. To be invited to participate in this project is an honor I could never have imagined for myself!

Transcriptionists need and will continue to need trusted up-to-date resources to help them research difficult terms quickly. In developing the *Dorland's Immunology and Endocrinology Word Book/Medical Transcriptionists*, I had access to the entire *Dorland's* terminology database for the book's foundation. In addition to this immense database, a context editor, Susan Pierce, CMT, RHIT, a recognized expert in the field of immunology and endocrinology transcription, was selected to review the material from the database, to contribute new and unique terms, and to remove outdated and obsolete ones. With Susan's extensive research and diligent work, I believe this to be the most up-to-date word book for the field of immunology and endocrinology.

In developing the immunology and endocrinology word book, I wanted the size to be manageable so the book would be easy to handle, provide a durable long-lasting binding, and use a type font large enough to read while providing extensive terminology.

Anatomical plates were added as well as identification of anatomical landmarks in the body. Additionally, a list of the most frequently prescribed drugs has been included.

Although I have tried to produce the most thorough word book for immunology and endocrinology available to medical transcriptionists, it is difficult to include every term as the field of medicine is constantly evolving. As you discover new terms, please feel free to share them with me for inclusion in the next edition of *the Dorland's Immunology/Endocrinology Word Book for Medical Transcriptionists.*

I may be reached at the following e-mail address: Sharon@TheRhodes.com

SHARON B. RHODES, CMT, RHIT
Brentwood, Tennessee

A
A cell
surfactant protein A

α
α-adrenergic blocker
α-globulins
α heavy chain
α heavy chain disease
α-methyldopa blocker

α_2
α.-globulin

Ab
antibody

abacavir sulfate

Abadie's sign

ABC
ATP-binding cassette
ABC proteins

aberrant
a. goiter
a. thyroids
a. tissue

ablastin

abnormal hormone

abnormality
growth a's
autosomal a's
perceptual a's
potential a. of glucose tolerance
previous a. of glucose tolerance

ABO
ABO blood group
ABO blood group antigens
ABO blood group system
ABO typing

abortion
chemical a.
clonal a.
surgical a.

abrin

abruptio placentae

abscess
brain a.
helminthic a.
metastatic tuberculous a.
verminous a.
worm a.

Absettarov virus

absolute lymphocyte count

absorptiometry
dual-photon a.
photon a.

absorption
agglutinin a.
calcium a.
a. method
sodium a.

absorptive hypercalciuria

abuse
sexual a.

ACAID
anterior chamber–associated immune deviation

acanthamebiasis

acanthocephaliasis

acanthocheilonemiasis

acanthosis nigricans

acariasis

acaridiasis

acarinosis

acariosis

acaulinosis

accelerated
a. arteriosclerosis
a. starvation

accelerator
C3b inactivator a.

1

accessory
   a. cells
   a. effector cells
   a. molecules
   a. pancreatic duct
   a. parotid gland
   a. suprarenal glands
   a. thyroids
   a. thyroid glands

accident
   cerebrovascular a. (CVA)

accidental membrane

acclimation
   cold a.

Acel-Imune

A cell

acellular
   a. pertussis vaccine
   a. vaccine

acetonuria

acetylcholine (Ach)
   a. breakdown
   a. exocytosis
   a. receptors
   a. receptor antibodies
   a. synthesis

acetylcholinesterase

acetyl glyceryl ether phos-
   phoryl choline

Achard-Thiers syndrome

Achilles
   A. reflex time
   A. tendon reflex time

achlorhydria

acid
   a. agglutination
   amino a.
   p-aminosalicylic a.
   bile a.
   hyaluronic a.
   a.-lability test

acid *(continued)*
   nicotinic a.
   palmitic a.
   para-aminosalicylic a.
   phosphotungstic a.
   sialic a.
   teichoic a.
   vanillylmandelic a. (VMA)

acidophil
   alpha a.
   epsilon a.
   a. granules
   a. stem-cell adenoma

acidophile

acidophilic adenoma

acidosis
   diabetic a.
   lactic a.
   metabolic a.
   renal tubular a.

aciduria

Acinetobacter
   A. anitratus
   A. calcoaceticus
   A. lwoffi

acinus *pl.* acini
   thyroid acini

acladiosis

acne

acquired
   a. agammaglobulinemia
   a. antigen
   a. cytomegalovirus
   a. hypogammaglobulinemia
   a. immune deficiency syn-
      drome (AIDS)
   a. immunity
   a. immunodeficiency
   a. immunodeficiency syn-
      drome (AIDS)
   a. neutropenia
   a. resistance
   a. specific immunity
   a. tolerance

acremoniosis

acrodermatitis
a. chronica atrophicans

acromegalia

acromegalic
a. gigantism

acromegalogigantism

acromegaloidism

acromegaly
eosinophil tumor with a.

acromicria

acro-osteolysis syndrome

acroparesthesia

ACTH
adrenocorticotropic hor-
mone
ACTH reserve
ACTH-secreting ade-
noma

actin

actinobacillosis

actinomycin D

actinomycoma

actinomycosis

actinomycotic
a. mycetoma

actinophage

actinophytosis

action
angiotensin a.
autocrine a.
corticotropin-releasing factor a.
paracrine a.
a. potential

activated
a. 7-dehydrocholesterol
a. lymphocyte
a. macrophages

activated *(continued)*
a. mast cells
a. partial thromboplastin
time (APTT)

activation
B cell a.
complement a.
cytotoxic a.
a.-induced cell death
(AICD)
kinin a.
lymphocyte a.
a. phase
polyclonal a.
steroid-site a.
T cell a.
transcription a.
transcriptional a.

activator
plasminogen a.
polyclonal a.
signal transducers and a's
of transcription (STAT)
a. surfaces
transcription a.

active
a. anaphylaxis
a. cutaneous anaphylaxis
a. domains
a. immunity
a. immunization
a. serum
a. vaccination
a. zones

activin

activity
aggressin a.
anaphylatoxin a.
antibody a.
antigen-bound phagocyte a.
assays of a.
endonuclease a.
macrophage pinocytotic a.
multiplication-stimulat-
ing a.
nonsuppressible insulin-
like a.

activity *(continued)*
  opsonic a.
  physical a.
  pinocytic a.
  plasma renin a. (PRA)
  protease a.
  reverse transcriptase a.
  transcriptional a.

acute
  a. anterior poliomyelitis
  a. articular rheumatism
  a. cellular rejection
  a. early rejection
  a. glomerulonephritis
  a. hyperphosphatemia
  a. idiopathic polyneuritis
  a. infectious lymphocytosis
  a. inflammatory response
  a. laryngotracheobronchi-
    tis virus
  a. lateral poliomyelitis
  a. late rejection
  a. lymphoblastic leukemia
    (ALL)
  a. lymphocytic leukemia
    (ALL)
  a. phase plasma proteins
  a. phase proteins
  a. phase reactants
  a. phase response
  a. posterior ganglionitis
  a. pseudomembranous can-
    didiasis
  a. pyogenic thyroiditis
  a. rejection
  a. suppurative thyroiditis

acylcarnitine

acyltransferase
  lecithin–cholesterol a.
    (LCAT)

ADA
  adenosine deaminase
    ADA deficiency

adamantinoma
  pituitary a.

adansonian classification

adaptive
  a. hormone
  a. immune response
  a. immunity

ADCC
  antibody-dependent cell-
    mediated cytotoxicity
  antibody-dependent cellu-
    lar cytotoxicity

addiction
  food a.

Addison's disease

addisonian
  a. crisis
  a. syndrome

addition
  haptenic a.

addressin
  mucinlike vascular a's
  vascular a's

Aden fever

adenine

adeno-associated virus

adenocarcinoma
  follicular a.
  mucinous a.
  papillary a.
  polypoid a.

adenocyte

adenohypophyseal

adenohypophysectomy

adenohypophysial
  a. hormones

adenohypophysis

adenoids

adenolipoma

adenoma
  acidophilic a.
  acidophil stem-cell a.

adenoma *(continued)*
ACTH-secreting a.
a. of the adrenal cortex
adrenocortical a.
adrenocorticotropic hor-
mone–secreting a.
aldosterone-producing a.
aldosterone-secreting a.
alpha subunit a.
basophil a.
basophilic a.
bronchial a.
chief cell a.
chromophobe a.
chromophobic a.
colloid a.
corticotrope a.
corticotrope cell a.
corticotroph a.
corticotroph cell a.
cortisol-producing a.
embryonal a.
endocrine-active a.
endocrine-inactive a.
eosinophil a.
eosinophilic a.
fetal a.
follicular a.
functional a.
functioning a.
glycoprotein a.
glycoprotein hormone a.
gonadotrope a.
gonadotroph a.
gonadotroph cell a.
growth hormone cell a.
growth hormone–secret-
ing a.
Hürthle cell a.
hyperfunctional a.
hyperfunctioning a.
islet cell a.
lactotrope a.
lactotroph a.
langerhansian a.
macrofollicular a.
mammosomatotroph a.
microfollicular a.
mixed-cell a.

adenoma *(continued)*
mixed somatotroph-lacto-
troph a.
multiple a.
nonfunctional a.
nonfunctioning a.
nonsecreting a.
nonsecretory a.
null-cell a.
oncocytic a.
oxyphilic a.
oxyphilic granular cell a.
papillary cystic a.
parathyroid a.
parathyroid a. of thymus
pituitary a.
plurihormonal a.
prolactin cell a.
prolactin-secreting a.
pseudomucinous cyst a.
renal a.
somatotrope a.
somatotroph a.
thyroid a.
thyroid-stimulating hor-
mone–secreting a.
thyrotrope a.
thyrotroph a.
thyrotroph cell a.
toxic a.
trabecular a.
TSH-secreting a.

adenomatosis
endocrine a.
familial multiple endo-
crine a.
multiple endocrine a.
(MEA)
pluriglandular a.
polyendocrine a.
type I multiple endocrine a.
type IIA multiple endo-
crine a.
type IIB multiple endo-
crine a.

adenomatous
a. goiter
a. hyperplasia

adenomectomy

adenomyoma

adenopathy
inguinal a.
regional a.

adenosine
cyclic a. monophosphate
(cyclic AMP)
a. deaminase (ADA)
a. deaminase deficiency

adenoviral

Adenoviridae

adenovirus
a. infection
mammalian a's
a. multiplication
a. virion

adenylate cyclase

adenyl cyclase

adenylyl cyclase

ADH
antidiuretic hormone

adherence
immune a.
opsonic a.

adherent cells

adherin

adhesion
a. molecules

adiaspiromycosis

adiasporosis

adipocyte hyperplasia

adipokinetic
a. hormone

adipokinin

adipose
a. cells
a. genital dystrophy

adipose *(continued)*
a. tissue

adiposis
a. cerebralis

adiposity
cerebral a.
pituitary a.

adiposogenital
a. degeneration
a. dystrophy
a. syndrome

adjunctive
a. therapy

Adjuvant 65

adjuvant
aluminum a.
bacterial a.
Freund's a.
mycobacterial a.

adjuvanticity

administration
nasal a.

adolescent
a. growth
a. growth spurt
a. gynecomastia
a. thyrotoxicosis

adoptive
a. cellular immunotherapy
a. immunity
a. immunization
a. immunotherapy
a. tolerance
a. transfer

adrenal
accessory a. glands
a. androgens
a. body
a. capsule
congenital a. hyperplasia
a. control
a. cortex
a. cortical hyperplasia

adrenal *(continued)*
    a. cortical steroid
    a. crisis
    a. dysfunction
    ectopic a. tissue
    a. estrogen
    fetal a. cortex
    a. gland
    a. hormone
    a. hyperplasia
    a. hypertension
    a. hypofunction
    a. hypoplasia
    a. insufficiency
    a. line
    lipoid a. hyperplasia
    a. medulla
    a. medullary function
    a. neuroblastoma
    nodular a. hyperplasia
    a. pheochromocytoma
    pituitary-a. suppression
    primary a. insufficiency
    a. pseudocyst
    a. reserve
    a. response
    a. rest
    a. rest tumor
    secondary a. insufficiency
    a. steroid inhibition
    a. tumor
    a. virilism

adrenalectomize

adrenalectomy

Adrenalin (epinephrine)

adrenaline (*same as* epineph-
    rine)
    a. release
    a. secretion
    a. synthesis

adrenalism

adrenalitis
    autoimmune a.
    infectious a.

adrenalopathy

adrenalotropic

adrenarche
    premature a.

adrenergic
    α-a.
    β-a.
    a. nervous system
    a. pathways
    a. receptors

adrenic

adrenitis

adrenoceptor

adrenocortical
    acute a. insufficiency
    a. adenoma
    a. carcinoma
    chronic a. insufficiency
    familial a. insufficiency
    a. function
    a. hormone
    a. hyperplasia
    a. hypersecretion
    a. insufficiency
    primary a. insufficiency
    a. reserve
    secondary a. insufficiency
    a. steroid
    a. tumor

adrenocorticohyperplasia

adrenocorticoid

adrenocorticomimetic

adrenocorticotrophic
    a. hormone (ACTH)

adrenocorticotrophin

adrenocorticotropic
    a. hormone (ACTH)
    a. hormone infusion test
    a. hormone reserve
    a. hormone–secreting ade-
        noma
    a. hormone secretion
    short a. hormone test

adrenocorticotropin

adrenodoxin

adrenogenic
    a. tissue

adrenogenital
    a. syndrome

adrenogenous

adrenokinetic

adrenoleukodystrophy

adrenolytic tests

adrenomedullary
    a. hormones
    a. opioids
    a. triad

adrenomedullotropic

adrenomegaly

adrenopathy

adrenoprival

adrenoreceptor

adrenostatic

adrenosterone

adrenotrophic

adrenotrophin

adrenotropic

adrenotropin

adsorption
    agglutinin a.
    immune a.

adult
    a. hypothyroidism
    a. stature prediction
    a. T cell leukemia
    a. T cell lymphoma

adult-onset
    a.-o. diabetes mellitus
    a.-o. obesity

advanced glycation end products

adynamic ileus

Aedes

AFC
    antibody-forming cell

afferent
    a. lymphatic duct
    a. lymph vessels

affinity
    antibody a.
    a. chromatography
    a. labeling of receptors
    a. maturation
    a. model
    receptor a.
    secondary antibody a.

AFLP
    amplification fragment length polymorphism

AFP
    alpha fetoprotein

African
    A. histoplasmosis
    A. horse sickness virus
    A. swine fever virus
    A. tick fever
    A. trypanosomiasis

Ag
    antigen

agammaglobulinemia
    acquired a.
    Bruton's a.
    Bruton-type agammaglobulinemia
    Bruton's X-linked a.
    common variable a.
    a. infections
    malignant Swiss-type a.
    Swiss-type a.
    X-linked a. (XLA)

agammaglobulinemia *(continued)*
   X-linked infantile a.

agar
   a. gel
   a. gel diffusion test

agarose
   a. gel electrophoresis

age
   bone a.
   maternal a.
   skeletal a.

agenesis
   gonadal a.
   Leydig cell a.
   müllerian a.
   ovarian a.
   testicular a.

agenitalism

agent
   anti-inflammatory a.
   antineoplastic a.
   antiserotonin a.
   antithyroid a's
   cholecystographic a's
   cytotoxic a.
   cytotoxic chemotherapeutic
    immunosuppressive a's
   delta a.
   hypoglycemic a.
   immunosuppressive a.
   infectious a.
   microbial a's
   progestational a.
   spermicidal a.

age-related
   a.-r. aneuploidy
   a.-r. aspects
   a.-r. osteoporosis

agglutinable

agglutination
   acid a.
   bacteriogenic a.
   cold a.
   cross a.

agglutination *(continued)*
   direct a.
   direct bacterial a.
   enhancing a.
   group a.
   H a.
   indirect a.
   a. inhibition
   latex a.
   O a.
   particle a.
   passive a.
   passive latex a.
   platelet a.
   rapid latex a.
   reverse passive a.
   salt a.
   sheep cell a.
   a. test
   a. titer
   Vi a.

agglutinative

agglutinator

agglutinin
   a. absorption
   a. adsorption
   anti-Rh a.
   chief a.
   cold a.
   complete a.
   cross a.
   cross-reacting a.
   febrile a's
   flagellar a.
   group a.
   H a.
   immune a.
   incomplete a.
   leukocyte a.
   major a.
   MG a.
   minor a.
   O a.
   partial a.
   platelet a.
   saline a.
   somatic a.

agglutinin *(continued)*
    streptococcus MG a.
    T a.
    warm a.

agglutinogen
    Bordetella pertussis a.

agglutinogenic

agglutinophilic

agglutogenic

aggregate anaphylaxis

aggregation

aggrephore

aggressin
    a. activity

aging
    a. ovary

α-globulins

α_2-globulin

aglycemia

agonad

agonadal

agonadism
    XY a.

agonist
    dopamine a's
    a. peptide
    peptide a.

agranular leukocyte

agranulocytosis

agretope

agricultural anthrax

Agrostis

AGT
    antiglobulin test

α heavy chain
    α h. c. disease

AHG
    antihuman globulin
        AHG test

AHO
    Albright hereditary osteo-
        dystrophy

AI
    anaphylatoxin inactivator

AICD
    activation-induced cell
        death

AIDS
    acquired immunodeficiency
        syndrome
        AIDS-related complex
           (ARC)

AIHA
    autoimmune hemolytic
        anemia

AILD
    angioimmunoblastic lym-
        phadenopathy with dys-
        proteinemia

airborne
    a. infection

Akabane virus

akamushi disease

akiyami

AL
    AL amyloidosis
    AL test

alanine aminotransferase (ALT)

alarm reaction

alastrim

Albers-Schönberg syndrome

Albright
    A. disease
    A. hereditary osteodystro-
        phy (AHO)

albumin
  bovine serum a. (BSA)
  a. index

albuminuria

Alcaligenes
  A. denitrificans
  A. faecalis
  A. odorans

alcoholism

aldosterone
  a. escape
  a. function
  a.-producing adenoma
  a.-producing carcinoma
  a.-producing tumor
  a.-secreting adenoma
  a.-secreting carcinoma
  a.-secreting tumor
  a. synthesis

aldosteronism
  primary a.
  pseudoprimary a.
  secondary a.

aldosteronogenesis

aldosteronoma

aldosteronopenia

aldosteronuria

Aldrich's syndrome

Aleutian mink disease virus

alexin

aleydigism

ALG
  antilymphocyte globulin

alimentary
  a. glycosuria
  a. hypoglycemia
  a. system

alkali
  sodium a.

alkaline phosphatase

alkalosis

ALL
  acute lymphoblastic leukemia
  acute lymphocytic leukemia

allele

allelic exclusion

Allen
  A.-Doisy test
  A.-Doisy unit

allergen
  ingested a.
  inhaled a.
  pollen a.

allergenic
  a. extract

allergic
  a. aspergillosis
  a. bronchopulmonary as-
  pergillosis
  a. conjunctivitis
  a. disease
  a. encephalomyelitis
  a. gastroenteropathy
  a. granulomatosis
  a. granulomatous angiitis
  a. neuritis
  nonseasonal a. rhinitis
  a. reaction
  a. rhinitis
  seasonal a. rhinitis
  a. vasculitis

allergist

allergization

allergize

allergoid

allergological

allergologist

allergology

allergosis

allergy
    anaphylactic a.
    atopic a.
    bacterial a.
    cold a.
    delayed a.
    drug a.
    food a.
    gastrointestinal a.
    hereditary a.
    immediate a.
    industrial a.
    latent a.
    papain a.
    penicillin a.
    physical a.
    pollen a.
    polyvalent a.
    spontaneous a.
    a. treatment
    vomiting in a's

allescheriasis

allescheriosis

alloantibody

alloantigen

alloantisera

alloantiserum

allogeneic
    a. antigen
    a. disease
    a. effect factor (AEF)
    a. fetus
    a. graft
    a. individuals
    a. MHC molecules
    a. mixed leukocyte reaction
    a. recognition
    a. transfusion
    a. transplantation

allogenic
    a. inhibition

allograft
    a. immunity
    a. reaction

allogroup

alloimmune

alloimmunization

allopregnane

allopregnanediol

allopurinol

alloreactive
    a. antibodies
    a. T lymphocytes

alloreactivity

allosensitization

allosteric effect

allotope

allotransplantation

allotype
    Am a's
    Gm a's
    Inv a's
    Km a's
    Oz a.

allotypic
    a. determinant
    a. group
    a. markers
    a. variation

allotypy

alloxan
    a. diabetes

alloxantin

Almeida's disease

alopecia
    temporal a.

alpha (α)
    a. acidophil

alpha *(continued)*
    a. beta T cell receptors
    a. blockade
    a. cell
    a. chain disease
    a. chain marker
    a. fetoprotein (AFP)
    a. globulins
    a. granules
    a. heavy chain disease
    a. hemolysin
    a. interferon
    a. macroglobulin
    a. receptors
    a. staphylolysin
    a. subunit
    a. subunit adenoma

$alpha_1$-antitrypsin

Alphaherpesvirinae

$alpha_2$-macroglobulin

Alphavirus

alphavirus

alprostadil

ALS (antilymphocyte serum)

Alström syndrome

ALT
    alanine aminotransferase

altered
    a. appetite
    a. ligand hypothesis
    a. peptide ligands
    a. self hypothesis

Alternaria

alternariosis

alternative
    a. pathway
    a. complement pathway

alum

aluminum
    a. adjuvant

aluminum *(continued)*
    a. hydrate
    a. hydroxide
    a. phosphate
    a. precipitation

alveolar
    a. hydatid disease
    a. macrophages

alveolitis
    extrinsic allergic a.

alymphocytosis

alymphoplasia
    thymic a.

Am
    alpha chain marker
        Am allotypes
        Am antigens
        Am factor

Amapari virus

amaurosis
    diabetic a.

ambiguous genitalia

ambisexual
    a. development

amboceptor
    a. unit

ambosexual

Ambrosia

ambrosterol

amebiasis
    a. cutis
    pulmonary a.

amebic
    a. granuloma
    a. meningoencephalitis
    a. pericarditis
    a. pneumonia

amebiosis

amebism

amebocyte
    phagocytic a.
ameloblastoma
    pituitary a.
amenorrhea
    chronic a.
    hypothalamic a.
    ovarian a.
    pituitary a.
    primary a.
    psychogenic a.
    secondary a.

American trypanosomiasis

AMH
    antimüllerian hormone
amine
    a. precursor uptake and de-
        carboxylation (APUD)
        cells
    biogenic a.
    sympathomimetic a's
    vasoactive a's

aminergic nervous system

amino acid
    a. a. analysis
    a. a.–induced hypoglyce-
        mia
    a. a. sequence

γ-aminobutyric acid

amino-chlorohydrin

aminoglutethimide

aminoheterocyclic compound

p-aminosalicylic acid

amniocentesis

amphibolic
    a. stage

amphigonadism

amphipathic helix

amphiregulin

amphistomiasis

amplification
    DNA a.
    a. fragment
    a. fragment length
    a. fragment length poly-
        morphism (AFLP)
    a. loop
    a. via phosphorylation

amplifier T lymphocyte

ampulla

amygdala

amylin

amyloid
    a. protein
    serum a. protein

amyloidosis
    AL a.
    cutaneous lichen a.
    immunocyte-derived a.
    immunocytic a.
    lichen a.
    light chain–related a.
    primary a.

amyloid transthyretin

amyotrophy

ANA
    antinuclear antibodies

anabolic
    a. steroid

anabolism

anadrenalism

anadrenia

anaerobic metabolism

analgesic
    narcotic a's
    a. nephropathy

anallergic

analogue (*spelled also* analog)
    folic acid a.

analogue *(continued)*
   purine a.
   pyrimidine a.

analysis *pl.* analyses
   amino acid a.
   clonal a.
   immunoprecipitation a.
   Scatchard a.
   ultracentrifugal a.
   Western blot a.

anamnesis

anamnestic
   amnestic antibody response
   a. reaction
   a. response

anaphylactic
   a. allergy
   a. antibody
   a. conjunctivitis
   a. hypersensitivity
   a. keratitis
   a. reaction
   a. rhinitis
   a. shock
   a.-type sensitivity

anaphylactogen

anaphylactogenesis

anaphylactogenic

anaphylactoid
   a. crisis
   a. reaction
   a. shock

anaphylatoxin
   a. II
   a. activity
   a. inactivator (AI)
   a. inhibitor

anaphylaxis
   active a.
   active cutaneous a.
   aggregate a.
   antiserum a.

anaphylaxis *(continued)*
   cutaneous a.
   cytotoxic a.
   cytotrophic a.
   generalized a.
   inverse a.
   local a.
   passive a.
   passive cutaneous a. (PCA)
   reverse a.
   slow-reacting substance of a. (SRS-A)
   systemic a.

anaphylotoxin

anaplastic
   a. carcinoma of thyroid gland
   a. thyroid carcinoma

anatoxic

anatoxin
   diphtheria a.
   a.-Ramon

ANCA
   antineutrophil cytoplasmic autoantibody

anchorage dependence

anchored messengers

anchor residue
   peptide a. r's

ancylostomiasis

Anderson's disease

androgalactozemia

androgen
   adrenal a's
   complete a. resistance
   a. deficiency
   a. effects
   fetal a.
   incomplete a. resistance
   a. insensitivity
   a. insensitivity syndrome
   maternal a.
   a. metabolism

androgen *(continued)*
  ovarian a.
  a. plasma levels
  a. production rates
  a. receptors
  a. replacement therapy
  a. resistance
  a. secretion
  urinary a.

androgenic
  a. hormone
  a. zone

androgenicity

androgenization
  fetal a.

androgenized

androgyne

androgynism

androgynoid

androgynous

androgyny

android
  a. obesity

androidal

andromimetic

andromorphous

andropathy

andropause

androstane

androstanediol
  a. glucuronide

androstene

androstenediol

androstenedione
  a. hormone

androsterone

anemia
  aplastic a.

anemia *(continued)*
  autoimmune hemolytic a.
   (AIHA)
  Bartonella a.
  drug-induced hemolytic a.
  drug-induced immune he-
   molytic a.
  ground itch a.
  hemolytic a.
  hemolytic autoimmune a.
  hookworm a.
  hypochromic a.
  immune hemolytic a.
  immunohemolytic a.
  infectious hemolytic a.
  miners' a.
  normocytic normochrom-
   ic a.
  pernicious a.
  refractory a.
  sickle cell a.
  warm autoimmune hemo-
   lytic a. (WAIHA)

anergia

anergic

anergy
  clonal a.
  negative a.
  positive a.

aneuploidy
  age-related a.

ANF
  antinuclear factor
  atrial natriuretic factor

angiitis *pl.* angiitides
  allergic granulomatous a.
  hypersensitivity a.
  leukocytoclastic a.
  necrotizing a.

angina
  herpes a.
  a. herpetica

angiocrine

angiocrinosis

angioedema

angiogenesis
    a. factor

angioimmunoblastic
    a. lymphadenopathy
    a. lymphadenopathy with
        dysproteinemia (AILD)

angiomatosis
    bacillary a.

angioneurotic edema

angiostrongyliasis

angiostrongylosis

angiotensin
    a. I
    a. II
    a. III
    a. action
    a. amide
    a. receptors

angiotensin-converting enzyme

angiotensinogen

angiotonin

anglicus sudor

angry back

anhydrohydroxyprogesterone

anicteric
    a. hepatitis
    a. leptospirosis

animal
    congenic a's
    Houssay a.
    knockout a.
    sensitized a.
    transgenic a.

anion
    superoxide a.

anisakiasis

anisomycin (ANM)

ankylosing spondylitis

ankylostomiasis

anlage
    thymic a.

ANM
    anisomycin

ANN
    artificial neural network

annexin

annular
    a. tubule
    a. tubule tumor

anomaly
    chromosome a's

Anopheles
    A. A virus
    A. B virus

anorchia
    congenital a.

anorexia
    a. nervosa
    a. treatment

anosmia

anovulation
    chronic a.

antagonism
    steroid hormone a.

antagonist
    calmodulin a's
    insulin a's
    a. peptide
    progesterone a.

antenatal

antepyretic

anterior
    a. border of body of pan-
        creas
    a. border of pancreas

anterior *(continued)*
    a. chamber–associated immune deviation (ACAID)
    a. lobe
    a. lobe of hypophysis
    a. lobe of pituitary gland
    a. pituitary
    a. pituitary hormones
    a. poliomyelitis
    a. surface of adrenal gland
    a. surface of pancreas
    a. surface of suprarenal gland

anterosuperior surface of body of pancreas

Anthoxium

anthracic

anthracoid

anthrax
    agricultural a.
    cerebral a.
    cutaneous a.
    gastrointestinal a.
    inhalational a.
    intestinal a.
    malignant a.
    meningeal a.
    pulmonary a.
    a. vaccine

anthropophilic

anthropozoophilic

anti–acetylcholine receptor (anti-AChR) antibodies

anti-AChR
    anti–acetylcholine receptor
        anti-AChR antibodies

antiadrenal antibody

anti-β-adrenergic effect

antiagglutinin

anti-allotype
    a.-a. antibody

antianaphylaxis

antiandrogen

antiantibody

antiantitoxin

antiautolysin

antibacterial immunity

antibiotic
    a. resistance

antibody (Ab)
    acetylcholine receptor a's
    a. activity
    a. affinity
    alloreactive a's
    anaphylactic a.
    anti–acetylcholine receptor (anti-AChR) a's
    antiadrenal a.
    anti-allotype a.
    anticardiolipin a.
    anti-CD3 a.
    anti-CD4 a.
    anti-CD18 a.
    anticentromere a.
    anti-cytokine a.
    anti-D a.
    anti-DNA a.
    a.-antigen complex
    anti–glomerular basement membrane (anti-GBM) a's
    anti-hapten a.
    anti-idiotype a.
    anti-idiotypic a.
    anti-IL4 a.
    anti-immunoglobulin a.
    anti-insulin receptor a.
    anti-isotype a.
    anti-La a.
    anti-M a.
    anti-MHC a.
    antimicrosomal a's
    antimitochondrial a's
    antineutrophil a.
    antineutrophil cytoplasmic a.
    antinuclear a's (ANA)
    antiphospholipid a's
    antireceptor a's

antibody *(continued)*
  anti-Rh a.
  anti-Ro a.
  anti–sheep red blood
    cell a.
  anti–SS-A a.
  anti–SS-B a.
  antithyroglobulin a.'s
  antithyroid a.'s
  anti-TNF α a.
  auto–anti-idiotypic a.'s
  autologous a.
  a. avidity
  bacteriolytic a.
  bivalent a.'s
  bispecific a.
  blocking a.
  a. catabolism
  cell-bound a.
  cell-fixed a.
  clonotypic a.'s
  cold a.
  cold-reactive a.
  complement-fixing a.
  complete a.
  cross-reacting a.
  a. cross-reactivity
  cytophilic a.
  cytotoxic a.
  cytotropic a.
  a.-dependent cell-mediated
    cytotoxicity (ADCC)
  a.-dependent cellular cyto-
    toxicity (ADCC)
  detecting a.
  a. detection
  diphtheria a.
  direct fluorescent a.
  a. diversity
  Donath-Landsteiner a.
  duck virus hepatitis yolk a.
  enhancing a.
  a. excess
  febrile a.
  a. feedback
  ferritin conjugated a.
  fluorescent a.
  a. formation
  a.-forming cell (AFC)
  Forssman a.

antibody *(continued)*
  a. function
  fungal a.
  gamma globulin a.'s
  globulin a.'s
  a. half-life
  heteroclitic a.
  heteroconjugate a.
  heterocytotropic a.
  heterogenetic a.
  heterologous a.'s
  heterophil a.
  heterophile a.
  high-affinity a.'s
  HIV a.'s
  homocytotropic a.
  humoral a.
  hybrid a.
  immune a.
  incomplete a.
  indirect fluorescent a. (IFA)
    test
  a. induction
  a. intoxication
  isophil a.
  Ku a.
  maternal a.
  a. measurement
  mitochondrial a.'s
  a. molecule
  monoclonal a. (MAb)
  natural a.'s
  neutralizing a.
  OKT3 monoclonal a.
  opsonizing a.
  panel-reactive a. (PRA)
  passive a.
  P-K (Prausnitz-Küstner) a.'s
  placental transfer a.
  polyclonal a.
  Prausnitz-Küstner (P-K) a.'s
  pre-existing a.
  a. production
  protective a.
  reagin a.
  reaginic a.
  a. repertoire
  a. response
  Rh a.'s

antibody *(continued)*
  saline a.
  secondary a. affinity
  secondary a. interactions
  secondary a. response
  a.-secreting plasma cells
  sensitizing a.
  serum a's
  a. site
  Smith a.
  a. specificity
  sperm-immobilizing a.
  streptococcal a.
  a. synthesis
  thyroid colloidal a's
  a. titer
  toxoplasma a.
  treponemal immobilizing a.
  TSH-displacing a. (TDA)
  TSH receptor a's
  a. variability
  variable a.
  viral a.
  warm a.
  warm-reactive a.
  Wassermann a.
  xenogeneic a's
  xenoreactive a.

antibody-binding
  a.-b. protein antigen
  a.-b. virus

antibody-mediated
  a.-m. cytotoxicity of cells
  a.-m. hypersensitivity
  a.-m. immunity
  a.-m. neutralization
  a.-m. protective immunity
  a.-m. stimulation
  a.-m. thrombocytopenia

anticardiolipin antibody

anti-CD3 antibody

anti-CD4 antibody

anti-CD18 antibody

anticentromere antibody

anticholinergic
  a. drugs

antichymosin

anticoagulant

anticomplement

anticomplementary
  a. serum

anticonvulsant
  a.-induced osteomalacia

anticore window

anti-cytokine antibody

anticytolysin

anticytotoxin

anti-D
  a.-D antibody

anti-deoxyribonuclease B test

antidiuresis

antidiuretic hormone (ADH)

anti-DNA antibody

antiestrogen
  a. binding site
  long-acting a.
  physiological a.
  pure a.
  short-acting a.

antiestrogenic

antifertility vaccine

anti-GBM
  anti–glomerular basement
  membrane
    anti-GBM antibodies

antigen (Ag)
  ABO a.
  ABO blood group a's
  acquired a.
  a.-activated B cells
  allogeneic a.
  Am a's

antigen *(continued)*
    antibody-binding protein a.
    Au a.
    Australia a.
    autologous a.
    a. binding
    a.-binding fragment
    a.-binding site
    blood group a's
    Boivin a.
    a.-bound phagocyte activ-
      ity
    a. C *(of poliovirus)*
    capsular a.
    a. capture assay
    carcinoembryonic a. (CEA)
    cardiolipin a.
    CD a.
    cell surface a.
    class I a's
    class II a's
    class III a's
    a.-combining site
    common a.
    common acute lymphoblas-
      tic leukemia a. (CALLA)
    common leukocyte a's
    a. competition
    complete a.
    a. concentration
    conjugated a.
    cross-reacting a.
    cross-reactive a.
    cutaneous lymphocyte a.
      (CLA)
    cutaneous lymphoid a.
    cytomegalovirus a.
    D a. *(of poliovirus)*
    delta a.
    a.-dependent differentiation
    a. determinant sites
    differentiation a's
    a. dose vs. immunization
    a. drift
    E a.
    early a. (EA)
    endogenous a.
    endogenous protein a.
    Epstein-Barr nuclear a.

antigen *(continued)*
    a. excess
    exogenous a.
    exogenous microbial a.
    exogenous protein a.
    extractable nuclear a's
    febrile a's
    flagella a.
    flagellar a.
    foreign a.
    Forssman a.
    Frei a.
    a. gain
    genetically identical trans-
      plantation a's
    Gm a's
    Goodpasture a.
    H a. *(of Salmonella typhi)*
    H-2 a's
    H chain a.
    heat-stabile a.
    hepatitis a.
    hepatitis A a.
    hepatitis-associated a.
      (HAA)
    hepatitis B a.
    hepatitis B core a. (HBcAg)
    hepatitis B e a. (HBeAg)
    hepatitis B surface a.
      (HBsAg)
    hepatitis D a.
    heterogeneic a.
    heterogenetic a.
    heterogenic a.
    heterologous a.
    heterophil a.
    heterophile a.
    high-frequency a's
    high-incidence a's
    high-titer, low-avidity a.
    histocompatibility a's
    histocompatibility a. sys-
      tem
    HLA a's
    homologous a.
    human immunodeficiency
      virus a.
    human leukocyte a's (HLA)

antigen *(continued)*
    human mucosal lympho-
      cyte a. (HML)
    H-Y a.
    I a.
    i a.
    Ia a's
    ICFA a.
    idiotypic a.
    immune-associated a.
    immunogenic a.
    a.-independent differentia-
      tion
    a.-induced proliferation
    inhaled a.
    a. interaction
    Inv group a.
    isogeneic a.
    isophile a.
    K a.
    Km a's
    Kveim a.
    La a.
    LD a's
    leukocyte a's
    leukocyte common a's
      (LCA)
    leukocyte culture a's
    leukocyte function–asso-
      ciated a. (LFA) (1–3)
    leu-M1 a.
    Lewis a.
    a.-liberated transfer factor
    low-frequency a's
    low-incidence a's
    Ly a's
    Lyb a's
    lymphocyte-defined (LD)
      a's
    lymphocyte function–asso-
      ciated a. (LFA)
    lymphocyte function–asso-
      ciated a.-3 (LFA-3)
    lymphocyte surface a.
    Lyt a's
    M a.
    Mac-1 a.
    major histocompatibility
      a's

antigen *(continued)*
    masking of a's
    melanoma a.
    microbial a's
    microbial test a.
    minor H a's
    minor histocompatibility
      a's
    minor lymphocyte stimu-
      lating a.
    minor lymphocyte stimula-
      tory a.
    Mitsuda a.
    MLC a's
    Mls a.
    MLS a.
    modified a.
    multivalent a.
    mumps skin test a.
    nuclear a's
    O a. *(of Salmonella typhi)*
    oncofetal a.
    organ-specific a.
    Oz a.
    P a. *(of adenovirus)*
    pancreatic oncofetal a.
      (POA)
    pan–T-cell a's
    partial a.
    particulate a.
    peptide a.
    Pl(A1) a.
    platelet a.
    pollen a.
    Pr a.
    a. presentation
    a.-presenting cells (APC)
    private a's
    a. processing (APC)
    proliferating cell nuclear a.
      (PCNA)
    prostate-specific a. (PSA)
    protein a.
    public a's
    Qa a.
    a.-reactive cells
    recall a.
    a. receptor

antigen *(continued)*
    a. receptor activation motif
      (ARAM)
    a. recognition
    a. recognition activation
      motif
    red cell a.
    Reiter a.
    retrogenic a's
    Rh a.
    Rh blood group a.
    RNP a.
    Ro a.
    SD a's
    second a.
    self-a.
    a.-sensitive cells
    a. sensitization
    a.-sensitized memory cells
    sequestered a's
    sero-defined (SD) a's
    serologically defined (SD)
      a's
    serum hepatitis a.
    SH a.
    shared a.
    a. shift
    shock a.
    Sm a.
    soluble a.
    somatic a's
    species-specific a's
    a.-specific B lymphocytes
    a.-specific depression
    a.-specific T-cell helper fac-
      tor
    a.-specific T-cell suppres-
      sor factor
    a.-specific T lymphocytes
    SS-A a.
    SS-B a.
    streptococcal a. cross reac-
      tivity
    surface a.
    synthetic a.
    T a.
    θ a.
    Tac a.
    T cell–dependent a.

antigen *(continued)*
    T cell–independent a.
    T cell a. receptor
    T-dependent a.
    theta a.
    Thomsen-Friedenreich a.
    Thy 1 a.
    thymus-dependent a.
    thymus-dependent pro-
      tein a.
    thymus-independent a.
    TI-1 a.
    T-independent a.
    tissue a.
    tissue-specific a.
    tolerogenic a.
    tolerogenic protein a.
    Tp4 a.
    transplant a.
    transplantation a's
    a. transplantation
    treponemal a's
    tumor a.
    tumor-associated a. (TAA)
    tumor rejection a.
    tumor-specific a. (TSA)
    tumor-specific transplanta-
      tion a. (TSTA)
    a. unit
    a. valency
    VDRL a.
    very late a's (VLA) (1–6)
    very late activation
      (VLA) a.
    Vi a.
    viral capsid a.
    Wassermann a.
    xenogeneic a.

antigen-antibody
    a.-a. binding
    a.-a. complex
    a.-a. interaction
    a.-a. reaction

antigenemia

antigenemic

antigenic
    a. competition

antigenic *(continued)*
   a. determinant
   a. drift
   a. modulation
   a. peptides
   a. shift
   a. specificity
   a. valency
   a. variation

antigenicity
   tumor a.

antiglobulin
   a. consumption test
   a. coprecipitation technique
   a. reaction
   a. test (AGT)

anti–glomerular basement membrane (anti-GBM) antibodies

antiglucocorticoid

antigoitrogenic

antigonadotropic

anti-hapten antibody

anti-HBc

anti-HBs

antihemagglutinin

antihemolysin

antiheterolysin

antihistamine

antihormone

antihuman globulin (AHG)
   a. g. reagent
   a. g. test

anti–human globulin serum

anti-hyaluronidase test

antihyperglycemic drug

antihypertensive drug

anti-idiotype
   a. antibody

anti-idiotype *(continued)*
   a.-i. vaccine

anti-idiotypic antibody

anti-IL4 antibody

anti-immunoglobulin antibody

anti-inflammatory
   a.-i. agent

anti-insulin
   a.-i. receptor antibody

anti-isolysin

anti-isotype antibody

anti-La antibody

antilymphocyte
   a. globulin (ALG)
   a. immunoglobulin
   a. serum (ALS)

antilysin

antilysis

antilytic

anti-M antibody

anti-MHC antibody

antimicrobial
   a. immunity
   a. mechanism
   Metchnikoff's theory of a. immunity

antimicrosomal antibodies

antimineralocorticoid

antimitochondrial antibodies

antimüllerian
   a. hormone (AMH)

antineoplastic agent

antineutrophil
   a. antibody
   a. cytoplasmic antibody
   a. cytoplasmic autoantibody (ANCA)

antinuclear
   a. antibodies (ANA)

antinuclear *(continued)*
    a. factor (ANF)

antinucleoprotein factor

antioncogene

antiopsonin

antiphagocytic

antiphospholipid antibodies

antiprecipitin

antipneumococcus serum

antiprogestin

antiprogestogen

antipsychotic

antirabies serum

antireceptor antibodies

anti-Rh agglutinin

anti-Rh antibody

antiricin

anti-Ro antibody

antisecretory

antisepsis
    physiologic a.

antiseptic
    a. paint

antiserotonin agent

antiserum *pl.* antiserums, anti-sera
    a. anaphylaxis

anti-sheep red blood cell anti-body

anti-SS-A antibody

anti-SS-B antibody

antistaphylohemolysin

antistaphylolysin

antistreptokinase

antistreptolysin
    a. O (ASO)

antistreptolysin *(continued)*
    a. O neutralization test
    a. O titer

antitetanic serum (ATS)

antithymocyte globulin (ATG)

antithyroglobulin antibodies

antithyroid
    a. agents
    a. antibodies

antithyrotoxic

antithyrotropic

antitissue
    a. immunity
    a. reaction

anti-TNF α antibody

antitoxic
    a. immunity
    a. serum
    a. unit

antitoxigen

antitoxin
    botulinal a.
    botulinum a.
    botulinus a.
    botulism a.
    bovine a.
    diphtheria a.
    equine a.
    pertussis a.
    tetanus a.
    toxin-a. (TA)
    von Behring a.

antitoxinogen

antitoxinum

antitropin

antitrypsin
    $alpha_1$-a.

antituberculin

antitumor vaccine

antivenin

antiviral
    a. immunity
    a. proteins
    a. state

antivirotic

antixenic

aortic arch

aortopulmonary window

aparathyroidism

aparathyrosis

APC
    antigen-presenting cells

aphrodisin

aphthous
    a. fever
    a. pharyngitis

aphylactic

aphylaxis

apical plasma membrane

apituitarism

aplasia
    thymic a.
    thymic-parathyroid a.

aplastic anemia

apocrine gland

apophysis *pl.* apophyses
    cerebral a.
    a. cerebri

apoplexy
    pituitary a.

apoptosis

apoptotic

apparent hyperprolactinemia
    syndrome

appendix *pl.* appendices

appestat

appetite
    altered a.
    a. regulation
    a.-suppressant drugs

application

AP-1 protein

APTT
    activated partial thrombo-
        plastin time

APUD
    amine precursor uptake
    and decarboxylation
        APUD cells
        APUD system

apudoma

aqueous vasopressin

arachidonic acid
    a. a. metabolites

arachnoid cyst

ARAM
    antigen receptor activation
        motif

arboviral

arbovirus
    group A a's
    group B a's

area *pl.* areae or areas
    B-dependent a.
    hypophysiotropic a.
    paracortical a.
    parafollicular a's
    T-dependent a.
    thymus-dependent a.
    thymus-independent a.
    T-independent a.

ARC
    AIDS-related complex

arch
    aortic a.

Arenaviridae

Arenavirus

arenavirus

argentaffin cells

Argentine
A. hemorrhagic fever
A. hemorrhagic fever virus

Argentinian hemorrhagic fever

arginine
a. vasopressin
a. vasotocin (AVT)

argininosuccinicaciduria

argipressin

argyrophilic cells

armed
a. effector cells
a. effector T cells
a. macrophages

arm-raising test

aromatase
a. deficiency
a. reaction

aromatic L-amino-acid decarboxylase

aromatization
extraglandular a.

arrest
maturational a.

arrestin

arrhenoblastoma

arrhythmia

Arroyo's sign

arsonate group structure

arsphenamine

arterenol

arterial blood gases

arteriogram
internal mammary a.

arteriography
penile a.

arteriopathy
cyclosporine-associated a.

arteriosclerosis
accelerated a.
graft a.

arteriosclerotic

arteritis

arterivirus

artery
inferior thyroid a.
parathyroid a's

arthralgia

arthritis *pl.* arthritides
collagen a.
juvenile rheumatoid a.
Lyme a.
reactive a.
Reiter's a.
rheumatoid a. (RA)
salmonella a.
septic a.
Yersinia a.

arthropathy
psoriatic a.

Arthus
A. phenomenon
A. reaction
reverse A. reaction
reverse passive A. reaction
A.-type reaction
A.-type reactivity

artifact

artificial neural network (ANN)

arylsulfatase

ASAT
aspartate aminotransferase

ascariasis
pulmonary a.

ascaridiasis

ascaridosis

Ascaris pneumonitis

ascending poliomyelitis

ascertainment artifact

Aselli's gland

aseptic
  a. meningitis
  a. technique

asexual dwarf

Asherman syndrome

Asian influenza

Asiatic cholera

Askanazy cells

ASO
    antistreptolysin O
        ASO neutralization test
        ASO titer

aspartate aminotransferase
  (ASAT)

aspecific

aspect
    age-related a's

aspergilloma

aspergillomycosis

aspergillosis
    allergic a.
    allergic bronchopulmo-
      nary a.
    aural a.
    chronic necrotizing a.
    invasive a.
    pulmonary a.

Aspergillus
    A. amstelodami
    A. clavatus
    A. flavus
    A. fumigatus

Aspergillus (continued)
    A. glaucus
    A. nidulans
    A. niger
    A. ochraceus
    A. oryzae
    A. restrictus
    A. terreus
    A. versicolor

assay
    a's of activity
    antigen capture a.
    blastogenesis a.
    cell-mediated lympholysis
      (CML) a.
    CH50 a.
    CH100 a.
    CML a.
    competitive binding a's
    competitive enzyme-linked
      immunosorbent a.
    competitive inhibition a.
    D-dimer a.
    EAC rosette a.
    ELISA SPOT a.
    ELISPOT a.
    enzyme immunoassay
    enzyme-linked immunosor-
      bent a. (ELISA)
    E rosette a.
    estradiol a.
    estradiol exchange a.
    exchange a.
    fluorescent antibody a.
    fluorescent antigen a.
    HeLa cell adherence a.
    hemagglutination a.
    hemagglutination inhibition
      (HI, HAI) a.
    hemolytic complement a.
    hemolytic plaque a.
    heterogeneous ligand a.
    homogeneous ligand a.
    HPLC–electrochemical de-
      tection a.
    immune a.
    immune adherence hemag-
      glutination a. (IAHA)

assay *(continued)*
  immunofluorescence a.
    (IFA)
  immunofluorescent a. (IFA)
  immunoradiometric a.
    (IRMA)
  Jerne plaque a.
  ligand a.
  limiting dilution a.
  lymphocyte-limiting dilu-
    tion a.
  lymphocyte proliferation a.
  microcytotoxicity a.
  microhemagglutination a.–
    Treponema pallidum
    (MHA-TP)
  micro-indirect immunoflu-
    orescence a.
  mixed lymphocyte cul-
    ture a.
  MLC a.
  Ouchterlony gel-diffusion a.
  physicochemical a.
  plaque a.
  radioenzymatic a.
  radioimmunoprecipita-
    tion a. (RIPA)
  radioimmunosorbent a.
  radioreceptor a.
  Raji cell a.
  sandwich a.
  serologic a.
  total complement a.
  Treponema pallidum hem-
    agglutination a. (TPHA)
  TUNEL a.
  a. validity test (AVT)
  Western blot a.
  whole complement a.

association
  a. constant
  genetic a.

astemizole

asthma
  bronchial a.
  intrinsic a.

asthenocoria

astrocyte

Astroviridae

Astrovirus

astrovirus

asymptomatic
  a. neurosyphilis

ataractics

ataxia
  a.-telangiectasia
  a.-telangiectasia syndrome

ateliotic dwarfism

ATG
  antithymocyte globulin

atherogenesis

atheroma

atherosclerosis
  a. etiology
  a. prevention
  a. treatment

atherosclerotic
  a. coronary heart disease

athlete's foot

athletic performance

athrepsia

athrophagocytosis

athymia

athymic mouse

athyrea

athyreosis

athyreotic
  a. cretinism

athyria

athyroidemia

athyroidism

athyroidosis

athyrosis

athyrotic
 a. cretinism

atopen

atopic
 a. allergy
 a. disease
 a. eczema
 a. rhinitis

atopy
 human a.

ATP-binding cassette (ABC)
 ATP-b. c. proteins

atresia
 cystic a.

atrial
 a. fibrillation
 a. natriuretic factor (ANF)
 a. natriuretic peptide
 a. peptides

atriopeptides

atriopeptin

atrophic
 a. autoimmune thyroiditis
 a. thyroiditis
 a. vulvovaginitis

atrophy
 compensatory a.
 endocrine a.
 idiopathic adrenal a.
 multiple system a.
 muscle a.
 optic a.
 progressive muscular a.
 toxic a.

atropine

ATS
 antitetanic serum

attenuate

attenuated
 a. live vaccine
 a. vaccine

attenuated *(continued)*
 a. virus

attenuation

attractiveness

atypical
 a. (reactive) lymphocytes
 a. measles
 a. pneumonia
 a. tuberculosis

Au antigen

Au antigenemia

Auerbach's plexus

aula

Aureobasidium

auscultation

Australia antigen

Australian
 A. Q fever
 A. tick typhus
 A. X disease virus

autacoid

autoactivation

autoagglutination

autoagglutinin

autoallergic

autoallergy

autoantibody
 antineutrophil cytoplas-
  mic a. (ANCA)
 collagen a's
 glomerular basement mem-
  brane a's
 intrinsic factor a's
 natural a's
 nonpathogenic a's
 organ-specific a's
 pathogen-generated a's
 receptor a's
 red cell a.
 a. tests

autoanticomplement

autoantigen

auto–anti-idiotypic antibodies

autoantisepsis

autoantitoxin

autobody

autochthonous
   a. graft

autocoid

autocoupling hapten

autocrine
   a. action
   a. function
   a. growth factors
   a. secretion
   a. stimulation

autocytolysin

autocytotoxin

autofluorescence

autogeneic

autogenous
   a. graft
   a. vaccine

autograft

autografting

autohemagglutination

autohemagglutinin

autohemolysin

autohemolysis

autohemolytic

autoimmune
   a. adrenalitis
   atrophic a. thyroiditis
   a. diabetes
   a. disease
   a. disorders
   a. exophthalmos
   a. hemolytic anemia (AIHA)

autoimmune *(continued)*
   a. hypersensitivity
   a. hypoglycemia
   a. nephropathy
   a. neutropenia
   nongoitrous a. thyroiditis
   a. polyendocrine-candidia-
      sis syndrome
   a. polyglandular syndrome
   a. purpura
   a. response
   a. testicular failure
   a. thrombocytic purpura
   a. thrombocytopenia
   a. thyroiditis

autoimmunity
   drug-induced a.
   endocrine a.
   non–organ-specific a.
   organ-specific a.
   systemic a.
   transient a.

autoimmunization

autoinfection

autoinoculable

autoinoculation

autointerference

autoisolysin

autoleukoagglutinin

autologous
   a. antibody
   a. antigen
   a. graft
   a. transplantation

autolymphocyte therapy

autolysin

autolysis

autonomic
   a. nervous system
   a. neuropathy

autophagosome

autopharmacologic

autopharmacology

autophosphorylation

autoplast

autoplastic
a. graft

autoplasty

autoradiography

autosensitization

autoreactive T cells

autoreactivity

autosensitized

autoserous

autoserum
a. therapy

autosomal
a. abnormalities
a. dominant gene
a. recessive gene
a. recessive immunodeficiency
a. severe combined immunodeficiency (SCID)

autospermotoxin

autostimulation

autotherapy

autothromboagglutinin

autotransplant

autotransplantation

autovaccination

autovaccine

autovaccinia

autovaccinotherapy

autumn fever

auxilytic

auxotype

avascular necrosis

avidin

avidity
antibody a.
a. hypothesis

avipoxvirus

avirulence

avirulent
a. staphylococcus

AVT
arginine vasotocin
assay validity test

axial
a. osteomalacia

axis pl. axes
cortical-hypothalamic-pituitary a.
hypothalamic-pituitary a.
hypothalamic-pituitary-adrenal a.
hypothalamic-pituitary-adrenocortical a.
hypothalamic-pituitary-gonadal a.
hypothalamic-pituitary-thyroid a.
hypothalamo-pituitary-Leydig cell a.
hypothalamo-pituitary-seminferous tubular a.
pituitary-thyroid a.
renal-adrenal a.

axon

azatadine maleate

azathioprine

3'azido-3'deoxythymidine
same as zidovudine

azidothymidine (AZT)
same as zidovudine

AZT
azidothymidine

B
  bursa-derived
    B cell
    B lymphocyte
    B lymphoblast
  B complex
  B virus

β
  β-adrenergic blocker
  β-endorphin
  β-lipotropin
  $β_2$-microglobulin

B7
  B7-1 (CD81)
  B7-2 (CD86)
  B7 protein

B19 virus

Babesia microti

Babinski-Fröhlich syndrome

bacillary angiomatosis

bacille
  b. Calmette-Guérin (BCG)

bacillemia

Bacillus
  B. anthracis

bacillus
  Döderlein b.
  tubercle b.

back
  angry b.

bacteremia

bacteria (*plural of* bacterium)

bacterial
  b. adjuvant
  b. allergy
  b. endotoxins
  b. infection
  b. polysaccharide
  b. polysaccharide immune
    globulin (BPIG)

bacterial (*continued*)
  b. products
  b. superantigen
  b. toxin
  b. vaccine
  b. virus

bactericidal permeability in-
  creasing protein (BPI)

bactericide
  specific b.

bactericidin

bacterin

bacteriocidin

bacteriogenic agglutination

bacteriolysin
  b. test

bacteriolytic
  b. antibody
  b. serum

bacterio-opsonin

bacteriophage
  b. plaque
  temperate b.
  b. titer

bacteriophagia

bacteriophagic

bacteriophagology

bacteriophagy

bacterioprecipitin

bacteriopsonic

bacteriopsonin

bacteriosis

bacteriotherapy

bacteriotoxemia

bacteriotropic

bacteriotropin

bacterium *pl.* bacteria
  encapsulated b.
  extracellular bacteria
  inactivated bacteria
  intracellular bacteria
  lysogenic b.
  pyogenic b.
  bacteria symbiosis with vi-
    ruses
  bacteria vs. mycoplasmas

Bacteroides
  B. thetaiotaomicron

bacteroidosis

Bakau virus

bakers' itch

balance
  mineral b.
  nitrogen b.

balanced pathogenicity

balantidiasis

balantidiosis

balantidosis

baldness
  male pattern b.

ball
  fungus b.

BALT
  bronchial-associated lym-
    phoid tissue

bancroftosis

Bannwarth's syndrome

barbers' itch

bare lymphocyte syndrome

baroreceptor

Barr body

barrel
  beta b's

barrel *(continued)*
  b. chest

barrier
  b. contraception
  host b's

Bartonella
  B. anemia
  B. bacilliformis
  B. henselae
  B. quintana

bartonelliasis

bartonellosis

Bartter's syndrome

basal
  b. granular cells
  b. metabolic rate (BMR)
  b. tuberculosis

basedoid

Basedow
  B's disease
  B's goiter

basedowiform

basement membrane
  glomerular b. m.
  glomerular b. m. autoanti-
    bodies
  glomerular b. m. autoim-
    mune disease

basidiobolomycosis

basis *pl.* bases
  b. glandulae suprarenalis

basophil
  b. adenoma
  beta b.
  b. chemotactic factor (BCF)
  b. count
  Crooke-Russell b's
  b. degranulation test
  delta b.
  b. granule
  b. progenitors

basophile

basophilic
    b. adenoma

basophilism
    Cushing's b.
    pituitary b.

batteyin

BAT
    brown adipose tissue

Bayou virus

B1 B cells (CD5 B cells)

B2 B cells (conventional B
  cells)

β-blocker

β1C

BCDF
    B cell differentiation fac-
      tors

B cell
    B c. activation
    antigen-activated B c's
    B c. antigen receptors
    B1 B c's (CD5 B cells)
    B2 B c's (conventional B
      cells)
    CD5 B c's
    B c. coreceptor complex
    B c. corona
    B c. defects
    B c. differentiation factors
      (BCDF)
    B c. growth factor
    immature B c.
    B c. interaction
    B c. lymphoma
    mature B c's
    memory B c's
    B c. mitogens
    polyclonal B c's
    B c. progenitor protein ki-
      nase
    proliferating B c's
    B c. receptor complex

B cell *(continued)*
    self-reactive B c's
    B c. tolerance
    B c. tumor

BCF
    basophil chemotactic factor

BCG
    bacille Calmette-Guérin
    BCG vaccine

BCGF
    B cell growth factors

Bcl-2

B complex

B-dependent area

bead
    paramagnetic b's

Becker
    B's phenomenon
    B's sign

Beckwith
    B. syndrome
    B.-Wiedemann syndrome

beclomethasone dipropionate

becquerel (Bq)

beer potomania

behavior
    eating b.
    maternal b.
    b. modification
    sexual b.

behavioral therapy

Behring's law

Beigel's disease

bejel

Belgrade virus

Bence Jones
    B. J. protein

Bence Jones *(continued)*
   B. J. proteinemia
   B. J. proteinuria

β-endorphin

beneficient virus

benign
   b. glycosuria
   b. infantile mammoplasia
   b. leptospirosis
   b. lymphoreticulosis
   b. monoclonal gammopathy
   b. thyroid tumor
   b. tumor

bentonite flocculation test

benzylpenicilloyl polylysine

Berger's disease

Bernard
   B's puncture
   B.-Sergent syndrome

Berne virus

berry cell

beta (β)
   b. barrels
   b. basophil
   b. cell
   b. cell dysfunction
   b. chain
   b. globulins
   b. granules
   b. hemolysin
   b. interferon
   b. lysin
   b. particles
   b. receptors
   b. sheets
   b. staphylolysin
   b. subunit

Betaherpesvirinae

beta-lysin

beta$_2$-microglobulin

BF
   blastogenic factor

BF *(continued)*
   lymphocyte blastogenic
      factor

β1F

BFA
   Brefeldin A

BFP
   biologic false-positive

β1H

bicarbonate

Biederman's sign

bilateral
   b. gynandromorphism
   b. hermaphroditism

bile
   b. acid

bilharziasis

bilharzioma

bilharziosis

biliary
   b. colic
   b. gland
   b. tract

bilirubin

Bilophila
   B. wadsworthia

binary fission

binding
   antigen b.
   antigen-antibody b.
   b. protein
   b. reagent

binucleated cells

bioactive hormone

bioassay
   calcitonin b.

biochemical messenger

biochemically recognizable osteomalacia

biogenic amine

biological
   b. amplification systems
   implanted b. insulin deliv-
      ery system
   b. insulin delivery system
   b. response modifiers

biologicals

biologic false-positive (BFP)

biopsy
   bone b.

biorhythm

biotherapy

biotin

Biozzi mouse

Birbeck granule

birnavirus

birth
   b. control
   b. defects

bisdiazopine

bisexual

bisexuality

bispecific antibody

bite
   insect b.

Bittner virus

bivalent
   b. antibodies
   b. attenuated vaccine

BK virus

black
   b. death
   b.-dot ringworm
   b. piedra

black *(continued)*
   b. plague

bladder dysfunction

blast
   b. formation
   b. transformation

blastocyst

blastogenesis
   b. assay

blastogenic
   b. factor (BF)
   b. inhibitor factor

Blastomyces
   B. dermatitidis

blastomycin

blastomycosis
   Brazilian b.
   cutaneous b.
   keloidal b.
   North American b.
   South American b.
   systemic b.

Blastoschizomyces

bleeding
   breakthrough b.
   estrogen breakthrough b.
   progesterone break-
      through b.
   uterine b.
   vaginal b.
   withdrawal b.

blennorrhagia

blepharoptosis

blindness
   river b.
   unilateral b.

B-lineage specific activator protein (BSAP)

blister
   fever b.

Blk kinase

blockade
  alpha b.
  reticuloendothelial b.
  virus b.

blocker
  α-adrenergic b.
  α-methyldopa b.
  β-b.
  β-adrenergic b.
  calcium channel b.
  sympathetic b.

blocking
  b. antibody
  b. factors

blood
  b. cell
  b. cell count
  fasting b. sugar (FBS)
  b. flow
  b. glucose
  b. group
  b. group antigens
  b. island
  b. phagocyte
  b. pressure
  red b. cells
  red b. cell destruction
  renal b. flow
  b. sugar (glucose)
  b. transfusion
  b. typing
  b. urea nitrogen (BUN)
  b. vessel
  b. volume
  white b. cells

blood-borne precursor stem cell

Bloom syndrome

blot
  Northern b.
  Southern b.
  Western b.

blotting
  Northern b.

blotting *(continued)*
  Southern b.
  Western b.

Blount disease

bluegrass

bluetongue disease of sheep

BLV-HTLV retroviruses

B lymphoblast

B lymphocyte
  activated B l.
  bystander B l's
  immature B l.
  B l. stimulatory factors
    (BSF)
  mature B l.

BMR
  basal metabolic rate

BNP
  brain natriuretic peptide

body
  adrenal b.
  Barr b.
  brassy b.
  Call-Exner b's
  chromaffin b.
  coccoid x b's
  b. composition
  Councilman's b's
  Cowdry type I inclusion b's
  elementary b.
  epithelial b's
  b. fat
  Gamna-Favre b's
  Guarnieri's b's
  b. image
  immune b.
  inclusion b's
  infundibular b.
  LCL b's
  Levinthal-Coles-Lillie b's
  Lipschütz b's
  Lostorfer's b's
  lyssa b's
  Mooser b's
  multivesicular b.

body *(continued)*
    Negri b's
    b. of pancreas
    parathyroid b's
    Paschen b's
    pheochrome b.
    pineal b.
    pituitary b.
    postbranchial b's
    pyknotic b's
    reticulate b.
    Ross's b's
    Sandström's b's
    suprarenal b.
    telobranchial b's
    b. temperature
    b. temperature mechanism
    thyroid b.
    Torres-Teixeira b's
    ultimobranchial b's
    Weibel-Palade b's
    b. weight
    Winkler's b's
    X b.
    Y b.

Boivin antigen

Bolivian
    B. hemorrhagic fever
    B. hemorrhagic fever virus

Bollinger's granules

bolster fingers

bombesin

bonding
    hydrogen b.

bonds
    hydrogen b.

bone
    b. age
    age-related b. loss
    b. biopsy
    b. calcium
    cancellous b.
    cortical b.
    b. densitometry
    b. dysplasia

bone *(continued)*
    b. formation
    b. growth
    lamellar b.
    b. loss
    b. marrow
    b. metabolism
    b. mineralization
    mineralization of b's
    b. proteoglycans
    b. resorption
    b. scan
    b. scanning
    b. structure
    trabecular b.
    woven b.

bone marrow
    b. m. chimera
    b. m.–derived cell
    b. m. transplantation

Bonferroni correction

Bonnevie-Ullrich syndrome

booster
    b. immunization
    b. injection
    b. response

border
    anterior b. of body of pancreas
    anterior b. of pancreas
    inferior b. of body of pancreas
    inferior b. of pancreas
    medial b. of adrenal gland
    medial b. of suprarenal gland
    superior b. of adrenal gland
    superior b. of body of pancreas
    superior b. of pancreas
    superior b. of suprarenal gland

Bordet
    B.-Gengou phenomenon
    B.-Gengou reaction

Bordetella
    B. parapertussis
    B. pertussis
    B. pertussis agglutinogen
    B. pertussis endotoxin

Borna disease virus

Bornaviridae

Bornavirus

Bornholm disease

Borrelia
    B. afzelii
    B. berbera
    B. burgdorferi
    B. carteri
    B. caucasica
    B. crocidurae
    B. dipodilli
    B. duttonii
    B. garinii
    B. hermsii
    B. hispanica
    B. kochii
    B. latyschewii
    B. mazzottii
    B. merionesi
    B. microti
    B. neotropicalis
    B. novyi
    B. obermeyeri
    B. parkeri
    B. recurrentis
    B. turicatae
    B. venezuelensis

borreliosis
    Lyme b.

Boston's sign

botryomycosis

botryomycotic

botulism

boutonneuse
    b. fever

bovine serum albumin (BSA)

bowel
    b. disease
    b. function in thyrotoxico-
      sis

box
    TATA b.
    W b.
    X b.
    Y b.

Boyden chamber

BPI
    bactericidal permeability
      increasing protein

BPIG
    bacterial polysaccharide
      immune globulin

B7 protein

Bq
    becquerel

bradykinin

bradyzoite

brain
    b. abscess
    b. natriuretic peptide
      (BNP)

brancher deficiency glycogenosis

Branhamella catarrhalis

brassy body

Brazilian
    B. blastomycosis
    B. spotted fever

breakbone fever

breakdown
    acetylcholine b.

breakthrough bleeding

breast
    b. budding
    b. cancer
    b. development

breast *(continued)*
    b. disease
    b. disorders
    endocrine b. cancer therapy
    b. enlargement
    b. feeding
    b. hypoplasia

Breda virus

Brenner tumor

bridge
    cytoplasmic b.

Brill
    B's disease
    B.-Zinsser disease

Brefeldin A (BFA)

Brion-Kayser disease

Brissaud
    B's dwarf
    B's infantilism

brittle
    b. bone disease
    b. bone syndrome
    b. diabetes

"broad-beta" disease

bromelain
    fruit b.
    stem b.

bromelin

bromergocriptine

bromocriptine mesylate

bronchial
    b. adenoma
    b.-associated lymphoid tissue (BALT)
    b. asthma
    b. challenge
    b. challenge test
    b. provocation

bronchiolitis

bronchoconstriction

bronchogenic
    b. cancer
    b. carcinoma

bronchomycosis

bronchopneumonia

bronchospasm

bronzed disease

bronze liver

brow
    olympian b.
    olympic b.

brown adipose tissue (BAT)

Brown-Séquard's treatment

Bruce effect

Brucella
    B. abortus
    B. bronchiseptica
    B. canis
    B. melitensis
    B. neotomae
    B. ovis
    B. rangiferi tarandi
    B. suis

Brucellergin skin test

brucellosis

Bruton
    B's agammaglobulinemia
    B's disease
    B.-type agammaglobulinemia
    B's tyrosine kinase (Btk)
    B's X-linked agammaglobulinemia

BSA
    bovine serum albumin

BSAP
    B-lineage specific activator protein

BSF
    B lymphocyte stimulatory factors

Btk
  Bruton's tyrosine kinase

bubble baby

bubo
  bullet b.
  chancroidal b.
  climatic b.
  malignant b.
  primary b.
  syphilitic b.
  tropical b.
  virulent b.

bubon
  b. d'emblée

bubonic
  b. plague

buccal
  b. mucosa
  b. smear

Buckley's syndrome

budding
  breast b.

budesonide

buffer

buffalo
  b. hump
  b. type

bulbar
  b. encephalitis
  b. poliomyelitis

bulging eyeballs

bulimia nervosa

bullet bubo

Bullis fever

bullneck

bullosis diabeticorum

bullous pemphigoid

bumps

BUN
  blood urea nitrogen

Bunyamwera
  B. group viruses
  B. virus

Bunyaviridae

Bunyavirus

bunyavirus

burimamide

Burkholderia
  B. cepacia

Burkitt's lymphoma

burn

bursa *pl.* bursae
  b.-equivalent
  b.-equivalent tissue
  b. of Fabricius

bursal
  b. equivalent tissue

bursectomy
  neonatal b.

burst
  respiratory b.

Buschke's disease

Busse-Buschke disease

Bussuquara virus

butyrophenone

B virus

B19 virus

Bwamba
  B. group viruses
  B. virus

bypass
  ileal b.
  jejunoileal b.

bystander
  b. B lymphocytes
  innocent b.
  b. lysis

C
  antigen C (*of poliovirus*)
  C cells
  complement component
  constant
    C domain
    C region
  C peptide
  C-reactive protein
  C receptor
  C virus

C_H
  C-terminal portion of an immunoglobulin heavy chain

C_L
  C-terminal portion of an immunoglobulin light chain

C1 (*complement component*)
  C1 esterase
  C1 esterase inhibitor
  C1 inhibitor (C1INH)
  C1q
  C1r
  C1s

C2 (*complement component*)
  C2a

C3 (*complement component*)
  C3a
  C3b
  C3b inactivator
  C3b inactivator accelerator
  C3 convertase
  C3d
  C3 nephritic factor (C3 NeF)
  C3 proactivator (C3PA)
  C3 proactivator convertase

C3/C5 convertase

C4 (*complement component*)
  C4a
  C4b
  C4 binding protein

C5 (*complement component*)
  C5a
  C5a receptor
  C5b
  C5 convertase

C6 (*complement component*)
  C6789

C7 (*complement component*)

C8 (*complement component*)

C9 (*complement component*)

CA
  croup-associated
    CA virus

CA_2 (*an antigen in thyroid colloid*)

Ca
  calcium

cachectin

cachexia
  hypophysial c.
  c. hypophysiopriva
  pituitary c.
  c. suprarenalis

cadaveric donor transplantation

caddy stool

Calabar
  C. edema
  C. swellings

calciferol

calcification
  dystrophic c.
  extraskeletal c.

calcineurin

calciosome

calcipenia

calciphylactic

calciphylaxis
  systemic c.
  topical c.

calcitonin (CT)
  c. bioassay
  c. deficiency
  c. gene–related peptide
  plasma c. levels
  c.-producing tumor
  c. radioimmunoassay
  c. receptors
  c. secretion

calcitoninoma
  pancreatic c.

calcitriol

calcium (Ca)
  c. absorption
  bone c.
  c. channel blocker
  c. chelators
  c. citrate
  c. homeostasis
  c. level
  c. metabolism
  c. plaques
  c. reabsorption
  serum c.
  urinary c.

calciuria

caliciviral

Caliciviridae

Calicivirus

calicivirus
  feline c.
  human c's

calculus
  renal calculi

California
  C. disease
  C. encephalitis virus
  C. group viruses

CALLA
  common acute lymphoblas-
    tic leukemia antigen

Call-Exner bodies

Calmette's vaccine

calmodulin
  c. antagonists
  c.-dependent multiprotein
    kinase

calnexin

calorigenesis

calreticulin

Calymmatobacterium
  C. granulomatis

CAM
  cell adhesion molecule

cAMP
  cyclic adenosine mono-
    phosphate
      cAMP-dependent pro-
        tein kinase

camp fever

Campylobacter
  C. cinaedi
  C. coli
  C. fecalis
  C. fennelliae
  C. fetus
  C. fetus subsp. *fetus*
  C. fetus subsp. *intestinalis*
  C. fetus subsp. *jejuni*
  C. fetus subsp. *veneralis*
  C. hyointestinalis
  C. jejuni
  C. pylori
  C. rectus
  C. sputorum
  C. sputorum subsp. *bubulus*
  C. sputorum subsp. *mucos-
    alis*
  C. sputorum subsp. *sputo-
    rum*

campylobacteriosis
   enteric c.

cancellous bone

cancer (*see also* carcinoma)
   breast c.
   bronchogenic c.
   c. cell
   colloid c.
   embryonal testicular c.
   endocrine responsive c.
   endometrial c.
   laryngeal c.
   medullary c.
   metastatic c.
   parathyroid c.
   prostate c.
   thyroid c.
   uterine c.
   c. vaccine

Candida
   C. albicans
   C. granuloma
   C. guilliermondii
   C. krusei
   C. lusitaniae
   C. parapsilosis
   C. pseudotropicalis
   C. stellatoidea
   C. tropicalis
   C. vaginitis
   C. vulvovaginitis

candidate tumor

candidemia

candidiasis
   acute pseudomembran-
      ous c.
   c. endocrinopathy syn-
      drome
   chronic mucocutaneous c.
   cutaneous c.
   mucocutaneous c.
   oral c.
   vaginal c.
   vulvovaginal c.

candidin

candidosis

Cannon
   C's theory
   C.-Bard theory

canthariasis

capacity
   genetic c.
   phagocytic c.
   virus neutralizing c.

capillariasis

capillary
   c. basement membrane
   c. thickening

Capim
   C. group viruses
   C. virus

capita (*plural of* caput)

Capnocytophaga
   C. canimorsus

capping
   c. phenomenon

capsid
   c. antigen

capsomer

capsomere

capsula *pl.* capsulae
   c. fibrosa glandulae thy-
      roideae
   c. glandulae thyroideae

capsular
   c. antigen
   c. polysaccharide
   c. polysaccharide vaccine

capsule
   adrenal c.
   fibrous c. of thyroid gland
   suprarenal c.

capsulorrhaphy

capture

caput *pl.* capita
   c. pancreatis

carbohydrate
   c. group
   c.-induced lipemia
   c. intolerance
   c. metabolism

carbon dioxide
   c. d. narcosis

carboxylate group structure

carboxypeptidase

carbuncle
   malignant c.

carcinoembryonic antigen
   (CEA)

carcinogen

carcinogenesis

carcinogenicity
   estrogen c.

carcinoid
   bronchial c. syndromes
   gastric c. syndromes
   gastric c. tumor
   c. syndrome
   c. tumor

carcinoma *pl.* carcinomas, car-
  cinomata (*see also* cancer)
   c. of adrenal cortex
   adrenocortical c.
   aldosterone-producing c.
   aldosterone-secreting c.
   anaplastic thyroid c.
   anaplastic c. of thyroid
    gland
   bronchogenic c.
   colloid c.
   cortisol-producing c.
   follicular thyroid c.
   follicular c. of thyroid
    gland
   gelatiniform c.

carcinoma (*continued*)
   gelatinous c.
   giant cell c. of thyroid
    gland
   Hürthle cell c.
   laryngeal c.
   medullary thyroid c.
   medullary c. of thyroid
    gland
   mucinous c.
   c. muciparum
   c. mucosum
   mucous c.
   papillary thyroid c.
   papillary c. of thyroid
    gland
   parathyroid c.
   thyroid c.
   undifferentiated c. of thy-
    roid gland

cardiac tissue

cardiodilatin

cardiolipin
   c. antigen

cardiomyopathy

cardionatrin

cardiothyrotoxicosis

cardiovascular
   diabetic c. neuropathy
   c. disease
   c. system

Cardiovirus

cardiovirus

carditis
   Lyme c.

carminophil

carnitine

carotid sinus

Carpenter syndrome

carrier
   gametocyte c.

carrier *(continued)*
   silent c.
   c. state

Carrión's disease

cartilage
   c.-derived growth factor
   c. grafting
   c. sulfation phenomenon
   thyroid c.

cascade
   complement c.
   peptide hormone c.

caseation necrosis

caseous
   c. pneumonia
   c. tubercle

cassette
   ATP-binding c.

Castellani-Low symptom

cast iron struma

castration
   chemical c.

castroid

cat
   c. flea typhus
   c.-scratch disease
   c.-scratch fever

catabolism
   antibody c.

catalase

cataphylaxis

cataract
   diabetic c.

catecholamine
   c. hormone
   plasma c.
   c. release
   c.-secreting tumor
   c. synthesis
   c. uptake

catecholaminergic

cathepsin G

cationic
   chemical c. growth factor
   c. growth factor
   c. proteins

Catu virus

cauda *pl.* caudae
   c. pancreatis

cavernosography

cavernosometry

CBG
   corticosteroid-binding globulin

C cells

CCAT
   conglutinating complement absorption test

CC-CCKR-5 cell surface receptor

CCF
   crystal-induced chemotactic factor

CCK
   cholecystokinin

CCP
   complement control protein

CD *(followed by a number)*
   cluster designation
      CD antigen
      CD marker
      CD molecule
      CD system
      CD2 receptor
      CD3 complex
      CD5 B cells
      CD45 (T-200)
      CD81 (TAPA-1)
      CD 117 (*c-kit*)

CDC
   Centers for Disease Control and Prevention

CD19:CR2:TAPA-1 complex

C (constant) domain

CDR (1–3)
    complement-determining
        region

CEA
    carcinoembryonic antigen
        CEA tumor

Cedecea

celiac disease

cell
    A c.
    accessory c's
    accessory effector c's
    activated mast c's
    adherent c's
    c. adhesion molecule
        (CAM)
    adipose c's
    alpha c.
    amine precursor uptake
        and decarboxylation
        (APUD) c's
    antibody-forming c. (AFC)
    antibody-secreting plasma
        c's
    antigen-activated B c's
    antigen-presenting c's
    antigen-reactive c's
    antigen-sensitive c's
    antigen-sensitized memory
        c's
    APUD c's
    argentaffin c's
    argyrophilic c's
    armed effector T c's
    Askanazy c's
    autoreactive T c's
    B c.
    basal granular c's
    B1 B c's
    B c. defects
    berry c.
    beta c.
    binucleated c's

cell *(continued)*
    blood c.
    blood-borne precursor
        stem c.
    blood c. count
    bone marrow–derived c.
    c.-bound antibody
    C c's
    cancer c.
    castration c's
    CD5 B c's
    chief c's
    chromaffin c's
    chromophobe c's
    chromophobic c's
    clear c.
    cleaved c.
    columnar epithelial c.
    committed c.
    contrasuppressor c's
    conventional B c's
    cortical stromal c.
    corticotrope c.
    corticotroph c.
    corticotroph-lipotroph c.
    corticotropic c.
    Crooke's c's
    c. cycle
    cytotoxic T c's
    D c.
    Daudi c's
    c. degeneration
    degranulation c's
    c. differentiation
    delta c.
    dendritic c.
    dendritic epidermal c.
        (dEC)
    dendritic epidermal T c.
        (dETC)
    dendritic phagocytic c.
        (DPC)
    Downey c's
    early pro-B c.
    effector c.
    effector T c's
    effector T c. function
    endocrine c's of the gut

cell *(continued)*
    endothelial c.
    enterochromaffin c's
    enteroendocrine c's
    epithelial c.
    epithelioid c.
    excitable c.
    exocrine c's
    F c.
    fat c's
    fetal c.
    c.-fixed antibody
    follicular center c.
    follicular dendritic c. (FDC)
    G c's
    gamma c's of hypophysis
    giant c.
    glial c.
    gonadotrope c.
    gonadotroph c.
    gonadotropic c.
    granulosa-theca c.
    grape c.
    helper c's
    helper CD4 T c's
    helper T c's
    hematopoietic c.
    hematopoietic stem c.
    hemopoietic stem c.
    high endothelial c's
    hilar c.
    homozygous typing c's (HTC)
    host c.
    Hürthle c's
    immature B c.
    immunologically competent c.
    inducer c.
    inflammatory c.
    inflammatory CD4 T c's (T$_H$1 cells)
    inflammatory T c's
    innocent bystander c.
    c. interaction
    c. interaction (CI) genes
    c. interaction (CI) molecules
    interdigitating c's

cell *(continued)*
    interdigitating dendritic c's
    interdigitating reticular c.
    interfollicular c's
    intermediate c.
    interstitial c's
    islet c's
    K c's
    killer c's
    killer T c's
    Kupffer's c.
    L c's
    lactotrope c.
    LAK (lymphokine-activated killer) c.
    Langerhans' c. (LC)
    large cleaved c.
    large cleaved follicular center c.
    large granule c's
    large noncleaved c.
    large noncleaved follicular center c.
    large uncleaved c.
    late pro-B c.
    LE c.
    Leishman's chrome c's
    leukemia c's
    Leydig c.
    light c's
    lymph c.
    lymphoid c's
    lymphokine-activated killer (LAK) c.
    M c's
    c. marker
    mast c.
    mature B c's
    mature T c's
    mediator c.
    c. membrane
    membranous c's
    memory c's
    memory B c's
    memory T c's
    mononuclear c.
    morular c.
    Mott c.

cell *(continued)*
- mulberry c.
- multinucleated c.
- multiple stem c. (MSC)
- multipotential stem c.
- myeloid c's
- myeloma c.
- naive c.
- naive B c's
- naive T c's
- natural killer (NK) c's
- natural suppressor c's
- neuroendocrine c's
- neurohormonal c's
- neurosecretory c.
- NK (natural killer) c's
- noncleaved c.
- nonphagocytic c.
- null c's
- nurse c.
- ovarian hilar c's
- oxyphil c's
- oxyphilic c's
- pancreatic clear c's
- pancreatic islet c's
- parafollicular c's
- passenger c's
- peripheral blood mononuclear c's
- peripheral blood progenitor c's (PBPC)
- peripheral blood stem c's
- phagocytic c.
- phagocytic Langerhans c.
- pheochrome c's
- pineal c.
- plaque-forming c. (PFC)
- plasma c.
- pluripotent stem c.
- polyhedral theca lutein-
  like c.
- PP c's
- pre-B c.
- precursor c.
- pregnancy c.
- pre-T c.
- primitive stem c.
- principal c's

cell *(continued)*
- pro-B c.
- professional antigen-presenting c.
- progenitor c.
- prolactin c.
- proliferating B c's
- c. proliferation
- RA c.
- Raji c.
- red c.
- red blood c.
- red blood c. destruction
- Reed-Sternberg c.
- resting wandering c.
- reticular c.
- reticuloendothelial c.
- rhagiocrine c.
- rod c.
- S c's
- scavenger c.
- secretory c's
- self-reactive B c's
- sensitized c.
- Sertoli c.
- sickle c. (SC)
- sickle c. anemia
- sickle c. disease
- SIF c's
- c. signaling
- small cleaved c.
- small cleaved follicular
  center c.
- small granule c's
- small noncleaved c.
- small noncleaved follicular
  center c.
- small pre-B c.
- small uncleaved c.
- somatostatin c's
- somatotrope c.
- somatotroph c.
- somatotropic c.
- superantigen-binding T c's
- stem c.
- suppressor c's
- suppressor T c's
- c. surface antigen
- c. surface immunoglobulin

cell *(continued)*
    c.-surface marker
    c. surface size
    T c.
    T_{DTH} c.
    T_H1 c's
    T c. activation
    T c. antigen receptor
    T c. clones
    T c. defects
    T c.–dependent antigen
    T c. diversity
    T c. function
    T c. growth factor
    T c. hybrids
    T c.–independent antigen
    T c. lines
    T c. lymphoma
    T c. memory
    T c. receptor complex
    T c. replacing factor
    T c. stimulation
    T c. subpopulation
    T c. subset
    superantigen-binding T c's
    T c. system
    target c.
    tart c.
    Tc c's
    Tc1 c's
    Tc2 c's
    TD c. *(same as* sensitized lymphocyte)
    $T\gamma$ c's
    TH c.
    theca c.
    thymic cortical epithelial c's
    thyroidectomy c's
    thyroid follicular c's
    thyrotrope c.
    thyrotroph c.
    thyrotropic c.
    tissue dendritic c's
    $T\mu$ c's
    transformed c.
    trophoblast c's
    trophoblastic c's
    TS c.

cell *(continued)*
    tumor c.
    tumor-infiltrating T c.
    ultimobranchial c's
    unipotent precursor T c.
    veil c's
    veiled c's
    Vero c's
    veto c's
    c. volume
    Warthin-Finkeldey c's
    wasserhelle c.
    water-clear c.
    white blood c's
    Xenopus cytotoxic c's

cell-mediated
    c.-m. cytotoxicity
    c.-m. hypersensitivity
    c.-m. hypersensitivity reaction
    c.-m. immunity (CMI)
    c.-m. lympholysis (CML)
    c.-m. lympholysis (CML) assay
    c.-m. secondary immune response

cellular
    c. cooperation
    c. growth
    c. immunity
    c. immunology
    c. receptor
    c. rejection
    c. resistance
    c. theory of immunity
    c. tolerance
    c. transfer

cellulitis

cellulose
    c. phosphate
    c. sodium phosphate

CELO virus

center
    C's for Disease Control and Prevention (CDC)

center *(continued)*
    Flemming c.
    germinal c.
    hypothalamic thirst c.
    reaction c.

central
    c. diabetes insipidus
    C. European encephalitis
        virus
    c. hypothyroidism
    c. lymphoid organs
    c. lymphoid tissues
    c. nervous system (CNS)
    c. nervous system tumor
    c. obesity
    c. pontine myelinolysis
    c. tolerance

centrifugation
    density gradient c.
    Ficoll-Hypaque gradient c.

centroblast

centrocyte

centromere

cephalic
    c. phase
    c. tetanus

cephalosporiosis

cephalotetanus

cercaria

cercosporamycosis

cerebral
    c. adiposity
    c. anthrax
    c. apophysis
    c. edema in diabetic keto-
        acidosis
    c. gigantism
    c. mucormycosis
    c. poliomyelitis
    c. rheumatism
    c. tetanus

cerebrospinal fluid (CSF)

cerebrovascular accident (CVA)

cerebrum

ceruloplasmin

cestode

cestodiasis

cestodic tuberculosis

cetirizine hydrochloride

c-fos gene

CG
    chorionic gonadotropin

CGD (chronic granulomatous
    disease)

CH50
    total hemolytic comple-
        ment
        CH50 assay
        CH50 unit

CH100 assay

Chagas' disease

Chagres virus

chain
    alpha (α) heavy c.
    alpha (α) heavy c. disease
    beta (β) c.
    delta (δ) c's
    DRa c.
    epsilon (ϵ) c.
    free heavy c. fragments
    gamma (γ) c.
    gamma (γ) heavy c.
    H (heavy) c.
    heavy c. disease
    heavy c. fragments
    invariant c.
    J (joining) c.
    kappa (κ) c.
    kappa (κ) light c's
    L (light) c.
    lambda (λ) c.

chain *(continued)*
  lambda (λ) group light c's
  lambda (λ) light c's
  lambda (λ) monoclonal
    light c's
  light (L) c.
  peptide c.
  surrogate light c's
  zeta (ζ) c.

challenge
  bronchial c.
  c. diet
  food c.
  histamine c.
  inhalational c.
  methacholine c.
  c. test

chamber
  Boyden c.
  Finn c.

chancre
  hard c.
  hunterian c.
  mixed c.
  monorecidive c.
  c. redux
  soft c.
  true c.
  tuberculous c.

chancriform

chancroid
  phagedenic c.
  serpiginous c.
  c. ulcer

chancroidal
  c. bubo

chancrous

change
  Crooke's c's
  Crooke-Russell c's
  genetic c's
  titer c's

Changuinola virus

channel
  ion c.

character
  primary sex c's
  secondary sex c's

characteristic
  immunoglobulin c's
  sexual c's

charbon

chart
  Liley c.

Chase-Sulzberger phenomenon

Chauffard
  C's syndrome
  C.-Still syndrome

Chédiak-Higashi syndrome

cheesy pneumonia

chelator
  calcium c's

chemical
  c. abortion
  c. castration
  c. cationic growth factor
  c. control
  c. diabetes
  c. hyperglycemia

chemiluminescence test

chemoattractant
  monocyte c's
  phagocyte c's

chemoendocrine

chemohormonal

chemoimmunology

chemokine
  RANTES c.
  c. receptor

chemoreceptor

chemotactic
  c. factor

chemotactic *(continued)*
    c. fragments

chemotaxis
    c. of leukocytes

chemotherapeutic drugs

chessboard titration

chest
    barrel c.

cheyletiellosis

Chiari-Frommel syndome

chiasm
    optic c.

chickenpox

Chicago disease

chick embryo interferon

chicken ovalbumin upstream promoter (COUP)

chief
    c. agglutinin
    c. cells
    c. cell adenoma
    c. cell hyperplasia

chigger
    c.-borne typhus
    c. dermatitis

chikungunya virus

chilomastigiasis

chilomastixiasis

chimera
    bone marrow c.
    radiation c.
    radiation bone marrow c's

chimpanzee

chlamydemia

Chlamydia
    C. pneumoniae
    C. psittaci
    C. trachomatis

chlamydiosis

chloasma

chloragocyte

chloroquine

chlorinated sugar

chlorotrianisene

Choix fever

cholecalciferol

cholecystographic agents

cholecystokinin (CCK)

cholelithiasis

cholera
    Asiatic c.
    dry c.
    c. enterotoxin
    pancreatic c.
    c. sicca
    c. toxin
    c. vaccine

choleragen

choleraic

choleraphage

choleriform

cholerigenic

cholerigenous

choleroid

cholestasis

cholestatic hepatitis

cholesterol
    c. desmolase deficiency
    c. side-chain cleavage deficiency

cholestyramine

choline
    acetyl glyceryl ether phosphoryl c.

cholinergic
   c. crisis
   c. pathways
   c. receptors

chondrocalcinosis

chondrocyte growth factor

chondrodysplasia

Chordopoxvirinae

choreoathetosis

choriocarcinoma
   pineal c.

chorioepithelioma

choriogonadotropin

choriomammotropin

choriomeningitis
   lymphocytic c. (LCM)

chorionic
   c. ACTH
   c. gonadotropin (CG)
   c. gonadotropin–secreting
      tumor
   c. somatomammotropin
   c. thyrotropin

chorioptic

chorioretinitis

Christopher's spots

chromaffin
   c. body
   c. cells
   c. cell tumor
   c. granules
   c. hormone
   c. reaction
   c. system
   c. tissue

chromaffinoma
   medullary c.

chromaffinopathy

chromaphil

chromatin
   X c.
   Y c.

chromatography
   affinity c.
   gel filtration c.
   high-pressure liquid c.
      (HPLC)
   steroid affinity c.

chromium

Chromobacterium
   C. violaceum

chromogen
   Porter-Silber c.

chromogranin

chromomycosis

chromophobe
   c. adenoma
   c. cells

chromophobic
   c. adenoma
   c. cells

chromosomal
   c. mosaicism
   c. rearrangement
   c. translocation

chromosome
   c. anomalies
   c. formation
   eukaryotic c.
   c. karyotype
   ring c.
   sex c.
   X c.
   Y c.

chronic
   c. active hepatitis
   c. amenorrhea
   c. anovulation
   c. carbon dioxide narcosis
   c. CO_2 narcosis

chronic *(continued)*
- c. diarrheal syndrome
- c. Epstein-Barr virus (EBV)
- c. essential pentosuria
- c. fatigue syndrome
- c. fibrous thyroiditis
- c. granulomatous disease (CGD)
- c. infection
- c. inflammatory bowel disease
- c. lymphadenoid thyroiditis
- c. lymphocytic leukemia (CLL)
- c. lymphocytic thyroiditis
- c. mucocutaneous candidiasis
- c. necrotizing aspergillosis
- c. obstructive pulmonary disease (COPD)
- c. progressive myelopathy
- c. rejection
- c. sclerosing thyroiditis
- c. thyroiditis
- c. viral hepatitis

Churg
- C.-Strauss syndrome
- C.-Strauss vasculitis

C21 hydroxylase

chylomicron
- c. remnants

chymase

chymopapain

CI
- cell interaction
    - CI genes
    - CI molecules

Ci
- curie

CID
- combined immunodeficiency

CIE
- counterimmunoelectrophoresis

CIITA
- class II MHC transactivator

ciliary neurotropic factor

cimicosis

cim locus

circadian rhythm

circulating
- c. immune complex
- c. neutrophils

circulation
- enterohepatic c.
- hypophysial portal c.
- hypophysioportal c.
- lymphocyte c.
- portal c.
- systemic c.

circumscribed myxedema

circumventricular organs

cirrhosis
- idiopathic biliary c.
- cryptogenic c.
- Laënnec's c.

citrate
- potassium c.

Citrobacter
- *C. amalonaticus*
- *C. diversus*
- *C. freundii*
- *C. intermedius*

C1INH
- C1 inhibitor

c-kit (CD117)
- *c-kit* oncogene

c-kit ligand

CLA
- cutaneous lymphocyte antigen

cladiosis

cladosporiosis
- c. epidermica

Cladosporium
   C. bantianum
   C. carrionii
   C. mansonii
   C. trichoides
   C. werneckii

clamping
   euglycemic c.

clamp technique

clap

clasmatocyte

class
   c. I antigens
   c. I restriction
   c. II antigens
   c. II-associated invariant
      chain peptide (CLIP)
   c. II restriction
   c. II transactivator
   c. III antigens
   heavy chain c's
   immunoglobulin c's
   c. switch
   c. switching

classic pathway

classical
   c. complement pathway
   c. pathway
   c. precipitin reactions

classification
   adansonian c.
   Bergey's c.
   Gell and Coombs c.
   Kauffman-White c.
   Lancefield c.
   Migula's c.
   numerical c.
   Runyon c.
   WHO c.

clavicular sign

clearance
   immune c.

clear cell
   pancreatic c. c's

clear plaque mutation

cleavage
   papain antibody c.
   pepsin antibody c.

cleaved cell

cleft
   Maurer's c's
   synaptic c.

clemastine
   c. fumarate

climacteric
   female c.
   male c.

climacterium

climate

climatic bubo

clinical
   c. endocrinology
   c. infection
   c. picture

Clinistix

Clinitest

CLIP
   class II-associated invariant
      chain peptide

clitorimegaly

clitoral hypertrophy

CLL (chronic lymphocytic leukemia)

clonal
   c. abortion
   c. analysis
   c. anergy
   c. deletion
   c. deletion theory
   c. expansion
   c. ignorance

clonal *(continued)*
    c. selection
    c. selection hypothesis
    c. selection theory

clone
    forbidden c.
    myeloma c.
    T cell c's

cloned T cell line

cloning
    oncogene c.

clonorchiasis

clonorchiosis

clonotype

clonotypic
    c. antibodies

closed-loop glycemic insulin delivery system

clostridial toxin

clostridiosis

Clostridium
    C. botulinum
    C. difficile
    C. histolyticum
    C. novyi
    C. oedematiens
    C. perfringens
    C. septicum
    C. tetani
    C. welchii

cloudy swelling

clump

clumping
    c. factor

cluster
    c's of differentiation (CD)
    c. designation (CD) *(followed by a number)*

clusterin

CMI
    cell-mediated immunity

CML
    cell-mediated lympholysis
    CML assay

CMN
    Clostridium, Mycobacterium, and *Nocardia*
    CMN group

c-myb gene

c-myc gene

C3 NeF
    C3 nephritic factor

CNS
    central nervous system

coagglutination

coagulase

coagulation
    disseminated intravascular c. (DIC)
    intravascular c.

coalesce

coat

coated
    c. pits
    c. vesicles

coast erysipelas

coccidioidal granuloma

Coccidioides

coccidioidin
    c. skin test
    c. test

coccidioidoma

coccidioidomycosis
    progressive c.
    secondary c.

coccidioidosis

coccidiosis

coccoid x bodies

cockade reaction

Cockayne syndrome

coctoantigen

cocto-immunogen

coctolabile

coctoprecipitin

coctostabile

coctostable

coding joint

Coe virus

coelomocyte

coenuriasis

coenurosis

cognitive phase

Cohen syndrome

coinfection

coisogenic

cold
    c. acclimation
    c. agglutination
    c. agglutinin
    c. agglutinin syndrome
    c. allergy
    c. antibody
    common c.
    c. exposure
    c. hemagglutinin
    c. hemoglobinuria
    c. nodule
    c.-reactive antibody
    c. sore
    c. target inhibition

colibacillemia

colibacillosis

colibacilluria

colic
    biliary c.
    renal c.

colicin

colic
    renal c.

coliphage

colitis
    ulcerative c.

coliuria

collagen
    c. arthritis
    c. autoantibodies
    c. disease

collagenase

collectin

collecting tubule

collision-coupling mechanism

Colliver's symptom

colloid
    c. adenoma
    bovine c.
    c. cancer
    c. carcinoma
    c. goiter
    thyroid c.

Colombian tick fever

colonic polyp

colonization infection

colony-stimulating factor (CSF)

Colorado
    C. tick fever
    C. tick fever virus

colostrum

colposcopy

Coltivirus

Columbia SK virus

columnar epithelial cell

coma
  diabetic c.
  hyperosmolar c.
  hyperosmolar nonketotic c.
  Kussmaul's c.
  myxedema c.
  nonketotic hyperosmolar c.
  posthypoglycemic c.

combinatorial diversity

combined
  c. anterior pituitary test
  c. B and T cell immunodeficiency
  c. hyperlipidemia
  c. immunodeficiency (CID)
  c. immunodeficiency disease
  severe c. immunodeficiency
  severe c. immunodeficiency disease
  c. vaccine

combining site

commensal

commensalism

commercially available vaccine

committed cell

common
  c. acute lymphoblastic leukemia antigen (CALLA)
  c. antigen
  c. bile duct
  c. cold
  c. cold viruses
  c. immunocyte
  c. leukocyte antigens
  c. lymphoid progenitors
  c. thymocyte
  c. variable agammaglobulinemia
  c. variable hypogammaglobulinemia
  c. variable immunodeficiency (CVID)

common (continued)
  c. variable unclassifiable immunodeficiency

communicable
  c. disease

community immunity

compartment
  class II MHC c. (MIIC)

compatibility

compatible

compensatory atrophy

competence
  immunologic c.

competition
  antigen c.
  antigenic c.

competitive
  c. binding assays
  c. enzyme-linked immunosorbent assay
  c. inhibition assay
  c. radioimmunoassay
  c. radioimmunosorbent test

complement
  c. activation
  c. cascade
  c. components (C1–C9)
  c. components and fragments
    C1
    C1q
    C1r
    C1s
    C2
    C2a
    C3
    C3a
    C3b
    C3d
    C4
    C4a
    C4b
    C5

complement *(continued)*
    C5a
    C5b
    C6
    C7
    C8
    C9
    c. control protein (CCP)
    c. control protein domains
    c.-determining region
      (CDR) (1–3)
    c. deviation
    c. fixation
    c. fixation inhibition test
    c. fixation reaction
    c. fixation test
    c.-fixing antibody
    c. inactivation
    c. pathways
    c. receptors
    c. regulation
    serum c.
    c. system
    total hemolytic c. (CH50)
    c. unit
    Xenopus c.

complementation

complementoid

complete
    c. agglutinin
    c. androgen insensitivity
    c. antibody
    c. antigen

complex
    AIDS-related c. (ARC)
    antibody-antigen c.
    antigen-antibody c.
    B c.
    B cell coreceptor c.
    B cell receptor c.
    CD3 c.
    CD19:CR2:TAPA-1 c.
    circulating immune c.
    Ghon c.
    H-2 c.
    hapten-carrier c.

complex *(continued)*
    histocompatibility c.
    HIV antibody binding c.
    HLA c.
    hormone receptor c.
    hypothalamic-pituitary-thy-
      roid c.
    immune c.
    immune stimulatory c.
      (ISCOM)
    inosinic-cytidylic acid c.
    LCMV-LASV c.
    major histocompatibility c.
      (MHC)
    c.-mediated hypersensitiv-
      ity
    membrane attack c. (MAC)
    polysaccharide c.
    primary c.
    primary inoculation c.
    primary tuberculous c.
    Ranke c.
    receptor-steroid c.
    signal recognition parti-
      cle c.
    Tacaribe c.
    T cell receptor c.
    Xenopus major histocom-
      patibility c.

complication
    diabetic c's
    primary c.
    secondary c's

component
    complement c's (C1–C9)
    costimulatory c.
    M c.
    secretory c. (SC)
    terminal complement c's

composite graft

composition
    body c.

compound
    aminoheterocyclic c.
    c. iodine solution

compulsive water drinking

computed tomography (CT)
  c. t. scan

concanavalin A (ConA)

concentration
  antigen c.
  immunoglobulin c.
  urine c.

concept
  threading c.

conceptus

concomitant immunity

concordant
  c. species
  c. xenograft

conditioning
  vasomotor c.

condyloma *pl.* condylomas,
  condylomata
    condylomata lata

configuration
  germline c.

confocal fluorescent microscope

conformational
  c. determinants
  c. epitopes

congenic
  c. animals
  MHC c.
  c. mice
  c. resistant strains

congenital
  c. adrenal hyperplasia
  c. adrenal hypoplasia
  c. anorchia
  c. cytomegalovirus infec-
    tion
  c. goiter
  c. hypothyroidism
  c. immunodeficiency
  c. myxedema
  c. rubella syndrome

congenital *(continued)*
  c. smallpox
  c. syphilis
  c. viral infection

conglutinating
  c. complement absorption
    test (CCAT)

conglutination
  c. reaction

conglutinin
  c. A
  immune c.

conglutinogen

Congo red fever

coniophage

conjugate
  c. heptavalent pneumococ-
    cal vaccine

conjugated
  c. antigen
  c. estrogens
  c. estrogen hormone

conjunctiva

conjunctivitis
  allergic c.
  anaphylactic c.

Conn's syndrome

connective tissue

connexon

Conor and Bruch's disease

consensus
  short c. repeat (SCR)

constant
  association c.
  dissociation c. (Kd)
  c. (C) domain
  c. (C) genes
  off-rate c's
  on-rate c's
  rate c.

constant *(continued)*
    c. region

constitution
    genetic c.

constitutional
    c. growth delay
    c. short stature

consumption

consumptive

contact
    c. dermatitis
    direct c.
    c. hypersensitivity
    immediate c.
    indirect c.
    c. inhibition
    mediate c.
    c. sensitivity
    c. tests

contactant

contagion

contagiosity

contagious
    c. disease

contaminated reagent

continuous
    c. epitopes
    c. subcutaneous insulin infusion

contraception
    barrier c.
    hormonal c.
    postcoital c.

contraceptive
    implanted c.
    injectable c.
    nonsteroidal c.
    oral c. (OC)
    vaginal c.

contraction
    volume c.

contrainsular

contrasexual
    c. precocity

contrast medium
    radiographic contrast media

contrasuppressor
    c. cells

contrasuppression

control
    adrenal c.
    birth c.
    chemical c.
    feedback c.
    metabolic c.
    paracrine c.
    secretomotor c.
    transcriptional c.

convalescence
    c. period
    c. serum

convalescent
    c. human serum
    c. serum

conventional B cells

conversion
    gene c.

convertase
    C3 c.
    C3 proactivator c.
    C5 c.

Coombs' test
    direct C. t.
    indirect C. t.

cooperation
    cellular c.

cooperativity
    negative c.
    positive c.

coprecipitin

coproantibody

coproporphyria
    hereditary c.

cord
    c. factor
    spinal c.

core
    c. polysaccharide

coreceptors

Cori's disease

cornea
    c. transplantation

Corner
    C.-Allen test
    C.-Allen unit

coronary heart disease

Coronaviridae

Coronavirus

coronavirus

corpus *pl.* corpora
    corpora albicantia
    corpora atretica
    c. callosum
    c. luteum
    c. luteum hormone
    c. pancreatis
    c. pineale

corpuscle
    Guarnieri's c's
    Lostorfer's c's
    Paschen's c's
    typhic c's

correction
    Bonferroni c.
    Yates' c.

correlation
    endocrine c.

cortex *pl.* cortices
    adrenal c.
    c. of adrenal gland

cortex *(continued)*
    fetal adrenal c.
    c. glandulae suprarenalis
    ovarian c.
    provisional c.
    suprarenal c.
    c. of suprarenal gland
    tertiary c.
    thymic c.

cortexone

cortical
    c. bone
    c. hormone
    c. stromal cell
    c. zone

cortical-hypothalamic-pituitary
  axis

cortices *(plural of* cortex)

corticoadrenal

corticoid

corticolipotrope

corticosteroid
    c.-binding globulin (CBG)
    17-OH-c's (17-hydroxycorti-
      costeroids)

corticosterone

corticosterone methyl oxidase
  deficiency

corticotrope
    c. adenoma
    c. cell
    c. cell adenoma
    c. tumor

corticotroph
    c. adenoma
    c. cell
    c. cell adenoma
    c.-lipotroph cell
    c. tumor

corticotrophic

corticotrophin

corticotroph-lipotroph

corticotropic
  c. cell

corticotropin
  c.-like intermediate lobe
    peptide
  c.-related peptide hor-
    mones
  c.-releasing factor (CRF)
  c.-releasing hormone (CRH)

corticotropinoma

cortisol
  c.-binding globulin
  c. hyperreactive syndrome
  c.-producing adenoma
  c.-producing carcinoma
  urinary c.

cortisone
  c. acetate
  c.-oral glucose tolerance
    test

Corynebacterium
  C. diphtheriae
  C. minutissimum
  C. parvum
  C. ulcerans
  C. xerosis

coryza virus

corzyme EIA test

cosensitize

cosmopolitan distribution

costimulation

costimulator

costimulatory
  c. component
  c. signals

cosyntropin

cotransmission

cottonpox

cotype

cough
  pertussis c.
  whooping c.

coulombic force

Councilman
  C's bodies
  C's lesion

counseling
  genetic c.

count
  absolute lymphocyte c.
  basophil c.
  eosinophil c.
  leukocyte c.
  lymphocyte c.
  monocyte c.
  neutrophil c.
  platelet c.

countercurrent
  c. hypothesis
  c. immunoelectrophoresis

counterelectrophoresis

counterimmunoelectrophoresis
  (CIE)

COUP
  chicken ovalbumin up-
    stream promoter
      COUP-transcription
        factor

coupling
  nonlinear c.

Cowdry type I inclusion bodies

Cowen's sign

cowpox
  c. virus

covalent

Coxiella
  C. burnetii

Coxsackie virus

coxsackievirus

C3PA

C peptide

CPP-32

CR (1–4)
    complement receptor

CRAF
    CD40 receptor–associated
    factor

cranial nerve neuritis

craniobuccal
    c. cysts
    c. pouch

craniopharyngeal
    c. cysts
    c. duct tumor
    c. pouch

craniopharyngioma

cranium

craw-craw

C-reactive protein

creatinine

CREB
    cyclic adenosine mono-
    phosphate response ele-
    ment–binding protein

creeping
    c. disease
    c. eruption
    c. myiasis

C (constant) region

Cre recombinase

CREST
    calcinosis, Raynaud's phe-
    nomenon, esophageal
    dysmotility, sclerodac-
    tyly, and telangiectases
        CREST syndrome

crest
    supraoptic c.

cretin
    c. dwarf

cretinism
    athyreotic c.
    athyrotic c.
    endemic c.
    infantile c.
    myxedematous c.
    neurologic c.
    spontaneous c.
    sporadic c.
    sporadic goitrous c.
    sporadic nongoitrous c.

cretinistic

cretinoid
    c. dysplasia
    c. idiocy

cretinous

Creutzfeldt-Jakob disease

CRF
    corticotropin-releasing fac-
    tor
        CRF action
        CRF regulation

CRH
    corticotropin-releasing hor-
    mone

Crimean
    C. hemorrhagic fever virus
    C.-Congo hemorrhagic fe-
    ver
    C.-Congo hemorrhagic fe-
    ver virus

crinophagy

crisis *pl.* crises
    addisonian c.
    adrenal c.
    anaphylactoid c.
    cholinergic c.
    hypercalcemic c.
    thyroid c.
    thyrotoxic c.

criterion *pl.* criteria
  Witebsky's criteria

CRM
  cross-reacting material

cRNA
  complementary RNA

cromolyn
  c. sodium

Crohn's disease

Crooke
  C's cells
  C's changes
  C's hyaline degeneration
  C's hyalinization
  C.-Russell basophils
  C.-Russell changes

cross
  c. agglutination
  c. agglutinin
  c. immunity
  c. infection
  c. matching
  phage c.

crossed immunoelectrophoresis

crosslinking
  c. of receptors

crossmatch

crossmatching

cross-reacting
  c.-r. agglutinin
  c.-r. antibody
  c.-r. antigen
  c.-r. material (CRM)

cross-reaction

cross-reactivation

cross-reactive antigen

cross-reactivity
  antibody c.-r.

cross-sensitization

croup-associated virus

croupous membrane

crusted scabies

cryofibrinogen

cryogammaglobulin

cryoglobulin (*types I, II, III*)

cryoglobulinemia
  essential mixed c.

cryptidin

cryptitope

cryptococcoma

cryptococcosis

Cryptococcus
  C. albidus
  C. histolyticus
  C. hominis
  C. meningitidis
  C. neoformans

cryptodeterminant

cryptogenic
  c. cirrhosis
  c. infection
  c. tetanus

cryptoplasmic

cryptorchid
  c. testis

cryptorchism

cryptosporidiosis

Cryptosporidium
  C. parvum

Cryptostroma

cryptozoite

crystal
  c.-induced chemotactic factor (CCF)

crystal *(continued)*
    c. scintillation

crystalline
    c. fragment receptor
    c. zinc insulin

crystallizable fragment

CSF
    cerebrospinal fluid
    colony stimulating factor
        CSF1

CT
    calcitonin
        CT bioassay
        CT deficiency
        CT radioimmunoassay
        CT receptors
        CT secretion
    computed tomography
        CT scan

CTL
    cytotoxic T lymphocyte

CTLA4 (CD152)

Cuban itch

cuffing

culture
    c. medium
    mixed lymphocyte c. (MLC)
    tissue c.

Cunninghamella

curare

curie (Ci)

current vaccine

Curvularia

Cushing
    C's basophilism
    C's disease
    iatrogenic C's syndrome
    C's syndrome
    C's syndrome medicamen-
        tosus

cushingoid
    c. facies

cutaneous
    c. anaphylaxis
    c. anthrax
    c. basophil hypersensitivity
    c. blastomycosis
    c. blowfly myiasis
    c. candidiasis
    c. diphtheria
    c. fungus
    c. immune system
    c. larva migrans
    c. lichen amyloidosis
    c. lupus erythematosus
    c. lymphocyte antigen
        (CLA)
    c. lymphoid antigen
    c. lymphoma
    c. mastocytosis
    c. myiasis
    c. reaction
    c. schistosomiasis
    c. T cell lymphoma

cutireaction

CVA
    cerebrovascular accident

CVID
    common variable immuno-
        deficiency

C virus

cyanoketone

cyanosis

cycle
    cell c.
    endometrial c.
    estrous c.
    hair c.
    HIV life c.
    menstrual c.
    reproductive c.

cyclic adenosine monophos-
    phate (cyclic AMP)

cyclic adenosine monophosphate *(continued)*
    c. a. m. response element–
    binding protein (CREB)

cyclic AMP
    cyclic adenosine mono-
    phosphate
        cyclic AMP–dependent
        protein kinase
        urinary cyclic AMP
        (UcAMP)

cyclin

cycling
    substrate c.

cyclooxygenase

cyclopentanoperhydrophen-
anthrene

cyclophilin

cyclophosphamide

cyclosporiasis

cyclosporin A

cyclosporine
    c. effect
    c.-associated arteriopathy

cynic
    c. spasm

Cynodon

cyproheptadine hydrochloride

cyproterone

cyst
    arachnoid c.
    craniobuccal c's
    craniopharyngeal c's
    intrapituitary c's
    müllerian duct c's
    ovarian c.
    Rathke's c's
    Rathke's cleft c's
    suprasellar c.

cystadenoma
    papillary c.

cystadenoma *(continued)*
    papillary c. of thyroid

cystic
    c. atresia
    c. fibrosis
    c. goiter

cysticercosis

Cysticercus cellulosae

cysticercus disease

cystine

cystinosis

cystinuria

cystocele

cystozoite

cytokine
    cytotoxic c's
    macrophage c's
    neurotoxic c.
    c. receptor
    Xenopus c's

cytology

cytolysin

cytolysis
    antibody-dependent cell-
    mediated c. (ADCC)
    immune c.

cytolytic
    c. T lymphocyte
    c. viral infection

cytomegalic
    c. inclusion disease
    c. inclusion disease virus

Cytomegalovirus

cytomegalovirus
    acquired c.
    c. antigen
    congenital c. infection
    c. infection
    latent c.

cytomegalovirus *(continued)*
  c. mononucleosis

cytometer
  flow c.

cytometry
  flow c.
  flow cell c.

cytopenic

cytophagocytosis

cytophagous

cytophagy

cytophil

cytophilic
  c. antibody

cytoplasmic
  c. inclusions
  c. proteins
  c. bridge

cytorrhyctes

cytoskeletal reorientation

cytosol

cytotaxigen

cytotoxic
  c. activation
  c. agent

cytotoxic *(continued)*
  c. agent sensitization
  c. anaphylaxis
  c. antibody
  c. chemotherapeutic immu-
    nosuppressive agents
  c. cytokines
  c. cytokine release
  c. drugs
  c. effector molecules
  c. hypersensitivity
  c. hypersensitivity reaction
  c. lytic granules
  c. memory
  c. reaction
  c. T cells
  c. T lymphocyte (CTL)
  c.-type hypersensitivity

cytotoxicity
  antibody-dependent cell-
    mediated c.
  antibody-dependent cellu-
    lar c. (ADCC)
  cell-mediated c.
  c. testing

cytotoxin

cytotrophic
  c. anaphylaxis

cytotropic
  c. antibody

D
  D antigen
  D cell
  D-dimer assay
  D-dimer test
  diversity
    D gene segments
    D region
    D segments
  surfactant protein D

daclizumab

Dactylaria

DAF
  decay accelerating factor

DAG
  diacylgylcerol

Dale
  D. phenomenon
  D. reaction

Dalrymple's sign

damage
  liver d.
  spinal cord d.
  tissue d.

dandy fever

Dane particle

D antigen (*of poliovirus*)

Danysz
  D. effect
  D. phenomenon

dapsone (DDS)

Darier sign

darkfield
  d. microscope
  d. microscopy

Darling's disease

Darlington plasmagene theory

DAT
  direct antiglobulin test

Daudi cells

Davidsohn differential test

dawn phenomenon

DBH
  dopamine β-hydroxylase

D cell

D-dimer
  D-d. assay
  D-d. test

DDS
  dapsone

dead vaccine

deallergization

Dean and Webb titration

death
  activation-induced cell d.
    (AICD)
  black d.
  programmed cell d.
  thymocyte d.

debilitated host

Debré's phenomenon

dEC
  dendritic epidermal cell

decarboxylase
  aromatic L-amino-acid d.

decay accelerating factor (DAF)

declining glucose tolerance

decomplementize

decrease
  volume-regulatory d. (VRD)

deer fly fever

default pathway

defect
  B cell d's
  birth d's
  DNA repair d.

defect *(continued)*
    iodotyrosine-coupling d.
    iodotyrosine dehaloge-
      nase d.
    Ir (immune response)
      gene d.
    metabolic d's
    organification d.
    side-chain cleavage d.
    T cell d's

defective
    d. endogenous retroviruses
    d. virus

defeminization

defense
    d. rupture

defensin

deficiency
    adenosine deaminase
      (ADA) d.
    adrenocorticotropic hor-
      mone (ACTH) d.
    androgen d.
    aromatase d.
    calcitonin d.
    cholesterol desmolase d.
    cholesterol side-chain
      cleavage d.
    corticosterone methyl oxi-
      dase d.
    estrogen d.
    familial hepatic lipase d.
    genetic d.
    11β-hydroxylase d.
    17α-hydroxylase d.
    18-hydroxylase d.
    21-hydroxylase d.
    3β-hydroxysteroid dehy-
      drogenase d.
    11β-hydroxysteroid dehy-
      drogenase d.
    17β-hydroxysteroid dehy-
      drogenase d.
    immune d.
    immunologic d.
    iodine d.
    isolated IgA d.

deficiency *(continued)*
    leukocyte adhesion d.
    17,20-lyase d.
    lymphocyte-inherited d's
    lymphopenic immuno-
      logic d.
    myeloperoxidase d.
    neutrophil cytochrome d.
    nucleoside phospho-
      rylase d.
    phagocytic cell d's
    placental sulfatase d.
    PNP (purine nucleoside
      phosphorylase) d.
    primary immunoglobulin d.
    properdin d.
    purine nucleoside phos-
      phorylase (PNP) d.
    secondary immunoglobu-
      lin d.
    secretory isotype d's
    selective IgA d.
    sex-linked lymphopenic im-
      munologic d.
    stem cell d.
    d. symptom
    vitamin B_{12} d.
    X-linked immune d.
    zinc d.

deficient
    d. phagocytosis

definitive
    d. host
    d. zone of adrenal cortex

degeneration
    adiposogenital d.
    Crooke's hyaline d.

degranulation
    d. cells

dehydration

dehydroandrosterone

7-dehydrocholesterol
    activated 7-d.

11-dehydrocorticosterone

dehydroepiandrosterone (DHEA)
    d. loading test
    d. sulfate

dehydroisoandrosterone

de Lange syndrome

delay
    constitutional growth d.
    growth d.

delayed
    d. allergy
    d. hypersensitivity (DH)
    d. hypersensitivity reaction
    d. hypersensitivity skin test
    d. menarche
    d. puberty
    d.-type hypersensitivity (DTH)

del Castillo's syndrome

deletion
    antigenic d.
    clonal d.
    functional d.

delta (δ)
    d. agent
    d. antigen
    d. basophil
    d. cell
    d. chains
    d. hepatitis
    hepatitis d.
    d. staphylolysin

Deltavirus

demasculinization

Dematium

dementia

demodectic

demodicidosis

demodicosis

de Morsier's syndrome

dendrite

dendritic
    d. cell
    d. epidermal cell (dEC)
    d. epidermal T cell (dETC)
    interdigitating d. cells
    d. phagocytic cell (DPC)

dengue
    d. fever
    hemorrhagic d.
    d. hemorrhagic fever
    d. shock syndrome
    d. virus

densitometry
    bone d.

density
    d. gradient centrifugation
    d. gradient ultracentrifugation

Denys-Leclef phenomenon

deoxycholate
    d. sodium

deoxycorticosterone
    d. acetate escape

11-deoxycorticosterone (DOC)
    11-d. acetate
    11-d. pivalate

11-deoxycortisol

deoxycortone

deoxynucleotidyl transferase
    terminal d. t. (Tdt)

deoxyribonucleic acid (DNA)

deoxyribonucleoprotein

deoxyribovirus

dependence
    anchorage d.

Dependovirus

depletion
    potassium d.

depletion *(continued)*
    sodium d.

depression
    antigen-specific d.

depressor substance

deprivation
    potassium d.
    water d.

de Quervain's thyroiditis

derangement
    hypertonic water bal-
        ance d.
    hypotonic water balance d.
    water balance d.

derivative
    purified protein d. (PPD)

dermal
    d. macrophage
    d. myiasis

dermamyiasis

dermatitis *pl.* dermatitides
    chigger d.
    contact d.
    exfoliative d.
    d. herpetiformis
    Pelodera d.
    rhabditic d.
    uncinarial d.

dermatobiasis

dermatocytis

dermatomyiasis

dermatomyositis (DM)

Dermatophagoides pteronyssinus

dermatophytic onychomycosis

dermis

dermoid
    d. tumor

dermopathy
    diabetic d.

dermopathy *(continued)*
    infiltrative d.

dermoreaction

DES
    diethylstilbestrol

desensitization
    heterologous d.
    homologous d.
    d. receptors
    rhodopsin d.
    d. therapy

desensitize

desert rheumatism

desetope

designation
    cluster d. (CD) *(followed by
        a number)*

desmopressin

desoxycorticosterone
    d. acetate
    d. pivalate

desoxycortone

despeciate

despeciated serum

despeciation

despecification

destruction
    extravascular d.
    red blood cell d.
    intravascular d.

dETC
    dendritic epidermal T cell

detecting antibody

detection
    antibody d.
    isotype d.

determinant
    allotypic d.

determinant *(continued)*
    antigenic d.
    conformational d's
    hidden d.
    immunogenic d.
    isotypic d's
    linear d's
    d. selection model
    sequential d.

determination
    quantitative d.
    sex d.

development
    ambisexual d.
    breast d.
    sexual d.

deviation
    anterior chamber–associated immune d. (ACAID)
    complement d.
    immune d.

device
    external vacuum tumescence d.
    intrauterine d. (IUD)

devil's grip

dexamethasone
    high-dose d. suppression test
    low-dose d. suppression test
    d. suppression test

dextroamphetamine

dextrose test

Dextrostix

dextrosuria

dextrothyroxine

DH
    delayed hypersensitivity

DHEA
    dehydroepiandrosterone
        DHEA loading test

DHEA *(continued)*
        DHEA sulfate

d'Herelle's phenomenon

dhobie itch

DHT
    dihydrotestosterone

diabetes
    adult-onset d. mellitus
    alloxan d.
    autoimmune d.
    brittle d.
    central d. insipidus
    chemical d.
    gestational d.
    gestational d. mellitus
    growth-onset d. mellitus
    d. insipidus (DI)
    d. insipidus–like syndrome
    insulin-dependent d. mellitus (IDDM)
    juvenile d. mellitus
    juvenile-onset d. mellitus
    ketosis-prone d. mellitus
    ketosis-resistant d. mellitus
    latent d.
    malnutrition-related d. mellitus
    maternal d.
    maturity-onset d. mellitus
    maturity-onset d. of youth
    d. mellitus (DM) *(types 1 and 2)*
    nephrogenic d. insipidus
    non–insulin-dependent d. mellitus (NIDDM)
    pituitary d. insipidus
    preclinical d.
    puncture d.
    renal d.
    severe d.
    steroid d.
    steroidogenic d.
    subclinical d.
    d. test
    thiazide d.
    tropical d. mellitus

diabetes *(continued)*
    tropical pancreatic d. mellitus
    type 1 d. mellitus
    type 2 d. mellitus

diabetic
    d. acidosis
    d. amaurosis
    d. cataract
    d. coma
    d. complications
    d. dermopathy
    d. foot syndrome
    d. gangrene
    d. ketoacidosis
    d. lipemia
    d. mononeuropathy
    d. myelopathy
    d. neuropathy
    d. puncture
    d. retinopathy
    d. sugar

diabeticorum
    bullosis d.
    necrobiosis lipoidica d.
    xanthoma d.

diabetogenic
    d. factor
    d. hormone

diabetogenous

diacylglycerol (DAG)

diagnosis
    differential d.
    tumor d.

diagnostic
    d. serology
    d. workup

dialysis
    equilibrium d.

diapedesis
    leukocyte d.

diaphragm
    vaginal d.

diarrhea
    infectious d.

diarrheogenic
    d. syndrome
    d. tumor

diarthrodial joint

Diastix

diathesis
    gouty d.

dibothriocephaliasis

DIC
        disseminated intravascular coagulation

DIDMOAD
        diabetes insipidus, diabetes mellitus, optic atrophy and nerve deafness
            DIDMOAD syndrome

diencephalic syndrome

diet
    challenge d.
    elimination d.
    provocative d.
    d. therapy

dietary
    d. management
    d. restrictions

diethylamine

diethylstilbestrol (DES)

differential signaling hypothesis

differentiation
    d. antigens
    antigen-dependent d.
    antigen-independent d.
    cell d.
    external genital d.
    psychosexual d.
    sex d.
    sexual d.

diffuse
  d. goiter
  d. nontoxic goiter
  d. toxic goiter

diffusion
  double d.
  double d. in one dimension
  double d. in two dimensions
  fluid phase d.
  gel d.
  single d.
  single radial d.

DiGeorge syndrome

digestive
  d. glycosuria
  d. system

digital clubbing

dihydrotestosterone (DHT)

dihydroxycholecalciferol
  1,25-d.

3,4-dihydroxyphenylalanine

1,25-dihydroxyvitamin D

dihydroxyvitamin D_3
  1,25-d. D.

3,5-diiodothyronine

diiodotyrosine

dikwakwadi

dilution
  point of d.

dimer

dimerization

diminished immunity

dimorphism
  sexual d.

dinitrobenzene hapten

dinitrochlorobenzene

dinitrofluorobenzene

dinitrophenyl
  DNP

dinoprost

dinoprostone

dipetalonemiasis

diphenhydramine
  d. hydrochloride

diphosphonate

diphtheria
  d. anatoxin
  d. antibody
  d. antitoxin
  cutaneous d.
  faucial d.
  d. immunization
  laryngeal d.
  laryngotracheal d.
  nasal d.
  nasopharyngeal d.
  d.-pertussis-tetanus vaccine (DPT)
  pharyngeal d.
  d. and tetanus toxoids (DT)
  d. and tetanus toxoids and acellular pertussis vaccine (DTaP)
  d. and tetanus toxoids and pertussis vaccine (DTP)
  d. toxin
  d. toxoid
  umbilical d.

diphtherial
  d. tonsillitis

diphtheric

diphtherin

diphtheritic
  d. laryngitis
  d. paralysis
  d. pharyngitis

diphtheroid

diphyllobothriasis

dipylidiasis

direct
  d. agglutination
  d. antiglobulin test (DAT)
  d. antihuman globulin test
  d. bacterial agglutination
  d. contact
  d. Coombs' test
  d. fluorescent antibody
  d. immunofluorescence
  d. immunofluorescence
    technique
  d. immunomicroscopy
  d. radioimmunoassay
  d. test of immunofluores-
    cence

dirofilariasis

discoid lupus erythematosus

discontinuous epitope

discordant
  d. species
  d. xenograft

disease
  Addison's d.
  α heavy chain d.
  akamushi d.
  Albright d.
  allergic d.
  allogeneic d.
  Almeida's d.
  alpha chain d.
  alpha heavy chain d.
  alveolar hydatid d.
  Anderson's d.
  atherosclerotic coronary
    heart d.
  atopic d.
  autoimmune d.
  Basedow's d.
  Beigel's d.
  Berger's d.
  Blount d.
  bluetongue d. of sheep

disease (continued)
  Bornholm d.
  bowel d.
  breast d.
  Brill's d.
  Brill-Zinsser d.
  Brion-Kayser d.
  brittle bone d.
  "broad-beta" d.
  bronzed d.
  Bruton's d.
  Buschke's d.
  Busse-Buschke d.
  California d.
  cardiovascular d.
  Carrión's d.
  cat-scratch d.
  celiac d.
  Chagas' d.
  Chicago d.
  chronic granulomatous d.
  chronic inflammatory bow-
    el d.
  chronic obstructive pulmo-
    nary d. (COPD)
  collagen d.
  combined immunodeficien-
    cy d.
  communicable d.
  Conor and Bruch's d.
  contagious d.
  Cori's d.
  coronary heart d.
  creeping d.
  Creutzfeldt-Jakob d.
  Crohn's d.
  Cushing's d.
  cysticercus d.
  cytomegalic inclusion d.
  Daae's d.
  Darling's d.
  Duncan's d.
  Durand-Nicolas-Favre d.
  Ebola d.
  Ebola virus d.
  echinococcus d.
  endocrine d.
  end-stage renal d.

disease *(continued)*

    English sweating d.

    Epstein's d.

    experiential autoallergic d.

    Fabry d.

    Favre-Durand-Nicolas d.

    febrile d.

    Fiedler's d.

    fifth d.

    Filatov's (Filatow's) d.

    Flajani's d.

    fluke d.

    foot-and-mouth d.

    fourth venereal d.

    Francis' d.

    Franklin's d.

    Frei's d.

    fungal d.

    gallbladder d.

    gamma chain d.

    gamma heavy chain d.

    gastrointestinal d.

    Gaucher d.

    γ heavy chain d.

    Gilchrist's d.

    glomerular basement membrane autoimmune d.

    graft-versus-host (GVH) d.

    granulomatous d.

    Graves' d.

    Gull's d.

    GVH d.

    Hand-Schüller-Christian d.

    Hartnup d.

    Hashimoto's d.

    heart d.

    heavy chain d's

    Heine-Medin d.

    hematological d.

    hemolytic d. of the newborn (HDN)

    hepatolenticular d.

    hereditary d.

    Hers' d.

    Hirschsprung's d.

    His' d.

    His-Werner d.

    Hodgkin's d.

disease *(continued)*

    hookworm d.

    hunger d.

    hungry d.

    hydatid d.

    hyperparathyroid bone d.

    hypersensitivity d's

    hypertrophic vascular d.

    immune complex d.

    immune deficiency d.

    immune-mediated d's

    immunodeficiency d's

    immunoproliferative small intestine d.

    infectious d.

    intestinal autoimmune d.

    iron storage d.

    ischemic heart d.

    island d.

    juvenile Paget d.

    Kahler's d.

    Katayama d.

    kidney d.

    kissing d.

    Krabbe d.

    Kyasanur Forest d.

    Lancereaux-Mathieu d.

    Landouzy's d.

    legionnaires' d.

    Leiner's d.

    light chain d.

    liver d.

    Lobo's d.

    Lorain's d.

    lung d.

    lung fluke d.

    Lutz-Splendore-Almeida d.

    Lyme d.

    lymphoproliferative d.

    MAC d.

    McArdle's d.

    macrovascular d.

    Manson's d.

    maple syrup urine d.

    marble bone d.

    Marburg d.

    Marburg virus d.

    Marie's d.

    Marsh's d.

disease *(continued)*
    Medin's d.
    metastatic d.
    metazoan d.
    μ heavy chain d.
    microvascular d.
    mixed connective tissue d.
    monoclonal immunoglobu-
      lin deposition d.
    mu chain d.
    mu heavy chain d.
    muscle autoimmune d.
    Mycobacterium avium com-
      plex d.
    myeloproliferative d.
    nanukayami d.
    neoplastic d.
    neuroendocrine d.
    neuropsychiatric d.
    newborn hemolytic d.
    Newcastle d.
    Nicolas-Favre d.
    Niemann-Pick d.
    oculocraniosomatic d.
    oculocraniosomatic muscu-
      lar d.
    Ohara's d.
    organ-specific d.
    organ-specific autoim-
      mune d.
    Oriental lung fluke d.
    ox-warble d.
    Paget d.
    paralytic d.
    Parkinson's d.
    parrot d.
    Parry's d.
    peripheral vascular d.
    Pfeiffer's d.
    Phocas' d.
    Plummer's d.
    poliomyelitis-like d's
    polyendocrine autoimmune
      d's
    polyglandular autoimmune
      d's

disease *(continued)*
    Pompe's d.
    Posadas' d.
    Posadas-Wernicke d.
    primary immunologic d's
    prion d.
    pulmonary hypersensitivi-
      ty d.
    ragpicker's d.
    ragsorter's d.
    rat-bite d.
    Raynaud d.
    Refsum d.
    renal d.
    renal parenchymal d.
    respiratory d.
    Rh d.
    rheumatic heart d.
    Ribas-Torres d.
    rickettsial d.
    Riedel d.
    salivary gland d.
    Sandhoff d.
    sandworm d.
    San Joaquin Valley d.
    SC (sickle cell) d.
    Schilder's d.
    Schottmüller's d.
    secondary d.
    serum d.
    severe combined immuno-
      deficiency d. (SCID)
    sex-linked lymphogenic im-
      munologic d.
    sexually transmitted d.
    shimamushi d.
    sickle cell (SC) d.
    Simmonds' d.
    Sjögren's d.
    spontaneous autoim-
      mune d.
    Sticker's d.
    Strümpell's d.
    Sylvest's d.
    systemic autoimmune d.
    Takayasu's d.

disease *(continued)*
    Tay-Sachs d.
    Teschen d.
    thromboembolic d.
    thyroid d.
    tissue-specific autoimmune d.
    transmissible neurodegenerative d.
    trophoblastic d.
    tsutsugamushi d.
    Tyzzer's d.
    unilocular hydatid d.
    vagabonds' d.
    vagrants' d.
    venereal d.
    viral d.
    von Gierke d.
    von Hippel-Lindau d.
    von Recklinghausen d.
    von Willebrand's d.
    wasting d.
    Weil's d.
    Werner-His d.
    Wesselsbron d.
    Whitmore's d.
    Wilson's d.
    Wolman's d.
    woolsorter's d.
    X-linked lymphoproliferative d.

disequilibrium
    linkage d.

dismutase
    superoxide d.

disodium chromoglycate

disorder
    autoimmune d's
    breast d's
    eating d's
    growth d's
    immune complex d.
    lymphoproliferative d.
    metabolic d.
    neurological d's
    neuromuscular d's

disorder *(continued)*
    phagocytic dysfunction d's
    plasma cell d's
    renal tubular d's
    XX d.
    YY d.

display
    phage d.

disseminated
    d. intravascular coagulation (DIC)
    d. tuberculosis

dissemination
    microorganism d.

dissociation constant (Kd)

distal
    d. renal tubule
    d. tubule

distomiasis
    pulmonary d.

distress
    psychic d.

distribution
    cosmopolitan d.
    extrahypothalamic d.
    isotype d.
    phosphorus d.
    Poisson d.

disulfide bond

diuresis
    osmotic d.
    sodium d.

diuretics

divasta

diversification
    N region d.

diversion
    antigenic d.

diversity
    antibody d.

diversity *(continued)*
    combinatorial d.
    d. (D) gene segments
    germline d.
    junctional d.
    d. (D) region
    d. (D) segments
    T cell d.

diverticulum *pl.* diverticula
    pituitary d.

diving goiter

Dixon Mann's sign

DM
    dermatomyositis
    diabetes mellitus

DM molecule

DNA
    deoxyribonucleic acid
        DNA amplification
        DNA binding domain
        DNA-binding protein
        DNA-dependent kinase
        DNA-dependent protein kinase
        DNA dot blot hybridization
        DNA footprinting
        DNA fragmentation
        DNA-like RNA
        DNA oncogenic virus
        DNA probe
        recombinant DNA
        DNA repair defect
        DNA sequence
        DNA vaccination
        DNA virus

DNP
    dinitrophenyl

Dobrava
    D. virus
    D.-Belgrade virus

DOC
    11-deoxycorticosterone

docking protein

Döderlein bacillus

domain
    active d's
    C (constant) d.
    complement control protein d's
    DNA binding d.
    Fc d.
    immunoglobulin d's
    immunoglobulinlike d's
    SH3 d.
    sushi d.
    V (variable) d.

dominant
    d. idiotype
    d. negative oncogene

DO molecule

Donath
    D.-Landsteiner antibody
    D.-Landsteiner test

donee

donor

donovanosis

dopa

dopamine
    d. agonists
    d. β-hydroxylase (DBH)

dopaminergic
    d. pathways
    d. receptors
    d. system

dopaquinone

dorsal kyphosis

dose
    infective d.
    L+ d.
    L0 d.
    Lf d.
    limes nul d.

dose *(continued)*
 limes zero d.
 Lr d.
 maximum tolerated d.
  (MTD)
 median immunizing d.
 median infective d.
 median tissue culture infective d.
 reacting d.
 sensitizing d.

dot
 Maurer's d's
 Schüffner's d's

dot blot
 DNA d. b. hybridization
 d. b. hybridization
 d. b. technique

double
 d. diffusion
 d. diffusion method
 d. diffusion in one dimension
 d. diffusion test
 d. diffusion in two dimensions
 d. glucagon test
 d. isotope derivative technique
 d.-negative thymocyte
 d.-positive thymocyte
 d.-stranded RNA
 d.-stranded virus

dowager's hump

Downey cells

downgrading reaction

Down syndrome

DPC
 dendritic phagocytic cell

DPT
 diphtheria-pertussis-tetanus
  DPT vaccine

dracontiasis

dracunculiasis

dracunculosis

Drash syndrome

D (diversity) region

Dressler's syndrome

Dreyer and Bennett hypothesis

drift
 antigen d.
 antigenic d.

drinking
 compulsive water d.
 psychogenic water d.

droplet
 d. infection
 d. nuclei

drug
 d. allergy
 anticholinergic d's
 antihyperglycemic d.
 antihypertensive d.
 appetite-suppressant d's
 chemotherapeutic d's
 cytotoxic d's
 immunosuppression d's
 immunosuppressive d's
 lipid-lowering d's
 nonsteroidal antiinflammatory d.
 d. resistance
 d. therapy

drug-induced
 d.-i. autoimmunity
 d.-i. hemolytic anemia
 d.-i. hypoglycemia
 d.-i. immune hemolytic anemia
 d.-i. impotence
 d.-i. tolerance

drusen

dry cholera

dryness
    vaginal d.
DT
    diphtheria and tetanus tox-
        oids
DTaP
    diphtheria and tetanus tox-
        oids and acellular pertus-
        sis vaccine
            DTaP vaccine
DTH
    delayed-type hypersensitiv-
        ity
DTP
    diphtheria and tetanus tox-
        oids and pertussis vac-
        cine
            DTP vaccine

dual-beam x-ray spectropho-
    tometry

dual energy radiography

dual-photon absorptiometry

dual recognition hypothesis

Duchenne muscular dystrophy

duct
    accessory pancreatic d.
    afferent lymphatic d.
    common bile d.
    genital d's
    müllerian d's
    pancreatic d.
    thoracic d.

ductless glands

Duffy receptor

dumb rabies

Duncan
    D's disease
    D's syndrome

duodenum

duplex scanning

Durand-Nicolas-Favre disease

Dürck's nodes

Du rosette test

dust-borne
    d.-b. infection

Dutton's relapsing fever

Duvenhage virus

dwarf
    asexual d.
    Brissaud's d.
    cretin d.
    hypophysial d.
    hypothyroid d.
    infantile d.
    Laron d.
    Lévi-Lorain d.
    Lorain-Lévi d.
    normal d.
    physiologic d.
    pituitary d.
    primordial d.
    pure d.
    Russell d.
    sexual d.
    Silver d.
    true d.

dwarfish

dwarfism
    ateliotic d.
    dysmorphic d.
    hypophysial d.
    hypopituitary d.
    idiopathic d.
    Laron d.
    Laron-type d.
    Lévi-Lorain d.
    Lorain-Lévi d.
    pituitary d.
    primordial d.
    psychosocial d.
    Russell d.
    Russell-Silver d.
    Silver-Russell d.
    symptomatic d.

dye
  fluorescent d.
  d. test

dynamic
  d. equilibrium
  d. test

dysadrenalism

dysautosomia
  familial d.

dysbetalipoproteinemia
  familial d.

dyscorticism

dyscrasia
  plasma cell d's

dysesthesia

dysfunction
  adrenal d.
  beta cell d.
  bladder d.
  immunologic d.
  liver d.
  luteal phase d.
  sexual d.

dysgammaglobulinemia
  hyper-IgM d.
  lymphopenic d.

dysgenic gonadectomy

dysgenesis
  gonadal d.
  mixed gonadal d.
  pure gonadal d.
  reticular d.
  seminiferous tubule d.
  XO gonadal d. (*same as* Turner syndrome)
  XX gonadal d.
  XY gonadal d.
  46,XY gonadal d.

dysgenitalism

dysgerminoma

dysglobulinemia

dysglycemia

dysgonesis

dysmenorrhea

dysmentation

dysmorphic dwarfism

dyspareunia

dysplasia
  bone d.
  cretinoid d.
  fibrous d.
  micronodular d.
  primary adrenocortical nodular d.
  septo-optic d.
  skeletal d.

dysplastic

dysproteinemia

dyspnea
  d. in thyrotoxicosis
  exertional d.

dysproteinemia

dysthyreosis

dysthyroid
  d. ophthalmopathy
  d. orbitopathy

dysthyroidal
  d. infantilism

dysthyroidism

dystrophia
  d. adiposogenitalis

dystrophic
  d. calcification
  d. ossification

dystrophin

dystrophy
  adipose genital d.
  adiposogenital d.
  Duchenne muscular d.
  muscular d.
  myotonic d.

E

E
  E antigen
  E rosette
  E rosette assay

EA
  early antigen

E1A
  E1A protein

EAC
  erythrocyte, antibody, and
  complement
    EAC rosette
    EAC rosette assay

EAE
  experimental autoimmune
  encephalitis
  experimental allergic encephalomyelitis

E antigen

E1A protein

early
  e. antigen (EA)
  e. B-cell factor (EBF)
  e. latent syphilis
  e.-onset nonlethal osteopetrosis
  e. pro-B cell
  e. syphilis
  e. thymocyte

East African trypanosomiasis

eastern
  e. equine encephalomyelitis virus
  e. schistosomiasis

eating
  e. behavior
  e. disorders

EBF
  early B-cell factor

echinococciasis

echinococcus disease

EB
  Epstein-Barr
    EB virus

Ebola
  E. disease
  E. hemorrhagic fever
  E. virus
  E. virus disease

EBV
  Epstein-Barr virus
    chronic EBV

ECF
  eosinophil chemotactic factor

ECF-A
  eosinophil chemotactic factor of anaphylaxis

echinococcosis

Echinococcus

echinostomiasis

echovirus

Echte-Immunität

eclipse

economy
  thyroid hormone e.

ecotaxis

ecotropic

ectocervix

ectogenous infection

ectoderm

ectohormone

ectoparasite

ectopic
  e. ACTH syndrome
  e. adrenal tissue
  e. corticotropin-releasing
  hormone syndrome

ectopic *(continued)*
    e. gastrin-releasing peptide
      secretion
    e. hormone
    e. hyperparathyroidism
    e. lymphoid tissue
    e. pinealoma
    e. pregnancy
    e. thyroids

eczema
    atopic e.
    e. marginatum

edema
    angioneurotic e.
    Calabar e.
    diabetic-induced e.
    hereditary angioneurotic e.
    idiopathic cyclical e.
    malignant e.
    mucous e.
    pulmonary e.
    solid e.

edetate (EDTA)

editing
    receptor e.

Edmonston
    E. measles virus vaccine
    E. strain (*of measles*)

EDTA
    ethylenediaminetetraacetic
      acid (edetate)

education of T cells

Edwardsiella
    E. hoshinae
    E. tarda

EEE
    eastern equine encephalitis
        EEE virus

effect
    allosteric e.
    androgen e's
    Bruce e.
    cyclosporine e.

effect *(continued)*
    Danysz e.
    immunomodulatory e's
    prozone e.
    Somogyi e.
    Staub-Traugott e.
    Whitten e.
    Wolff-Chaikoff e.

effector
    armed e. cells
    e. cell
    e. functions of antibodies
    e. mechanism
    e. molecules
    e. phase of immune re-
      sponse
    e. T cells
    e. T cell function

effemination

efferent lymph vessels

EGF
    epidermal growth factor

Ehrlich
    E's side-chain theory
    E's theory

Ehrlichia
    E. canis
    E. chaffeensis
    E. sennetsu

ehrlichiosis
    human granulocytic e.
    human monocytic e.

EIA
    enzyme immunoassay

eicosanoid

Eikenella
    E. corrodens

ELAM
    endothelial leukocyte adhe-
      sion molecule

electrogenic transport

electroimmunodiffusion

electrolyte
    e. levels
    serum e.

electroneutral transport

electron microscope

electrophoresis
    agarose gel e.
    polyacrylamide gel e.
      (PAGE)
    rocket e.
    serum e.
    two-dimensional gel e.

electrophoretic mobility

electrostatic force

Elek
    E's diffusion test
    E's double diffusion test

element
    glucocorticoid response e's
      (GREs)
    negatively regulated ster-
      oid response e.
    phorbol ester response e.
    progesterone response e.
      (PRE)
    steroid response e. (SRE)
    transactivating response e.

elementary body

elephantiasis

elimination
    e. diet
    immune e.

ELISA
    enzyme-linked immunosor-
      bent assay
        sandwich ELISA
        ELISA SPOT assay
        ELISA test

Ellis-van Creveld syndrome

ELISPOT assay

El Tor strain (of Vibrio cholerae)

eluate

embedding

embryogenesis

embryonal
    e. adenoma
    e. testicular cancer

embryonic
    e. stem cell lines
    e. testicular regression syn-
      drome

EMC
    encephalomyocarditis
        EMC virus

emergency theory

emesis

eminence
    omental e. of body of pan-
      creas

emission
    gamma e.

EMIT
    enzyme-multiplied immuno-
      assay technique

emotion

emphysema

empty sella syndrome

encapsulated bacterium

encapsulation

encephalitis pl. encephalitides
    bulbar e.
    eastern equine e. (EEE)
    experimental autoim-
      mune e. (EAE)
    granulomatous amebic e.
    Japanese e.
    St. Louis e.
    tick-borne e. (TBE)
    western equine e. (WEE)

encephalitogenic protein

encephalitozoonosis

encephalomyelitis
    allergic e.
    western equine e. (WEE)
    Venezuelan equine e.

encephalomyocarditis
    e. virus

encephalopathy
    hypertonic e.
    subacute spongiform e.
    transmissible spongiform e.

end-binder

endemic
    e. cretinism
    e. goiter
    e. hematuria
    e. hemoptysis
    e. influenza
    e. poliomyelitis
    e. syphilis
    e. typhus

ending
    nerve e's

endocarditis

endocervical
    e. glands
    e. mucus
    e. polyp

endocrine
    e.-active adenoma
    e. adenomatosis
    e. atrophy
    e. autoimmunity
    e. breast cancer therapy
    e. cells of the gut
    e. correlation
    e. disease
    e. exophthalmos
    e. fracture
    e. glands
    e.-inactive adenoma
    e. manipulation
    multiple e. adenomatosis
    e. pancreas

endocrine *(continued)*
    e. part of pancreas
    e. responsive cancer
    e. system
    e. therapy

endocrinologic
    e. impotence
    e. sex

endocrinologist

endocrinology
    clinical e.

endocrinopathic

endocrinopathy

endocrinosis

endocrinotherapy

endocytosis
    receptor-mediated e.

endodermal

endogenous
    e. antigen
    e. hyperinsulinemia
    e. infection
    e. lipemia
    e. obesity
    e. opiate
    e. protein antigen
    e. pyrogen
    e. viral superantigen

endometrial
    e. cancer
    e. cycle
    e. hyperplasia
    e. polyp

endometrium

endonuclease
    e. activity
    restriction e's

endoparasite

endoplasmic reticulum

endorphin
    β-e.

endorphin *(continued)*
    humoral e.

endosecretory

endosome

endosymbiosis

endothelial
    e. cell
    e. leukocyte adhesion molecule (ELAM)
    e. system

endotheliolysin

endotheliolytic

endothelium

endotoxemia

endotoxic
    e. shock

endotoxin
    bacterial e's
    Bordella pertussis e.
    e.-induced fever
    Salmonella typhi e.
    e. tolerance

endovaccination

endpoint
    e. diffusion test
    nephelometric e.

end-stage renal disease

engineering
    genetic e.
    tissue e.

English sweating disease

englobe

engraftment

enhancement

enhancer

enhancing
    e. agglutination
    e. antibody

enkephalin

enlargement
    breast e.

Enroth's sign

entamebiasis

Entamoeba

enteric
    e. campylobacteriosis
    e. fever
    e. hyperoxaluria
    e. nervous system
    e. orphan viruses
    e. viruses

enterically transmitted non-A, non-B hepatitis

entericoid fever

Enterobacter
    E. aerogenes
    E. agglomerans
    E. cloacae
    E. gergoviae
    E. sakazakii

enterobiasis

enterochromaffin
    e. cells

enterococcemia

Enterococcus
    E. avium
    E. faecalis
    E. faecium

enterocolitis

enteroendocrine
    e. cells

enterogastrone

enteroglucagon

enterohepatic circulation

enteroidea

enteropathy
    gluten-sensitive e.

enterotoxin
    cholera e.
    staphylococcal e.
    Staphylococcus aureus e.
    streptococcal e.

enteroviral

Enterovirus

enterovirus

Entomophthora
    E. coronata

entomophthoramycosis

entomophthoromycosis
    e. basidiobolae
    e. conidiobolae

envelope
    HIV e.
    viral e.

enveloped virus

env gene (*of HIV*)

enzyme
    angiotensin-converting e.
    granule-associated e.
    e. immunoassay (EIA)
    e.-linked immunoassay
    e.-linked immunosorbent
      assay (ELISA)
    e.-multiplied immunoassay
      technique
    lysosomal e.
    proteolytic e.
    receptor-destroying e.

eosinophil
    e. adenoma
    e. cationic protein
    e. chemotactic factor (ECF)
    e. chemotactic factor of an-
      aphylaxis (ECF-A)
    e. count
    e. tumor with acromegaly

eosinophilia

eosinophilic
    e. adenoma
    e. gastroenteropathy
    e. granuloma
    e. meningitis
    e. meningoencephalitis

eotaxin

epiallopregnanolone

epiandrosterone

epidemiologic

epidemiology

epidemic
    e. arthritic erythema
    e. hemorrhagic fever
    e. hepatitis
    e. jaundice
    e. keratoconjunctivitis vi-
      rus
    e. myalgia
    e. parotitis
    e. pleurodynia
    e. poliomyelitis
    e. polyarthritis
    e. typhus

epidermal
    e. growth factor (EGF)
    human e. growth factor

epidermis

epidermolysin

epididymis

epiestriol

epi-illumination fluorescence
  microscope

epilepsy

epimastigote

epimestrol

epinephrine

epinephros

epiphyseal syndrome

epiphysitis

epiphysis
  e. cerebri

epithelial
  e. bodies
  e. cell
  e. growth factor
  e. interferon

epithelioid cell

epitheliolysin

epitheliotoxin

epithelium *pl.* epithelia
  follicular e.
  squamous e.
  surface e.
  vaginal e.

epitope
  conformational e's
  continuous e's
  discontinuous e.
  linear e.
  monomorphic e.
  e. spreading

epituberculosis

epituberculous infiltration

epitype

epoetin

epoprostenol

epsilon (ϵ)
  e. acidophil
  e. chain
  e. staphylolysin

Epstein
  E's disease
  E.-Barr latent infection
  E.-Barr nuclear antigen

Epstein *(continued)*
  E.-Barr virus (EB virus,
    EBV)
  E.-Barr virus superantigen

equilibrium
  e. analysis
  e. dialysis
  dynamic e.

equilin

equine
  e. antitoxin
  e. encephalomyelitis virus

equivalence
  e. point
  zone of e.
  e. zone reaction

erb-B oncogene

erection
  penile e.

E rosette
  E r. assay

error
  laboratory e.

eruption
  creeping e.

Erwinia
  E. amylovora
  E. carotovora
  E. herbicola

erysipelas
  coast e.

Erysipelothrix
  E. insidiosa
  E. rhusiopathiae

erythema
  e. arthriticum epidemicum
  e. chronicum migrans
  epidemic arthritic e.
  e. infectiosum

erythritol
  erythroblastosis fetalis

erythrocyte
  e. count
  e. sedimentation rate (ESR)
  papain-treated e.

erythrocyto-opsonin

erythrocytosis

erythrophage

erythrophagocytic
  e. lymphohistiocytosis

erythropoiesis

erythropoietic stimulating factor (ESF)

erythropoietin
  recombinant human e.

Erythrovirus

escape
  aldosterone e.
  deoxycorticosterone acetate e.
  iodine e.
  sodium e.
  tumor e.

Escherichia
  E. aurescens
  E. coli
  E. fergusonii
  E. vulneris

E-selectin

ESF
  erythropoietic stimulating factor

esophagostomiasis

ESR
  erythrocyte sedimentation rate

essential
  e. fructosuria
  e. hypertension
  e. mixed cryoglobulinemia

established virulence

ester
  phorbol e.

esterase
  C1 e.
  serine e.
  Staphylococcus aureus e.

esterified estrogens

estetrol

estradiol
  e. assay
  e. benzoate
  e. cypionate
  e. dipropionate
  e. enanthate
  ethinyl e.
  e. exchange assay
  e. production
  e. secretion
  e. undecylate
  e. valerate

estrane

estriasis

estrin

estriol

estrogen
  adrenal e.
  e. breakthrough bleeding
  e. carcinogenicity
  conjugated e's
  e. deficiency
  esterified e's
  e.-induced hypertension
  e. metabolism
  e. receptor
  e. therapy

estrogenic
  e. hormone

estrogenicity

estrogenous

estrone

estrophilin

estrous cycle

ether sensitivity

ethinyl
e. estradiol
e. testosterone

ethisterone

ethnic polymorphism

ethylenediaminetetraacetic acid (EDTA) (edetate)

ethylenedinitrilotetraacetic acid

ethylestrenol

ethynodiol diacetate

etiocholanolone

etiology
atherosclerosis e.

euadrenocorticism

Eubacterium
E. alactolyticum
E. lentum
E. limosum

euglycemia

euglycemic
e. clamping

eugonadotropic
e. hypogonadism

eukaryotic chromosome

eumycetoma

eumycotic mycetoma

eunuch

eunuchism

eunuchoid
e. gigantism

eunuchoidism
female e.

eunuchoidism *(continued)*
hypergonadotropic e.
hypogonadotropic e.

European typhus

eutrophic ossification

euthymism

euthyroid
e. hyperthyroxinemia
e. hypothyroxinemia
e. sick syndrome

euthyroidism
liothyronine e.

eutopic
e. hormone

event
signal e's

Everglades virus

eviration

Ewingella

examination
seminal fluid e.

exanthematic typhus of São Paulo

exanthematous
e. disease virus
e. typhus

excess
antibody e.
antigen e.
hormone e.

exchange
e. assay
ion e.
e. transfusion

excitable cell

excited skin syndrome

exclusion
allelic e.
isotype e.

exclusion *(continued)*
  isotypic e.

excretion

exertional dyspnea

exfoliatin

exfoliative
  e. dermatitis

exocrine
  e. cells
  e. glands

exocytosis
  acetylcholine e.

exogenous
  e. antigen
  e. hormonosis
  e. infection
  e. insulin hypoglycemia
  e. interferon
  e. microbial antigen
  e. obesity
  e. protein antigen
  e. pyrogens

exon

exonuclease

Exophiala

exophthalmia

exophthalmic goiter

exophthalmometry

exophthalmos
  autoimmune e.
  endocrine e.
  malignant e.
  thyrotoxic e.
  thyrotropic e.

exotoxin

expansion
  clonal e.

experiential autoallergic disease

experiment
  skin graft e.

experimental
  e. allergic encephalomyelitis (EAE)
  e. allergic neuritis
  e. autoimmune encephalitis (EAE)
  e. autoimmune myocarditis
  e. hyperglycemia
  e. obesity

exposure
  cold e.

external
  e. scintiscanning
  e. secretion
  e. secretory system
  e. vacuum tumescence device

extra-adrenal

extracellular
  e. bacteria
  e. matrix molecule
  e. parasite
  e. pathogen

extract
  allergenic e.
  poison ivy e.
  poison oak e.
  pollen e.

extractable nuclear antigens

extraction
  menstrual e.

extraembryonic membranes

extragenital

extraglandular aromatization

extrahypothalamic distribution

extramedullary hematopoiesis

extraparotid
  e. lymph gland

extraskeletal
  e. calcification
  e. ossification

extrasuprarenal

extravasation
  leukocyte e.
  neutrophil e.

extravascular
  e. destruction

extravascular *(continued)*
  e. hemolysis

extrinsic allergic alveolitis

exudate

exudative tuberculosis

eye

eyeball
  bulging e's

F

F cell

F1

F1 hybrid

FAB

fluorescent antibody
FAB test

Fab

fragment, antigen-binding
Fab fragment
Fab region

F(ab')$_2$ fragment

Fabricius
bursa of F.

Fabry disease

Facb

fragment, antigen and complement binding

face

moon f.
moon-shaped f.

facies *pl.* facies
f. anterior corporis pancreatis
f. anterior glandulae suprarenalis
f. anteroinferior corporis pancreatis
f. anterosuperior corporis pancreatis
cushingoid f.
f. inferior pancreatis
moon f.
f. posterior corporis pancreatis
f. posterior glandulae suprarenalis
f. renalis glandulae suprarenalis

facilitator neuron

FACS
fluorescence-activated cell sorter

FACS *(continued)*
fluorescence-activated cell sorting

factitial hypoglycemia

factitious
f. hypoglycemia
f. precocious puberty

factor
f. A
allogeneic effect f. (AEF)
Am f.
angiogenesis f.
antigen-liberated transfer f.
antigen-specific T-cell helper f.
antigen-specific T-cell suppressor f.
antinuclear f. (ANF)
antinucleoprotein f.
atrial natriuretic f. (ANF)
autocrine growth f's
f. B
basophil chemotactic f. (BCF)
B cell differentiation f's (BCDF)
B cell growth f's (BCGF)
blastogenic f. (BF)
blastogenic inhibitor f.
blocking f's
B lymphocyte stimulatory f's (BSF)
cartilage-derived growth f.
cationic growth f.
CD40 receptor–associated f. (CRAF)
chemical cationic growth f.
chemotactic f.
chondrocyte growth f.
ciliary neurotropic f.
clumping f.
C3 nephritic f. (C3 NeF)
colony-stimulating f. (CSF)
cord f.
corticotropin-releasing f. (CRF)

97

factor *(continued)*
 crystal-induced chemotactic f. (CCF)
 f. D
 decay accelerating f. (DAF)
 diabetogenic f.
 early B-cell f. (EBF)
 eosinophil chemotactic f. (ECF)
 eosinophil chemotactic f. of anaphylaxis (ECF-A)
 epidermal growth f. (EGF)
 epithelial growth f.
 erythropoietic stimulating f. (ESF)
 fibroblast growth f.
 gamma-activated f. (GAF)
 genetic f's
 glucose tolerance f.
 granulocyte colony-stimulating f. (G-CSF)
 granulocyte-macrophage colony-stimulating f. (GM-CSF)
 growth f.
 f. H
 Hageman f.
 heat-labile f's
 helper f's
 hematopoietic growth f's
 hepatocyte-stimulating f.
 high-molecular-weight neutrophil chemotactic f. (HMW-NCF)
 histamine-releasing f. (HRF)
 homologous restriction f. (HRF)
 hormonal f's
 human epidermal growth f.
 human serum f.
 humoral f.
 hydrazine-sensitive f. (HSF)
 hyperglycemic-glycogenolytic f. (HGF)
 f. I
 immunoglobulin-binding f. (IBF)
 inhibiting f's

factor *(continued)*
 insulin-like growth f's (IGF) (I and II)
 intrinsic f. (IF)
 Lawrence's transfer f.
 Lawrence-type dialyzable transfer f.
 LE f.
 leukemia inhibitory f.
 leukocyte inhibitory f. (LIF)
 leukotactic f.
 lymph node permeability f. (LNPF)
 lymphocyte-activating f.
 lymphocyte blastogenic f. (BF)
 lymphocyte migration–enhancing f. (LMEF)
 lymphocyte migration–inhibiting f. (LMIF)
 lymphocyte mitogenic f. (LMF)
 lymphocyte-promoting f.
 lymphocyte-transforming f. (LTF)
 macrophage-activating f. (MAF)
 macrophage aggregating f.
 macrophage chemoattractant and activating f./protein
 macrophage chemotactic f. (MCF)
 macrophage colony-stimulating f. (M-CSF)
 macrophage growth f. (MGF)
 macrophage inhibitory f.
 macrophage migration inhibitory f.
 microbial virulence f's
 migration-inhibiting f. (MIF)
 migration inhibition f. (MIF)
 migration inhibitory f. (MIF)
 mitogenic f.
 monocyte chemotactic f.
 MSH-inhibitory f. (MIF)

factor *(continued)*
    müllerian duct inhibitory f.
    müllerian inhibiting f.
    müllerian regression f.
    multicolony stimulating f.
    multilineage colony-stimu-
      lating f.
    nerve growth f. (NGF)
    neutrophil chemotactic f.
      (NCF)
    neutrophil f. in cytokine ac-
      tions
    nuclear f. of activated T
      cells (NFAT)
    nucleocapsid core f.
    osteoclast-activating f.
      (OAF)
    ovarian growth f.
    Oz f.
    f. P
    peptide growth f's
    platelet f. (1–4)
    platelet-activating f. (PAF)
    platelet-derived growth f.
      (PDGF)
    polypeptide growth f's
    prolactin-inhibiting f. (PIF)
    prolactin-releasing f. (PRF)
    proliferative inhibitory f.
    psychological f's
    psychosocial f's
    recruitment f.
    releasing f's
    Rh f.
    Rhesus f.
    rheumatoid f. (RF)
    sensitizing f.
    skeletal growth f.
    skin reactive f. (SRF)
    somatotropin release–in-
      hibiting f. (SRIF)
    spreading f.
    Steel f.
    stem cell f. (SCF)
    sulfation f's
    T cell growth f.
    T cell replacing f.
    thymic f.

factor *(continued)*
    thymic humoral f.
    trans-acting f.
    transcription f.
    transcription-activating f.
    transfer f. (TF)
    transforming growth f.
      (TGF)
    transforming growth f. a
      (TGF a)
    transforming growth f. β
      (TGF β)
    tumor angiogenesis f.
      (TAF)
    tumor necrosis f. (TNF)
    tumor necrosis f.-α
    tumor necrosis f.-β
    vasopermeability f.
    virulence f's
    von Willebrand's f.

Fahey test

failure
    autoimmune testicular f.
    heart f.
    kidney f.
    lactation f.
    Leydig cell f.
    liver f.
    lung f.
    multiple organ f.
    ovarian premature f.
    pituitary f.
    renal f.

fallopian tube

false
    f. hermaphroditism
    f. membrane

false-positive
    biologic f.-p. (BFP)

familial
    f. adrenocortical insuffi-
      ciency
    f. dysalbuminemic hyper-
      thyroxinemia
    f. dysautosomia

familial *(continued)*
- f. dysbetalipoproteinemia (follicular goiter)
- f. hepatic lipase deficiency
- f. hypercalcemia
- f. hypercalcitoninemia
- f. hypercholesterolemia
- f. hypertriglyceridemia
- f. hypocalciuric hypercalcemia
- f. hypoglycemia
- f. hypophosphatemia
- f. immunity
- f. isolated hyperthyroxinemia
- f. medullary thyroid carcinoma–pheochromocytoma syndrome
- f. perineal hypospadias
- f. pheochromocytoma
- f. precocious puberty
- f. testotoxicosis

family
- immunoglobulin supergene f. (IgSF)
- Janus f. of kinases (JAK)
- f. screening
- tachykinin f.

family planning
- natural f. p.
- symptothermal method of natural f. p.

Fanconi syndrome

Far East hemorrhagic fever

farmer's lung

Farr
- F. technique
- F. test

Fas (CD95)
- F. ligand
- F. protein

fascicular
- f. zone

Fasciola

fascioliasis

fasciolopsiasis

fasting
- f. blood sugar (FBS)
- f. hypoglycemia
- f. plasma glucose

fat
- body f.
- f. cells
- f.-mobilizing hormones

fatty acid
- f. a. synthase
- f. a. synthesis

faucial diphtheria

FA virus

favorable
- f. microenvironment

Favre-Durand-Nicolas disease

favus

FBS
- fasting blood sugar

Fc
- fragment, crystallizable
  - Fc domain
  - Fc fragment
  - Fc receptors
  - Fc region

Fc'

F cell

FcR
- Fc receptor
  - FcRN

Fd
- heavy chain portion of the Fab fragment
  - Fd fragment

FDC
- follicular dendritic cell

febrile
- f. agglutinins
- f. antibody
- f. antigens
- f. disease

febris
- f. melitensis

feedback
- antibody f.
- f. control
- hypothalamic-pituitary f. system

Felton's unit

female
- f. climacteric
- f. eunuchoidism
- f. homosexuality
- f. infertility
- f. intersex
- f. pseudohermaphrodism
- f. pseudohermaphrodite
- f. pseudohermaphroditism
- f. puberty
- f. reproduction
- f. sex hormone

feminine

femininity

feminism

feminization
- male f.
- incomplete testicular f.
- testicular f.

feminizing
- f. mesenchyma
- f. testes syndrome
- f. tumor

fermentation test

Fernandez reaction

ferritin conjugated antibody

fertile eunuch syndrome

fertilization
- in vitro f. (IVF)

fetal
- f. adenoma
- f. androgen
- f. androgenization
- f. cell
- f. gigantism
- f. gonad
- f. hyperglycemia
- f. macrosomia
- f. neurohypophysis
- f. pancreas
- f. protein
- f. tolerance
- f. vaccinia
- f. zone of adrenal cortex

fetoprotein
- alpha f. (AFP)

fetus
- allogeneic f.

fever
- Aden f.
- African tick f.
- aphthous f.
- Argentine hemorrhagic f.
- Argentinian hemorrhagic f.
- Australian Q f.
- autumn f.
- f. blister
- Bolivian hemorrhagic f.
- boutonneuse f.
- Brazilian spotted f.
- breakbone f.
- Bullis f.
- camp f.
- cane-field f.
- cat-scratch f.
- Choix f.
- Colombian tick f.
- Colorado tick f.
- Congo red f.
- Crimean-Congo hemorrhagic f.
- dandy f.
- deer fly f.
- dengue f.
- dengue hemorrhagic f.
- Dutton's relapsing f.

fever *(continued)*
    Ebola hemorrhagic f.
    endotoxin-induced f.
    enteric f.
    entericoid f.
    epidemic hemorrhagic f.
    Far East hemorrhagic f.
    field f.
    five-day f.
    Flinders Island spotted f.
    Fort Bragg f.
    glandular f.
    Hankow f.
    harvest f.
    Hasami f.
    Haverhill f.
    hay f.
    hemorrhagic f's
    hemorrhagic f. with renal
        syndrome
    herpetic f.
    hormonal f.
    f. index
    inundation f.
    island f.
    jail f.
    Japanese flood f.
    Japanese river f.
    Junin f.
    Katayama f.
    Kedani f.
    Kew Gardens spotted f.
    Kinkiang f.
    Korean hemorrhagic f.
    Korin f.
    Lassa f.
    Lone Star f.
    Malta f.
    Marburg hemorrhagic f.
    Marseilles f.
    marsh f.
    Mediterranean f.
    Meuse f.
    Mossman f.
    mountain tick f.
    mud f.
    nanukayami f.
    nine-mile f.
    nonseasonal hay f.

fever *(continued)*
    Omsk hemorrhagic f.
    Oriental spotted f.
    Oroya f.
    Pahvant Valley f.
    pappataci f.
    paratyphoid f.
    parenteric f.
    parrot f.
    Pfeiffer's glandular f.
    pharyngoconjunctival f.
    Philippine hemorrhagic f.
    phlebotomus f.
    pinta f.
    Pomona f.
    Pontiac f.
    pretibial f.
    Q f.
    quintan f.
    rabbit f.
    rat-bite f.
    recurrent f.
    relapsing f.
    rheumatic f.
    rice-field f.
    Rocky Mountain spotted f.
    rose f.
    sandfly f.
    scarlet f.
    Schottmüller's f.
    seasonal hay f.
    Sennetsu f.
    seven-day f.
    shin bone f.
    ship f.
    Sindbis f.
    slime f.
    Songo f.
    South African tickbite f.
    spirillum f.
    splenic f.
    spotted f.
    swamp f.
    Texas tick f.
    Thai hemorrhagic f.
    three-day f.
    tick f.
    Tobia f.
    trench f.

fever *(continued)*
    tsutsugamushi f.
    typhoid f.
    typhus f.
    undulant f.
    Venezuelan hemorrhagic f.
    viral hemorrhagic f's
    war f.
    Whitmore's f.
    Wolhynia f.
    Yangtze Valley f.
    yellow f.

fexofenadine hydrochloride

FIA
    fluorescence immunoassay
    fluorescent immunoassay
    fluoroimmunoassay

fiber
    neurosecretory f's
    Reissner f.
    secretomotor f's

fibrillation
    atrial f.

fibrin

fibrinogen

fibrinoid necrosis

fibroblast
    f. growth factor
    f. growth hormone
    f. interferon

fibrodysplasia

fibroepithelial
    f. interferon

fibrogenesis imperfecta ossium

fibromyoma *pl.* fibromyomas, fi-
bromyomata

fibrosis
    cystic f.
    pipestem f.
    Symmers' f.

fibrous
    f. capsule of thyroid gland

fibrous *(continued)*
    f. dysplasia
    f. goiter
    f. tubercle

Ficoll
    F. gradient
    F.-Hypaque gradient cen-
      trifugation

Fiedler's disease

field fever

fièvre
    f. boutonneuse

fifth disease

fight-or-flight reaction

filarial

filariasis
    Ozzard's f.

Filatov's (Filatow's) disease

Filipovitch's (Filipowicz's) sign

Filoviridae

Filovirus

filterable

filtrable

fimbria *pl.* fimbriae

finger
    bolster f's
    Madonna f's

Finn
    F. chamber
    F. chamber test

first
    f. messenger
    f.-set phenomenon
    f.-set rejection

Fisher-Race theory

fission
    binary f.

FITC (fluorescein isothiocyanate)

Fitz-Hugh–Curtis syndrome

five-day fever

fixation
 complement f.
 f. of complement
 latex f.
 Zamboni f.

fixed
 f. macrophage
 f. virus

FK506 (tacrolimus)

flagella antigen

flagellar
 f. agglutinin
 f. antigen

flagellin

flagellosis

flagellum *pl.* flagella

Flajani's disease

flare

Flaviviridae

Flavivirus

flavivirus

Flavobacterium
 F. meningosepticum

flea-borne typhus

fleckfieber

Flemming center

Flinders Island spotted fever

flocculation
 f. test

floccule
 toxoid-antitoxin f.

flora
 intestinal f.
 normal f.

flora *(continued)*
 vaginal f.

flow
 blood f.
 f. cell cytometry
 f. cell cytometry laser
 f. cytometer
 f. cytometry
 renal blood f.

flu

fluid
 cerebrospinal f. (CSF)
 interstitial f.
 f. phase diffusion
 seminal f.

fluke disease

flulike

flunisolide

Fluogen

fluorescein
 f. isothiocyanate (FITC)
 f.-labeled antihuman globulin

fluorescence
 f.-activated cell sorter (FACS)
 heterogeneous f. immunoassay
 homogeneous f. immunoassay
 f. immunoassay (FIA)
 f. quenching

fluorescent
 f. antibody (FA)
 f. antibody assay
 f. antibody technique
 f. antibody test
 f. antigen assay
 f. dye
 f. labels
 f. immunoassay (FIA)
 f. microscope

fluorescent *(continued)*
  f. microscopy
  f. scanning
  f. treponemal antibody absorption test (FTA-ABS)

fluoride

fluorochrome

fluoroimmunoassay (FIA)

fluticasone propionate

flush

flushing

flying squirrel
  f. s. typhus
  f. s.–associated typhus

foamy viruses

focal necrosis

focus
  f. formation
  primary f.

focusing
  isoelectric f.

fold
  immunoglobulin f.

folding of proteins

folic acid analogue

follicle
  lymph f's
  lymphoid f's
  ovarian f's
  primary f's
  secondary f's
  f. of Stannius
  thyroid f's
  f's of thyroid gland

follicle-stimulating hormone (FSH)
  human f.-s. h.
  f.-s. h.–releasing hormone

follicular
  f. adenocarcinoma

follicular *(continued)*
  f. adenoma
  f. carcinoma of thyroid gland
  f. center cell
  f. center cell lymphoma
  f. dendritic cells (FDC)
  f. epithelium
  f. goiter
  large cleaved f. center cell
  large noncleaved f. center cell
  small cleaved f. center cell
  small noncleaved f. center cell
  f. thyroid carcinoma

folliculostatin

folliculus
  folliculi glandulae thyroideae

follistatin

follitropin

fomes *pl.* fomites

fomite

fomites *(plural of* fomes)

Fonsecaea

food
  f. addiction
  f. allergy
  f. challenge
  f. challenge test
  f. poisoning

foot
  athlete's f.
  f. fungus
  Hong Kong f.
  Madura f.

foot-and-mouth disease

footprinting
  DNA f.

Forbes-Albright syndrome

forbidden clone
  f. c. theory

force
　　coulombic f.
　　electrostatic f.
　　hydrophobic f.
　　intermolecular f.
　　van der Waals f's

foreign
　　f. antigen
　　f. body reaction
　　f. serum

form
　　L f.

formalin

formation
　　antibody f.
　　blast f.
　　bone f.
　　chromosome f.
　　focus f.
　　granuloma f.
　　lattice f.
　　rouleaux f.

formazan

fornix *pl.* fornices

Forschheimer spots

Forssman
　　F. antibody
　　F. antigen

Fort Bragg fever

Foshay's test

four-peptide structure

fourth venereal disease

fowlpox
　　f. virus

fracture
　　endocrine f.

Fraenkel's nodules

fragile X syndrome

fragment
　　amplification f.

fragment *(continued)*
　　antigen-binding f.
　　chemotactic f's
　　crystallizable f.
　　Fab f.
　　F(ab')$_2$ f.
　　Fc f.
　　Fd f.
　　free heavy chain f's
　　heavy chain f's
　　parathyroid hormone
　　　(PTH) f's
　　restriction f.
　　Spengler's f's

fragmentation
　　DNA f.

fragmentin

framework
　　f. hypothesis
　　f. regions
　　f. segments

Framingham follow-up study

Francis
　　F's disease
　　F's test

Francisella
　　F. tularensis

Franklin's disease

Fraser syndrome

free
　　f. heavy chain fragments
　　f. hormone hypothesis
　　f. macrophage
　　f. thyroxine
　　f. thyroxine index
　　f. triiodothyronine
　　f. triiodothyronine index

Frei
　　F. antigen
　　F's disease
　　F. skin test
　　F. test

Freund's adjuvant

Fröhlich's syndrome

fructose
    f.-induced hypoglycemia

fructosuria
    essential f.

fruit bromelain

FSH
    follicle-stimulating hor-
        mone

FTA-ABS
    fluorescent treponemal an-
        tibody absorption test
        (FTA-ABS)

fulminant smallpox

function
    adrenal medullary f.
    adrenocortical f.
    aldosterone f.
    antibody f.
    autocrine f.
    bowel f. in thyrotoxicosis
    effector f's of antibodies
    effector T cell f.
    immunoadjuvant f.
    isotype f.
    kidney f.
    monocyte f.
    placental lactogen f.
    sexual f.
    T cell f.
    testicular f.

functional
    f. adenoma
    f. deletion
    f. hypopituitarism
    f. prepubertal castrate syn-
        drome
    f. tumor

functioning
    f. adenoma
    f. tumor

fundus

fungal
    f. antibody
    f. disease
    f. peritonitis

fungemia

fungoma

fungus pl. fungi
    f. ball
    cutaneous f.
    foot f.
    generalized f.
    localized f.
    opportunistic f.
    subcutaneous f.
    systemic f.

furious rabies

furunculosis
    f. blastomycetica
    f. cryptococcica

Fusarium
    F. poae
    F. sporotrichiella
    F. sporotrichioides
    F. tricinctum

fusin

fusion
    somatic cell f.

Fusobacterium
    F. gonidiaformans
    F. mortiferum
    F. naviforme
    F. nucleatum
    F. russii
    F. varium

fusospirochetosis

Fv
    fragment variable
        single chain Fv

fya receptor

Fyn (see tyrosine kinase)
    F. kinase

G

G
- G cells
- G protein
- protein G

γ
- γ heavy chain
- γ heavy chain disease

GAF
- gamma-activated factor

Gaffky
- G. scale
- G. table

gag gene (*of HIV*)

gain
- antigen g.

gait
- parkinsonian g.

galactagogin

galactokinase

galactopoietic hormone

galactorrhea
- g.-amenorrhea syndrome
- idiopathic g.

galactose-induced hypoglycemia

galactosemia

gallbladder disease

gallstone

GALT
- gut-associated lymphoid tissue

Gambian trypanosomiasis

gametocyte
- g. carrier

gametocytemia

gamma
- g.-activated factor (GAF)

gamma *(continued)*
- g. cells of hypophysis
- g. chain
- g. chain disease
- g. chain marker (Gm)
- g. delta T receptors
- g. emission
- g. globulins
- g. globulin antibodies
- g. heavy chain
- g. heavy chain disease
- g. interferon
- g. staphylolysin

gamma-aminobutyric acid

gammaglobulinopathy

Gammaherpesvirinae

gammopathy
- monoclonal g's
- benign monoclonal g.
- polyclonal g.

Gamna-Favre bodies

gamone

Gamulin Rh

ganglioneuroma

ganglionitis
- acute posterior g.

ganglioside

gangosa

gangrene
- diabetic g.

gap junction

Gardnerella
- *G. vaginalis*

gas
- arterial blood g's

gastric
- g. acid secretion
- g. glands
- g. inhibitory peptide (GIP)

gastric
  g. inhibitory polypeptide
  g. phase

gastrin
  g.-releasing peptide
  g. secretion

gastrinoma

gastritis

gastrodisciasis

gastroenteritis

gastroenteropancreatic, non–
  insulin-secreting tumor

gastroenteropathy
  allergic g.
  eosinophilic g.

gastrointestinal
  g. allergy
  g. anthrax
  g. disease
  g. hormones
  g. infection
  g. manifestations
  g. symptom
  g. system
  g. tract
  g. tularemia

gastrone

gastroparesis

GATA-2

Gaucher disease

gay bowel syndrome

GBG
  glycine-rich β glycoprotein

G cells

G-CSF
  granulocyte colony-stimu-
    lating factor

gel
  agar g.

gel (continued)
  g. diffusion
  g. diffusion test

gelatiniform carcinoma

gelatinous carcinoma

Gell and Coombs classification

γ emission

gender

gene
  autosomal dominant g.
  autosomal recessive g.
  c-fos g.
  C (constant) g's
  cell interaction (CI) g's
  class IB MHC g's
  class III MHC g's
  c-myb g.
  c-myc g.
  constant g's
  g. conversion
  D (diversity) g. segments
  env g. (of HIV)
  gag g. (of HIV)
  germline g.
  H g.
  histocompatibility g.
  HIV g's
  21-hydroxylase g.
  g. identification
  Ig g.
  immune response (Ir) g's
  immune suppressor (Is) g's
  immunoglobulin g's
  Ir (immune response) g's
  Is (immune suppressor) g's
  J (joining) g. segments
  g. knockout
  g. knockout mouse
  g. knockout techniques
  lethal g.
  MAGE-1 g. (melanoma anti-
    gen gene)
  melanoma antigen g.
  minor lymphocyte stimu-
    lating g.

gene *(continued)*
    minor lymphocyte stimulatory g.
    Mls g.
    MLS g.
    nef g.
    neomycin resistance (*neor*) g.
    pol g. (*of HIV*)
    polymorphic g.
    Qa g's
    recessive g.
    recessive lethal g.
    recombination activating g's
    reporter g's
    rev g. (*of HIV*)
    S g.
    g. segments
    seven-up g.
    smcy g.
    sor g.
    suppressor g.
    g. targeting
    tat g. (of HIV virus)
    g. therapy
    TLA g.
    tumor-suppressor g's
    variable g's
    V (variable) g. segments
    vpr g. (*of HIV*)
    vpu g. (*of HIV*)
    vpx g. (*of HIV-2*)
    Y chromosome g's

generalized
    g. anaphylaxis
    g. fungus
    g. glycogenosis
    g. vaccinia
    g. viral infection

generation time

generative lymphoid organs

genetic
    g. association
    g. capacity
    g. changes

genetic *(continued)*
    g. constitution
    g. counseling
    g. deficiency
    g. engineering
    g. factors
    g. immunity
    g. immunization
    g. markers
    g. restriction
    g. transformation

genetically identical transplantation antigens

genetics
    molecular g.
    reverse g.

Gengou phenomenon

genital
    g. ducts
    g. gland
    g. herpes
    g. sex
    g. tract
    g. tuberculosis
    g. ulcer syndrome

genitalia
    ambiguous g.

genitourinary
    g. schistosomiasis
    g. tuberculosis

genome

genomic organization

genotype

geotrichosis

German measles

germ cell mutation

germinal center

Germisten virus

germline
    g. configuration
    g. diversity

germline *(continued)*
  g. genes
  g. theory

germ theory

gestagen

gestation

gestational
  g. diabetes
  g. diabetes mellitus

γ heavy chain disease

GH
  growth hormone

Ghon complex

GHRH
  growth hormone–releasing
    hormone

giant
  g. cell
  g. cell carcinoma of thyroid
    gland
  g. cell thyroiditis
  g. follicular thyroiditis

Giardia lamblia

giardiasis

gigantism
  acromegalic g.
  cerebral g.
  eunuchoid g.
  fetal g.
  hyperpituitary g.
  normal g.
  pituitary g.

gikiyami

Gilchrist
  G's disease
  G's mycosis

GIP
  gastric inhibitory polypep-
    tide

Gitelman's syndrome

gland
  accessory adrenal g's
  accessory parotid g.
  accessory suprarenal g's
  accessory thyroid g's
  adrenal g.
  apocrine g.
  Aselli's g.
  biliary g.
  ductless g's
  endocervical g's
  endocrine g's
  exocrine g's
  extraparotid lymph g.
  gastric g's
  genital g.
  Gley's g's
  hemal g's
  heterocrine g.
  lacrimal g.
  mixed g.
  pancreatic g.
  parafrenal g's
  parathyroid g's
  parotid g.
  Philip's g's
  pineal g.
  pituitary g.
  posterior pituitary g.
  pregnancy g.
  prehyoid g's
  prostate g.
  Sandström's g's
  sebaceous g's
  secretory g's
  sentinel g.
  suprarenal g.
  sweat g's
  target g.
  thymus g.
  thyroid g.
  Virchow's g.
  Wölfler's g.

glandula *pl.* glandulae
  g. adrenalis
  glandulae endocrinae
  g. parathyroidea inferior
  g. parathyroidea superior
  g. pinealis

glandula *(continued)*
  g. pituitaria
  glandulae sine ductibus
  g. suprarenalis
  glandulae suprarenales accessoriae
  g. thyroidea
  glandulae thyroideae accessoriae

glandular
  g. fever
  g. plague
  g. tissue
  g. tularemia

Gley's glands

glial cell

glicentin

globi

globulin
  α-g's
  α_2-g.
  alpha g's
  g. antibodies
  antihuman g. (AHG)
  anti–human g. serum
  antilymphocyte g. (ALG)
  antithymocyte g. (ATG)
  β-g's
  bacterial polysaccharide immune g. (BPIG)
  beta g's
  corticosteroid-binding g. (CBG)
  cortisol-binding g.
  fluorescein-labeled antihuman g.
  γ-g's
  gamma g's
  hepatitis B immune g.
  immune g.
  immune human serum g.
  immune serum g.
  intravenous immune g.
  lymphocyte immune g.
  pertussis immune g.
  rabies immune g.

globulin *(continued)*
  $Rh_0(D)$ immune g.
  serum g's
  sex hormone–binding g. (SHBG)
  sex steroid–binding g.
  specific immune g.
  specific immune serum g. (SIG)
  testosterone-binding g. (TeBG)
  testosterone-estradiol–binding g.
  testosterone-estrogen–binding g.
  tetanus immune g.
  thyronine-binding g.
  thyroxine-binding g. (TBG)
  vaccinia immune g.
  varicella-zoster immune g.
  zoster immune g. (ZIG)

globus *pl.* globi

glomerular
  g. basement membrane
  g. basement membrane autoantibodies
  g. basement membrane autoimmune disease
  g. zone

glomerulonephritis
  acute g.
  immune complex g.
  membranous g.
  poststreptococcal g.

glomerulosclerosis

glomerulus *pl.* glomeruli

glucagon
  gut g.
  g. immunoreactant
  g.-like immunoreactivity
  g. stimulation test

glucagonoma
  g. syndrome

glucocorticoid
  g. receptor

glucocorticoid *(continued)*
  g. response elements
    (GREs)

glucogenesis

glucokinetic

gluconeogenesis

glucoregulation

glucose
  blood g.
  declining g. tolerance
  g.-dependent insulinotropic
    polypeptide
  fasting plasma g.
  impaired g. tolerance
  g.-induced hypoglycemia
  g. intolerance
  intravenous g.
  g. level
  oral g.
  oral g. tolerance test (OGTT)
  g.-6-phosphate dehydrogen-
    ase (G6PD)
  g.-sparing
  g. test
  g. tolerance
  g. tolerance factor
  g. tolerance test (GTT)
  g. transport system

glucosuria

glutaraldehyde

gluten
  g.-sensitive enteropathy
  g. sensitivity

glycan-bearing cell adhesion
  molecule-1 (GlyCAM-1)

glycate

glycation

glycemia

glycentin

glycine-rich β glycoprotein
  (GBG)

glycogen

glycogenesis

glycogenetic

glycogenolysis

glycogenosis
  brancher deficiency g.
  generalized g.
  hepatophosphorylase g.
  hepatorenal g.
  myophosphorylase defi-
    ciency g.

glycogenous

glycolipid

glycolytic pathway

glycophilia

glycoprotein
  g. adenoma
  glycine-rich β g. (GBG)
  g. hormone
  g. hormone adenoma
  g. Mac-1
  g. p150,95
  variable surface g. (VSG)

glycorrhea

glycostatic

glycosuria
  alimentary g.
  benign g.
  digestive g.
  hyperglycemic g.
  nondiabetic g.
  nonhyperglycemic g.
  normoglycemic g.
  orthoglycemic g.
  pathologic g.
  renal g.

glycosylated
  g. hemoglobin

glycosylation
  nonenzymatic g.

glycotropic

glycuresis

Gm
    gamma chain marker
        Gm allotypes
        Gm antigens
        Gm group

GM-1

GM-CSF
    granulocyte-macrophage
        colony-stimulating factor

GMK
    green monkey kidney (*culture medium*)

gnathostomiasis

GnRH
    gonadotropin-releasing
        hormone (GnRH)
            GnRH test

Godélier's law

goiter
    aberrant g.
    adenomatous g.
    Basedow's g.
    colloid g.
    congenital g.
    cystic g.
    diffuse g.
    diffuse nontoxic g.
    diffuse toxic g.
    diving g.
    endemic g.
    exophthalmic g.
    familial g.
    fibrous g.
    follicular g.
    intrathoracic g.
    iodide g.
    lingual g.
    lymphadenoid g.
    multinodular g.
    multinodular nontoxic g.
    nodular g.
    nontoxic g.
    parenchymatous g.
    perivascular g.
    plunging g.

goiter *(continued)*
    retrovascular g.
    simple g.
    substernal g.
    suffocative g.
    toxic g.
    toxic multinodular g.
    vascular g.
    wandering g.

goitre

goitrin

goitrogen

goitrogenic

goitrogenicity

goitrogenous

goitrous
    g. hypothyroidism
    g. thyroiditis

Golgi
    G. apparatus
    G. complex
    G's law

gonad
    fetal g.
    streak g's

gonadal
    g. agenesis
    g. dysgenesis
    g. mesenchyma
    mixed g. dysgenesis
    pure g. dysgenesis
    g. sex
    g. steroid
    XO g. dysgenesis (*same as*
        Turner syndrome)
    46,XY g. dysgenesis

gonadarche

gonadectomy
    dysgenic g.
    prophylactic g.

gonadoblastoma

gonadoinhibitory

gonadokinetic

gonadoliberin

gonadopathy

gonadotrope
  g. adenoma
  g. cell

gonadotroph
  g. adenoma
  g. cell
  g. cell adenoma

gonadotrophic

gonadotrophin

gonadotropic
  g. cell
  g. hormone

gonadotropin
  chorionic g. (CG)
  equine g.
  human chorionic g. (hCG)
  human menopausal g.
  pregnant mare serum g.
  g.-releasing hormone
    (GnRH)
  gonodotropin-resistant
    ovary

gonadotropinoma

gonane

gongylonemiasis

gonochorism

gonococcal urethritis

gonococcus *pl.* gonococci
  streptomycin-resistant gon-
    ococci

gonophage

gonorrhea

gonorrheal
  g. rheumatism
  g. urethritis

Good's syndrome

goodness of fit

Goodpasture
  G. antigen
  G's syndrome

Gordon's syndrome

gouty diathesis

G6PD
  glucose-6-phosphate dehy-
    drogenase

gp39

gp41

gp120

G protein

gradient
  Ficoll g.
  Ficoll-Hypaque g. centrifu-
    gation
  ion g.
  pH g.

Graefe's sign

Graffi virus

graft
  allogeneic g.
  allograft
  g. arteriosclerosis
  autochthonous g.
  autogenous g.
  autologous g.
  autoplastic g.
  composite g.
  heterologous g.
  heteroplastic g.
  homologous g.
  homoplastic g.
  homostatic g.
  homovital g.
  isogeneic g.
  isologous g.
  isoplastic g.
  lymphoreticular tissue g.
  g. rejection
  second-set g. rejection

graft *(continued)*
    skin g.
    skin g. experiment
    skin g. rejection
    syngeneic g.
    syngraft
    tissue g's
    g.-versus-host disease (GVHD)
    g.-versus-host (GVH) reaction
    xenogeneic g.
    xenograft

graftectomy

grafting
    cartilage g.

graft-versus-host
    g.-v.-h. disease
    g.-v.-h. reaction

Grancher's triad

granule
    acidophil g's
    alpha g's
    g.-associated enzyme
    basophil g.
    beta g's
    Birbeck g.
    Bollinger's g's
    chromaffin g's
    cytotoxic lytic g's
    Much's g's
    neurosecretory g. (NSG)
    Paschen's g's
    Schrön-Much g's
    Schüffner's g's
    secretory g's
    sulfur g's

granulocorpuscle

granulocyte
    g. colony-stimulating factor (G-CSF)
    g.-macrophage colony-stimulating factor (GM-CSF)
    polymorphonuclear g.

granulocytic
    g. pyrogen

granulocytopenia

granuloma *pl.* granulomas, granulomata
    amebic g.
    Candida g.
    candidal g.
    coccidioidal g.
    eosinophilic g.
    g. formation
    infectious g.
    g. inguinale
    Majocchi's g.
    monilial g.
    paracoccidioidal g.
    g. pudendi
    g. pudens tropicum
    umbilical g.
    g. venereum

granulomata *(plural of* granuloma*)*

granulomatosis
    allergic g.
    Wegener's g.

granulomatous
    g. amebic encephalitis
    g. disease
    g. hypersensitivity
    g. lesion
    g. reaction
    g. thyroiditis

granulosa-theca cell
    g.-t. c. tumor

grape cell

Graphium

grass

Graves
    G's disease
    G's ophthalmopathy
    G's orbitopathy

gray
    g. tubercle
    g.-patch ringworm

GREs
  glucocorticoid response elements

Griffith's sign

grip
  devil's g.

grippal

Gross virus

ground
  g. itch
  g. itch anemia
  g. substance

group
  ABO blood g.
  ABO blood g. antigens
  ABO blood g. system
  ABO typing
  g. agglutination
  g. agglutinin
  allotypic g.
  g. A streptococci
  blood g.
  Bunyamwera g. viruses
  Bwamba g. viruses
  California g. viruses
  Capim g. viruses
  carbohydrate g.
  carboxylate g.
  CMN g.
  Gm g.
  Guama g. viruses
  hydrophobic g.
  immunodominant g.
  platelet g.
  g. precipitation
  g. reaction

grouping
  haptenic g.

group-specific

growth
  g. abnormalities
  adolescent g.
  bone g.
  cellular g.

growth *(continued)*
  g. delay
  g. disorders
  fetal g.
  g. inhibition method
  longitudinal g.
  g.-onset diabetes mellitus
  organ g.
  paracrine g. factor
  pubertal g. spurt
  skeletal g.

growth factor
  autocrine g. f.
  B cell g. f's (BCGF)
  epidermal g. f. (EGF)
  epithelial g. f.
  fibroblast g. f.
  hematopoietic g. f's
  human epidermal g. f.
  insulin-like g. f's (IGF) (I and II)
  macrophage g. f. (MGF)
  nerve g. f. (NGF)
  ovarian g. f.
  peptide g. f's
  platelet-derived g. f. (PDGF)
  polypeptide g. f's
  skeletal g. f.
  T cell g. f.
  transforming g. f. (TGF)

growth hormone (GH)
  g. h. cell adenoma
  g. h.–producing tumor
  g. h. release–inhibiting hormone
  g. h.–releasing hormone (GHRH)
  g. h.–releasing hormone releasing tumor
  g. h.–secreting adenoma

GTP
  guanosine triphosphate

GTT
  glucose tolerance test

Guama
  G. group viruses
  G. virus

Guanarito virus

guanosine triphosphate (GTP)

guanylate kinase

Guarnieri
    G's bodies
    G's corpuscles
    G's inclusions

Guaroa virus

Gubler-Robin typhus

Guillain-Barré syndrome

Gull's disease

gumma *pl.* gummas, gummata
    syphilitic gummata
    tuberculous g.

gummatous
    g. syphilis
    g. ulcer

gummy
    g. tumor

gut
    g.-associated lymphoid tissue (GALT)
    g. glucagon

GVH
    graft-versus-host
        GVH disease
        GVH reaction

Gymnoascus

gynander

gynandria

gynandrism

gynandroblastoma

gynandroid

gynandromorph

gynandromorphism
    bilateral g.

gynandromorphous

gynandry

gynecic

gynecogen

gynecogenic

gynecoid

gynecomastia
    adolescent g.
    idiopathic g.
    nutritional g.
    pathologic g.
    physiological g.
    refeeding g.
    rehabilitation g.

gynecomastism

gynecomasty

gynogamone

gynoid obesity

H
  H agglutination
  H agglutinin
  H antigen (*of Salmonella ty-phi*)
  H chain
  H chain antigen
  H gene
  H receptor
  H substance

H-2
  H-2 antigens
  H-2 antigen system
  H-2 locus

HAA
  hepatitis-associated anti-gen

Habronema

habronemiasis

Haemophilus
  H. aegyptius
  H. aphrophilus
  H. b conjugate vaccine (HbCV)
  H. b polysaccharide vac-cine (HbPV)
  H. ducreyi
  H. influenzae
  H. parainfluenzae
  H. paraphrophilus
  H. parasuis
  H. somnus

haemozoin

Hageman factor

H agglutination

H agglutinin

HAI
  hemagglutination inhibition
    HAI assay
    HAI test

hair
  h. cycle

hair *(continued)*
  h. pattern
  pubic h.

hairpin structures

hairy cell leukemia

HAI test

Hajdu-Cheney syndrome

half-life
  antibody h.-l.

halzoun

hamartoma
  hypothalamic h.

hamburger thyrotoxicosis

hand
  spade h.

Hand-Schüller-Christian disease

Hankow fever

Hantaan virus

Hantavirus

hantavirus
  h. pulmonary syndrome

H antigen (*of Salmonella typhi*)
  minor H a's

H-2 antigens

H-2 antigen system

Hanzalova virus

haplomycosis

haplosporangin

haplotype
  MHC h.

hapten
  autocoupling h.
  h. inhibition test
  h.-carrier complex

haptene

haptenic
  h. addition
  h. grouping

haptoglobin

hard
  h. chancre
  h. sore

Harris' syndrome

hartmannelliasis

Hartnup disease

harvest
  h. fever

Hasami fever

Hashimoto
  H's disease
  H's struma
  H's thyroiditis

hashitoxicosis

Haverhill fever

hay fever
  nonseasonal h. f.
  seasonal h. f.

HBcAg
  hepatitis B core antigen

HbCV
  Haemophilus b conjugate
    vaccine

HBeAg
  hepatitis B e antigen

HbPV
  Haemophilus b polysaccha-
    ride vaccine

HBsAg
  hepatitis B surface antigen

H chain
  H c. antigen

hCG
  human chorionic gonado-
    tropin
      hCG secretion

hCG *(continued)*
      hCG test

H-2 complex

HCP
  hereditary coproporphyria

hCS
  human chorionic somato-
    mammotropin

hCT
  human chorionic thyrotro-
    pin

HDCV
  human diploid cell vaccine

HDL
  high-density lipoprotein

HDN
  hemolytic disease of the
    newborn

head
  h. of pancreas
  white h.

headache manifestation of pituitary tumor

healing
  wound h.

heart
  h. disease
  h. failure
  myxedema h.
  h. transplantation

heat
  h. inactivation
  h. intolerance
  h.-labile factors
  h.-labile toxin
  h. prostration
  h. shock protein
  h. stabile
  h.-stabile antigen

heavy chain
  h. c. classes
  h. c. diseases

heavy chain *(continued)*
    free h. c. fragments
    gamma h. c. disease
    h. c. portion of the Fab
      fragment

Heberden's nodes

height

Heine-Medin disease

Hektoen phenomenon

HEL
    hen egg-white lysozyme

HeLa cell adherence assay

helenine

Helicobacter
    H. cinaedi
    H. pylori

helix
    amphipathic h.

helminth
    h. infections

helminthemesis

helminthiasis

helminthic abscess

helminthism

helminthoma

helper
    h. CD4 T cells
    h. cells
    h. factors
    h. T cells
    h. T lymphocytes
    h. virus

helper/inducer subset

hemadsorption
    h. test
    h. virus *(types 1 and 2)*

hemagglutination
    h. assay

hemagglutination *(continued)*
    indirect h.
    h. inhibition (HAI, HI)
    h. inhibition assay
    h. inhibition reaction
    h. inhibition technique
    h. inhibition test
    passive h.
    h. reaction
    reverse passive h.
    h. test
    viral h.

hemagglutinative

hemagglutinin
    cold h.
    influenza h.
    warm h.

hemal glands

hemangioblastomatosis
    retinal cerebellar h.

hematemesis

hematocrit

hematogenous tuberculosis

hematological disease

hematopoiesis
    extramedullary h.

hematopoietic
    h. cell
    h. growth factors
    h. lineage
    h. stem cell
    h. system

hematopoietin
    receptor family h's

hematuria
    endemic h.

hemithyroidectomy

hemoagglutination

hemoagglutinin

hemoblast

hemochromatosis
  primary h.
  secondary h.

hemodynamic
  h. hypothesis
  h. shock

hemoflagellate

hemoglobin
  glycosylated h.
  h. synthesis

hemoglobinuria
  cold h.
  nocturnal h.
  paroxysmal cold h. (PCH)
  paroxysmal nocturnal h.
    (PNH)

hemolysin
  alpha h.
  beta h.
  hot-cold h.
  immune h.

hemolysis
  extravascular h.
  immune h.
  intravascular h.
  passive h.

hemolytic
  h. anemia
  autoimmune h. anemia
  h. autoimmune anemia
  h. complement assay
  h. disease of the newborn
    (HDN)
  drug-induced immune h.
    anemia
  immune h. anemia
  infectious h. anemia
  h. plaque assay
  h. unit
  warm autoimmune h. ane-
    mia (WAIHA)

hemolyzed

hemophagocytic
  h. lymphohistiocytosis

hemophagocytic *(continued)*
  h. syndrome

hemophiliac

hemopoiesis

hemopoietic stem cell

hemopoietin

hemoprecipitin

hemopsonin

hemoptysis
  endemic h.
  Manson's h.
  Oriental h.
  parasitic h.

hemorrhagic
  h. dengue
  h. fevers
  h. fever with renal syn-
    drome
  h. measles
  h. nephrosonephritis
  h. pian
  h. plague

hemorrhage
  transplacental h.

hemostasis

hemostatic

hemozoin

Henle's reaction

Henoch-Schönlein purpura

Hepacivirus

Hepadnaviridae

Hepadnavirus

hepadnavirus

heparin

hepaticoliasis

hepatic lipase
  familial h. l. deficiency

hepatic schistosomiasis

hepatitis *pl.* hepatitides
    h. A
    h. A antigen
    anicteric h.
    h. antigen
    h.-associated antigen
      (HAA)
    h. A vaccine inactivated
    h. A virus
    h. B
    h. B antigen
    h. B core antigen (HBcAg)
    h. B e antigen (HBeAg)
    h. B immune globulin
    h. B surface antigen
      (HBsAg)
    h. B vaccine
    h. B vaccine (recombinant)
    h. B virion
    h. B virus
    h. C
    cholangiolitic h.
    cholangitic h.
    cholestatic h.
    chronic active h.
    chronic viral h.
    h. C–like viruses
    h. C virus
    h. D
    h. D antigen
    delta h.
    h. delta
    h. delta virus
    h. D virus
    h. E
    enterically transmitted
      non-A, non-B h.
    epidemic h.
    h. E virus
    h. GB virus
    h. G virus
    homologous serum h.
    infectious h.
    inoculation h.
    long-incubation h.
    MS-1 h.
    MS-2 h.
    non-A–E h.

hepatitis *(continued)*
    non-A, non-B h.
    posttransfusion h.
    serum h.
    short-incubation h.
    transfusion h.
    h. vaccine
    viral h.
    h. virus

hepatocyte
    h.-stimulating factor

hepatolenticular disease

hepatolysin

hepatomegaly

hepatophosphorylase glycoge-
    nosis

hepatorenal glycogenosis

hepatosplenomegaly

heptamer

Heptavax-B

herd immunity

hereditary
    h. allergy
    h. angioneurotic edema
    h. coproporphyria
    h. disease
    h. fructose intolerance
    h. short stature

heredity

hermaphrodism

hermaphrodite
    pseudo-h.
    true h.

hermaphroditic

hermaphroditism
    bilateral h.
    false h.
    lateral h.
    spurious h.
    transverse h.

hermaphroditism *(continued)*
    true h.
    unilateral h.
    XX true hemaphroditism
    XY true hemaphroditism

hermaphroditismus
    h. verus
    h. verus bilateralis
    h. verus lateralis
    h. verus unilateralis

hernia
    h. uteri inguinalis

herpangina
    h. virus

herpes
    h. digitalis
    h. facialis
    h. febrilis
    genital h.
    h. genitalis
    h. gladiatorum
    h. labialis
    h.-like particles
    h. progenitalis
    h. simplex
    h. simplex virus
    traumatic h.
    h. virus
    wrestler's h.
    h. zoster

herpesviral

Herpesviridae

herpesvirus
    human h. 1
    human h. 2
    human h. 3
    human h. 4
    human h. 5
    human h. 6
    human h. 7
    human h. 8
    Kaposi's sarcoma–associated h.

herpetic
    h. fever

herpetiformis
    dermatitis h.

Hers' disease

Herxheimer
    H's reaction

heteroagglutination

heteroagglutinin

heteroantibody

heteroantigen

heterochromatization

heteroclitic
    h. antibody

heteroconjugate
    h. antibody

heterocytotropic
    h. antibody

heterodimer

heterogeneic
    h. antigen

heterogeneous
    h. fluorescence immunoassay
    h. immunoassay
    h. ligand assay

heterogenetic
    h. antibody
    h. antigen

heterogenic antigen

heterogenous

heterohemagglutination

heterohemagglutinin

heterohemolysin

heteroimmune

heteroimmunity

heteroimmunization

heterologous
    h. antibodies
    h. antigen
    h. desensitization
    h. graft
    h. serum
    h. vaccine

heterolysin

heterolysis

heterolytic

heterophil (*spelled also* hetero-phile)
    h. antibody
    h. antigen

heterophilic

heterophydiasis

heterophyiasis

heteroplastic
    h. graft

heterosexual

heterotopic
    h. liver transplantation
    h. transplantation

heterotransplantation

heterotypic
    h. vaccine

heterovaccine
    h. therapy

heterozygous

HEV
    high endothelial venule

hexamer

hexamitiasis

hexon

Heymann's nephritis

H gene

HGF
    hyperglycemic-glycogenoly-tic factor

hGH
    human growth hormone
        hGH-recombinant

HGPRT
    hypoxanthine-guanine phosphoribosyltransfer-ase

H1 histone protein

HHV8 virus

HI
    hemagglutination inhibition
        HI assay
        HI test

Hib-Imune

Hickey-Hare test

hidden determinant

HIE
    hyperimmunoglobulin E syndrome

high
    h.-affinity antibodies
    h.-density lipoprotein (HDL)
    h.-dose dexamethasone suppression test
    h.-dose tolerance
    h. endothelial cells
    h. endothelial venule (HEV)
    h.-frequency antigens
    h.-incidence antigens
    h.-molecular-weight neutro-phil chemotactic factor (HMW-NCF)
    h.-titer, low-avidity antigen
    h.-pressure liquid chroma-tography (HPLC)
    h. responder
    h.-zone tolerance

Higouménaki's sign

hilar
    h. cell
    h. cell hyperplasia
    ovarian h. cells
    h. cell tumor

hilum *pl.* hila
    h. of adrenal gland
    h. glandulae suprarenalis
    ovarian h.
    h. of suprarenal gland

hindrance
    steric h.

hinge region

hippocampus

Hirschsprung's disease

hirsute

hirsuties

hirsutism

hirudiniasis

His
    H's disease
    H.-Werner disease

histamine
    h.$_1$
    h.$_2$
    h. challenge
    h. flare test
    h.-releasing factor (HRF)
    h. sensitivity
    h. shock
    h. test

histioblast

histiocyte
    wandering h.

histiocytic

histiocytosis
    Langerhans' cell h.

histochemical antibody methods

histocompatibility
    h. antigens
    h. antigen system
    h. complex
    h. gene
    major h. antigens
    minor h. antigens

histocompatible

histocyte

histoincompatibility

histoincompatible

histologic section

histology

histone

Histoplasma
    H. capsulatum
    H. capsulatum var. *duboisii*

histoplasmin
    h. skin test

histoplasmoma

histoplasmosis
    African h.
    h. capsulatum
    h. duboisii
    progressive disseminated h.

histosensitive pneumonitis

histotope

HI test

HIV
    human immunodeficiency virus
        HIV-1
        HIV antibodies
        HIV antibody binding complex
        HIV drug resistance
        HIV envelope
        HIV genes
        HIV immune response
        HIV infection

HIV *(continued)*
    HIV life cycle
    HIV mutant peptides
    HIV opsonization
    HIV proteins
    HIV provirus
    HIV replication
    HIV seroconversion
    HIV structure
    HIV transmission
    HIV vaccination

hives

HLA
    human leukocyte antigens
        HLA-A11
        HLA antigens
        HLA-B53
        HLA complex
        HLA-DM
        HLA-DQ
        HLA-DR2
        HLA-DR3/DR4
        HLA-G
        HLA system
        HLA typing

HLT
    heat-labile toxin

H-2 locus

H-2M

H-2M3

hMG
    human menopausal gonad-
        otropin

HML
    human mucosal lympho-
        cyte antigen

HMW-NCF
    high-molecular-weight neu-
        trophil chemotactic factor

hnRNA
    heteronuclear RNA

Hodgkin
    H's disease

Hodgkin *(continued)*
    H's lymphoma

Hoffman syndrome

holoantigen

homeostasis
    calcium h.
    ionic h.
    osmotic h.

homing
    h. of basophils
    h. receptor

homobody

homocystinuria

homocytotropic
    h. antibody

homogeneous
    h. fluorescence immunoas-
        say
    h. immunoassay
    h. ligand assay
    h. rejection

homogenous

homograft
    h. reaction
    h. rejection

homologous
    h. antibodies
    h. antigen
    h. desensitization
    h. graft
    h. recombination
    h. restriction factor (HRF)
    h. serum
    h. serum hepatitis
    h. serum jaundice

homology
    h. regions

homolysin

homolysis

homophil

homophilic

homoplastic
   h. graft

homoplasty

homosexual

homosexuality
   female h.
   male h.

homostatic graft

Homo-Tet

homotopic
   h. transplantation

homotransplant

homovital graft

homozygous
   h. typing cells (HTC)

homunculus

honeycomb ringworm

Hong Kong
   H. K. foot
   H. K. influenza

hookworm
   h. anemia
   h. disease

horizontal
   h. transmission

hormonagogue

hormonal
   h. contraception
   h. factors
   h. fever
   h. imprinting
   h. manipulation
   h. specificity
   h. therapy

hormone
   abnormal h.
   adaptive h.
   adenohypophysial h's
   adipokinetic h.

hormone *(continued)*
   adrenal h.
   adrenocortical h.
   adrenocorticotrophic h.
     (ACTH)
   adrenocorticotropic h.
     (ACTH)
   adrenomedullary h's
   androgenic h.
   androstenedione h.
   anterior pituitary h's
   antidiuretic h. (ADH)
   antimüllerian h. (AMH)
   bioactive h.
   catecholamine h.
   chromaffin h.
   conjugated estrogen h.
   corpus luteum h.
   cortical h.
   corticotropin-releasing h.
     (CRH)
   diabetogenic h.
   ectopic h.
   estrogenic h.
   eutopic h.
   h. excess
   fat-mobilizing h's
   female sex h.
   fibroblast growth h.
   follicle-stimulating h. (FSH)
   follicle-stimulating h.–
     releasing h. (FSH-RH)
   galactopoietic h.
   gastrointestinal h's
   glycoprotein h.
   gonadotropic h.
   gonadotropin-releasing h.
   growth h. (GH)
   growth h. release–inhibi-
     ting h.
   growth h.–releasing h.
     (GHRH)
   human chorionic gonado-
     tropin h.
   human follicle-stimula-
     ting h.
   human growth h. (hGH)
   human pituitary growth h.
   hypophyseotropic h.

hormone *(continued)*
    hypophysiotropic h's
    immunoactive h.
    inhibiting h's
    insulin counteracting h.
    interstitial cell–stimula-
      ting h.
    islet h.
    lactation h.
    lactogenic h.
    lipolytic h's
    lipotropic h. (LPH)
    local h.
    luteal h.
    luteinizing h. (LH)
    luteinizing h.–releasing h.
      (LHRH)
    male sex h.
    luteotropic h.
    melanocyte-stimulating h.
      (MSH)
    melanophore-stimulating h.
    h. metabolism
    multiple h.
    neurohypophysial h's
    ovarian h's
    h. pairs
    parathyroid h. (PTH)
    peptide h's
    pituitary h.
    placental h's
    placental growth h.
    placental peptide h.
    polypeptide h.
    posterior pituitary h's
    prenatal h.
    h.-producing tumor
    progestational h.
    prolactin-inhibiting h.
    prolactin-releasing h.
    proparathyroid h.
    protein h.
    prothoracicotropic h.
    h. receptor
    h. receptor complex
    h. receptor interaction
    releasing h's
    h. resistance
    h. response elements

hormone *(continued)*
    h. secretion
    serum growth h.
    sex h's
    somatotrophic h.
    somatotropic h.
    somatotropin release–inhi-
      biting h.
    somatotropin-releasing h.
    steroid h's
    syndrome of inappropriate
      antidiuretic h. (SIADH)
    h. synthesis
    testicular h.
    testis h.
    h. therapy
    thyroid h's
    thyroid-stimulating h.
      (TSH)
    thyrotropic h.
    thyrotropin-releasing h.
      (TRH)
    TSH-releasing h. (TRH)
    vasodilator h's

hormonic

hormonogen

hormonogenesis

hormonogenic

hormonology

hormonopoiesis

hormonopoietic

hormonoprivia

hormonosis
    exogenous h.

hormonotherapy

horror
    h. autotoxicus

horseradish peroxidase technique

host
    h. barriers
    h. cell

host *(continued)*
    debilitated h.
    h. defense mechanisms
    definitive h.
    h. immune systems
    h. immunity
    immunocompetent h.
    intermediate h.
    h.-parasite interactions
    h. protective immunity
    h. range
    h. reactions
    reservoir h.
    h. resistance
    h. specificity
    three h. cascade systems

hot
    h.-cold hemolysin
    h.-cold lysis
    h. nodule

house dust mite

Houssay
    H. animal
    H. phenomenon

HPA axis

hPL
    human placental lactogen

HPLC
    high performance liquid
        chromatography
            HPLC–electrochemical
            detection assay

HPV
    human papilloma virus

H receptor

HRF
    histamine-releasing factor
    homologous restriction fac-
        tor

HSF
    hydrazine-sensitive factor

HSP
    heat shock protein

H substance

HTACS
    human thyroid adenylate
        cyclase stimulators

HTC
    homozygous typing cells

HTLV
    human T-lymphotropic vi-
        rus 1
            HTLV-1
            HTLV-1–associated
                myelopathy
            HTLV III

human
    h. atopy
    h. caliciviruses
    h. chorionic gonadotropin
        (hCG)
    h. chorionic gonadotropin
        hormone
    h. chorionic somatomam-
        motropin (hCS)
    h. chorionic thyrotropin
        (hCT)
    h. diploid cell vaccine
        (HDCV)
    h. follicle-stimulating hor-
        mone
    h. granulocytic ehrlichiosis
    h. growth hormone (hGH)
    h. herpesvirus (1–8)
    h. immunodeficiency virus
        (HIV)
    h. immunodeficiency virus
        antigen
    h. leukocyte antigens
        (HLA)
    h. menopausal gonadotro-
        pin
    h. monocytic ehrlichiosis
    h. mucosal lymphocyte an-
        tigen
    h. papillomavirus
    h. parainfluenza virus
        (1–4)
    h. parvovirus B19

human *(continued)*
    h. parvovirus RA-1
    h. pituitary growth hormone
    h. placental lactogen (hPL)
    h. respiratory syncytial virus
    h. serum factor
    h. serum jaundice
    h. T-cell leukemia virus
    h. T-cell lymphotropic virus (*types I, II, III*)
    h. thyroid adenylate cyclase stimulators (HTACS)
    h. T-lymphotropic virus (1, 2)
    h. toxocariasis

humanization

humanized monoclonal antibodies

humoral
    h. amplification systems
    h. antibody
    h. endorphin
    h. factor
    h. immune response
    h. immunity
    h. secondary immune response
    h. synthesis
    h. theory of immunity

hump
    buffalo h.
    dowager's h.

hunger disease

hungry
    h. bone syndrome
    h. disease

hunterian chancre

Hunter syndrome

Hurler syndrome

Hürthle
    H. cells

Hürthle *(continued)*
    H. cell adenoma
    H. cell carcinoma
    H. cell tumor

Hutchinson-Gilford syndrome

hutchinsonian triad

Hu-Tet

HV region

hyalinization
    Crooke's h.

hyalohyphomycosis

hyaluronic acid

hyaluronidase

H-Y antigen

hybrid
    h. antibody
    T cell h's
    h. virus

hybridization
    DNA dot blot h.
    dot blot h.
    in situ h.
    molecular probe h.
    Northern blot h.
    oligonucleotide probe h.
    Southern blot h.
    subtractive h.
    Western blot h.

hybridoma
    murine h.
    T lymphocyte h.

hydatid
    alveolar h. disease
    h. disease
    h. toxemia
    unilocular h. disease

hydatidosis

hydration

hydrazine-sensitive factor (HSF)

hydrocephalus

hydrochlorothiazide

hydrocortisone
  h. acetate
  h. butyrate
  h. cypionate
  h. hemisuccinate
  h. sodium phosphate
  h. sodium succinate
  h. valerate

hydrogen
  h. bonds
  h. bonding
  h. peroxide

hydroperoxyeicosatetraenoic
  acid

hydrophagocytosis

hydrophilic

hydrophobia
  paralytic h.

hydrophobic
  h. force
  h. group
  h. interactions

4-hydroxyandrostenedione

hydroxycorticosteroid
  17-h.

17β-hydroxycorticosterone

hydroxyeicosatetraenoic acid

5-hydroxyindoleacetic acid

hydroxylase
  11β-h. deficiency
  17α-h. deficiency
  18-h. deficiency
  21-h. deficiency
  21-h. gene
  phenylalanine h.

hydroxypregnenolone

17α-hydroxyprogesterone

hydroxyproline

hydroxysteroid
  17-h.

hydroxysteroid dehydrogenase
  3β-h. d. deficiency
  11β-h. d. deficiency
  17β-h. d. deficiency

5-hydroxytryptamine

3-hydroxytyramine

hymenolepiasis

hyperacute rejection

hyperadrenalism

hyperadrenocorticism

hyperaldosteronemia

hyperaldosteronism
  primary h.
  pseudoprimary h.
  secondary h.

hyperaldosteronuria

hyperandrogenism

hyperapobetalipoproteinemia

hyperbetalipoproteinemia

hypercalcemia
  familial h.
  familial hypocalciuric h.
  idiopathic h.
  postmenopausal h.

hypercalcemic
  h. crisis
  h. keratopathy

hypercalcitoninemia
  familial h.

hypercalcitoninism

hypercalciuria
  absorptive h.
  renal h.
  type I h.

hyperchloremia

hypercholesterolemia
  familial h.

hyperchromaffinism

hypercorticalism

hypercorticism

hypercortisolism

hypercreatinemia

hyperdefecation

hyperdynamic β-adrenergic syndrome

hyperemesis gravidarum

hyperemia

hypereosinophilic syndromes

hyperepinephrinemia

hyperergia

hyperestrogenemia

hyperestrogenism

hyperestrogenosis

hyperexcretory

hyperfunction

hyperfunctional adenoma

hyperfunctioning adenoma

hypergammaglobulinemia
   monoclonal h's
   polyclonal h.

hypergastrinemia

hypergenitalism

hyperglandular

hyperglobulinemia

hyperglucagonemia

hyperglycemia
   chemical h.
   experimental h.
   fetal h.
   rebound h.
   stress h.

hyperglycemic
   h. glycosuria

hyperglycemic *(continued)*
   h.-glycogenolytic factor (HGF)

hyperglycosemia

hyperglycosuria

hypergonadism

hypergonadotropic
   h. eunuchoidism
   h. hypogonadism

hyper-IgM
   h.-IgM dysgammaglobuline-mia
   h.-IgM syndrome

hyperimmune
   h. serum

hyperimmunity

hyperimmunization

hyperimmunoglobulinemia
   h. E

hyperimmunoglobulin E syn-drome (HIE)

hyperimmunoglobulin M (hy-per-IgM) syndrome

hyperinsulinar
   h. obesity

hyperinsulinemia
   endogenous h.

hyperinsulinism

hyperkalemia

hyperkeratosis

hyperketonuria

hyperkinesia

hyperleydigism

hyperlipidemia
   combined h.

hyperlipoproteinemia

hypermagnesemia

hypermetabolism

hypermineralocorticoidism

hypermutation
    somatic h.

hypernatremia
    essential h.

hyperorchidism

hyperosmolar
    h. coma
    h. nonketotic coma

hyperovarianism

hyperovarism

hyperoxaluria
    enteric h.

hyperpancreorrhea

hyperparathyroid bone disease

hyperparathyroidism
    ectopic h.
    h. incidence
    neonatal h.
    primary h.
    secondary h.
    tertiary h.

hyperphagia

hyperphosphatasia

hyperphosphatemia
    acute h.

hyperphosphatemic osteomala-
    cia

hyperphosphaturia

hyperpigmentation

hyperpinealism

hyperpituitarism

hyperpituitary
    h. gigantism

hyperplasia
    adenomatous h.
    adipocyte h.

hyperplasia *(continued)*
    adrenal h.
    adrenal cortical h.
    adrenocortical h.
    chief cell h.
    congenital adrenal h.
    endometrial h.
    hilar cell h.
    juxtaglomerular cell h.
    lipoid adrenal h.
    nodular adrenal h.
    nodular adrenocortical h.
    parathyroid h.
    somatotrope h.
    stromal h.
    water-clear cell h.

hyperpotassemia

hyperproinsulinemia

hyperprolactinemia

hyperprolactinemic

hyperproteinemia

hypersecretion
    adrenocortical h.
    insulin h.

hypersensitive
    h. pneumonitis

hypersensitivity
    anaphylactic h.
    h. angiitis
    antibody-mediated h.
    antibody-mediated cytotox-
        ic h.
    autoimmune h.
    cell-mediated h.
    complex-mediated h.
    congenital adrenal hyper-
        plasia
    contact h.
    cutaneous basophil h.
    cytotoxic h.
    cytotoxic-type h.
    delayed h. (DH)
    delayed-type h. (DTH)

hypersensitivity *(continued)*
   h. diseases
   granulomatous h.
   immediate h.
   immune complex–medi-
    ated h.
   insulin h.
   penicillin h.
   h. pneumonitis
   h. reaction
   stimulatory h.
   T cell–mediated h.
   tuberculin-type h.
   type I h.
   type II h.
   type III h.
   type IV h.
   h. vasculitis

hypersensitization

hypersomatotropism

hypersomia

hypersuprarenalism

hypertension
   adrenal h.
   essential h.
   estrogen-induced h.
   malignant h.
   pregnancy-induced h.
   renal h.
   renovascular h.
   stress h.
   volume h.
   volume-mediated h.

Hyper-Tet

hyperthyrea

hyperthyroid

hyperthyroidism
   apathetic h.
   iodine-induced h.
   masked h.
   secondary h.

hyperthyroiditis

hyperthyroidosis

hyperthyroxinemia
   euthyroid h.
   familial dysalbuminemic h.
   (FDH)
   familial isolated h.

hypertonic
   h. encephalopathy
   h. water balance derange-
    ment

hypertrichosis

hypertriglyceridemia
   familial h.

hypertrophic
   h. osteoarthritis
   h. vascular disease

hypertrophy
   clitoral h.
   lymphoid h.

Hypertussis

hyperuricemia

hyperuricosuria

hypervaccination

hypervariable
   h. regions

hyperviscosity syndrome

hypervitaminosis A

hypervolemia

hyphae

hyphomycosis

hypoadrenalism

hypoadrenocorticism
   neonatal h.

hypoaldosteronemia

hypoaldosteronism
  hyporeninemic h.
  isolated h.

hypoaldosteronuria

hypoandrogenism

hypocalcemia
  neonatal h.

hypochromic anemia

hypocitraturia

hypocomplementemia

hypocomplementemic
  h. vasculitis

hypocorticalism

hypocorticism

hypodermiasis

hypodermosis

hypoepinephrinemia

hypoergia

hypoergic

hypoergy

hypoestrogenemia

hypofertile

hypofertility

hypofunction
  adrenal h.

hypofunctioning

hypogammaglobulinemia
  acquired h.
  common variable h.
  physiologic h.
  transient h. of infancy
  X-linked h.
  X-linked infantile h.

hypogenitalism

hypoglandular

hypoglucagonemia

hypoglycemia
  alimentary h.
  amino acid–induced h.
  autoimmune h.
  drug-induced h.
  exogenous insulin h.
  factitial h.
  factitious h.
  familial h.
  fasting h.
  fructose-induced h.
  galactose-induced h.
  glucose-induced h.
  idiopathic h.
  insulin-induced h.
  ketotic h.
  leucine-induced h.
  mixed h.
  neonatal h.
  postabsorptive h.
  postprandial h.
  reactive h.

hypoglycemic
  h. agent
  h. shock

hypoglycemosis

hypogonadal
  h. obesity

hypogonadism
  eugonadotropic h.
  hypergonadotropic h.
  hypogonadotropic h.
  male h.
  neurogenic h.
  pituitary h.
  primary h.
  secondary h.

hypogonadotropic
  h. eunuchoidism
  h. hypogonadism

hypoinsulinemia

hypoinsulinism

hypokalemia

hypokalemic
h. polyuria

hypoleydigism

hypolipidemia

hypolymphemia

hypomagnesemia

hypomagnesuria

hyponatremia

hypo-orchidism

hypo-ovarianism

hypopancreatism

hypopancreorrhea

hypoparathyroid

hypoparathyroidism
idiopathic h.

hypophamine

hypophosphatemia
familial h.
X-linked h.
X-linked familial h.

hypophyseal
h. portal system

hypophysectomize

hypophysectomy

hypophyseoportal
h. system
h. veins

hypophyseoprivic

hypophyseotropic
h. hormone

hypophysial
h. cachexia
h. dwarf
h. dwarfism
h. infantilism

hypophysial *(continued)*
h. portal circulation
h. stalk

hypophysioportal
h. circulation
h. system

hypophysioprivic

hypophysiotropic
h. area
h. hormones

hypophysis
h. cerebri

hypophysitis
lymphocytic h.

hypopigmentation

hypopinealism

hypopituitarism
functional h.
idiopathic h.

hypopituitary dwarfism

hypoplasia
adrenal h.
breast h.
congenital adrenal h.
Leydig cell h.
thymic h.

hypoplastic

hypoproteinemia

hyporeninemic
h. hypoaldosteronism

hyporesponder

hyposensitive

hyposensitivity

hyposensitization

hyposomatotropinemia
hypothalamic h.

hyposomatotropism

hyposomia

hypospadias
  familial perineal h.
  pseudovaginal perineoscrotal h.

hyposthenuria
  persistent h.

hyposuprarenalism

hypotension
  orthostatic h.

hypothalamic
  h. amenorrhea
  h.-pituitary feedback system
  h. hamartoma
  h. hypophysial portal system
  h. hyposomatotropinemia
  h. hypothyroidism
  h.-pituitary-adrenal axis
  h.-pituitary-adrenocortical axis
  h.-pituitary axis
  h.-pituitary-gonadal axis
  h.-pituitary portal system
  h.-pituitary system
  h.-pituitary-thyroid axis
  h.-pituitary-thyroid complex
  h.-pituitary unit
  h. thirst center

hypothalamo-hypophysial portal system

hypothalamo-pituitary-Leydig cell axis

hypothalamo-pituitary-seminferous tubular axis

hypothalamus

hypothermia

hypothesis
  altered ligand h.
  altered self h.
  avidity h.
  clonal selection h.

hypothesis *(continued)*
  countercurrent h.
  differential signaling h.
  Dreyer and Bennett h.
  dual recognition h.
  framework h.
  free hormone h.
  hemodynamic h.
  lattice h.
  Lyon h.
  mass action h.
  network h.
  occlusion h.
  passenger leukocyte h.
  quantitative h.
  side-chain h.
  signal h.
  somatomedin h.
  statistical mechanical h.
  unitarian h.
  von Pirquet h.

hypothyrea

hypothyroid
  h. dwarf
  h. obesity

hypothyroidism
  adult h.
  central h.
  congenital h.
  goitrous h.
  hypothalamic h.
  infantile h.
  juvenile h.
  juvenile acquired h.
  mild h.
  pituitary h.
  postablative h.
  postradioiodine h.
  primary h.
  secondary h.
  subclinical h.
  tertiary h.
  thyroidal h.
  thyroprivic h.
  trophoprivic h.

hypothyrosis

hypothyroxinemia
    euthyroid h.

hypotonic
    h. plasma
    h. saline
    h. syndromes
    h. water balance derange-
      ment

hypotonicity

hypovarianism

hypovolemia

hypoxanthine-guanine phospho-
    ribosyltransferase (HGPRT)

hypoxia

HypRho-D

Hypr virus

hysterectomy

hysterotomy

I
    I antigen
    I region

Ia antigens

IAHA
    immune adherence hemag-
        glutination assay

I antigen

i antigen

iatrogenic infection

IBF
    immunoglobulin-binding
        factor

ICAM (1 *and* 2)
    intercellular adhesion mol-
        ecule

iccosome

ICFA antigen

icteric

icterus

IDDM
    insulin-dependent diabetes
        mellitus

identification
    gene i.

identity
    partial i.

idioagglutinin

idiocy
    cretinoid i.

idioheteroagglutinin

idioheterolysin

idioisoagglutinin

idioisolysin

idiolysin

idiopathic
    i. adrenal atrophy
    i. biliary cirrhosis
    i. calcium urolithiasis
    i. cyclical edema
    i. dwarfism
    i. galactorrhea
    i. gynecomastia
    i. hypercalcemia
    i. hypoglycemia
    i. hypoparathyroidism
    i. hypopituitarism
    i. infertility
    i. polyneuritis
    i. postprandial syndrome
    i. puberty
    i. thrombocytopenic pur-
        pura

idiosyncrasy

idiosyncratic

idiotope

idiotype
    i.–anti-i. network
    dominant i.
    immunoglobulin i's

idiotypic
    i. antigen
    i. network
    i. variation

IEP
    immunoelectrophoresis

IF
    intrinsic factor

IFA
    immunofluorescence assay
        IFA test
    immunofluorescent assay
    indirect fluorescent anti-
        body

IFIX
    immunofixation

IFN
  interferon
Ig
  immunoglobulin
    Ig gene
    Ig gene transcription
IgA
  immunoglobulin A
    isolated IgA deficiency
    secretory IgA
    selective IgA deficiency

igbo-ora virus

IgE receptors

IGF
  insulin-like growth factors
    IGF-I
    IGF-II
    IGF-binding protein
      (IGFBP)

IGFBP
  IGF-binding protein

ignorance
  clonal i.
  immunologic i.

IgSF
  immunoglobulin supergene
    family

IL (*specific interleukins are designated by an Arabic numeral, as IL-1, IL-2*)
  interleukin

ileal bypass
  partial i. b.

ileitis
  regional i.

ileus
  adynamic i.
  myxedema i.

Ilheus virus

iliac nodes

image
  body i.
  internal i.

immature B cell

immediate
  i. allergy
  i. contact
  i. hemolytic reactions
  i. hypersensitivity
  i. hypersensitivity reaction
  systemic i. hypersensitivity

immobile cilia syndrome

immobilization test

immortalization

immune
  i. adherence
  i. adherence hemagglutination assay (IAHA)
  i. adsorption
  i. agglutinin
  i. antibody
  i. assay
  i.-associated antigen
  i. body
  cell-mediated secondary i. response
  i. clearance
  i. complex
  i. complex disease
  i. complex disorder
  i. complex glomerulonephritis
  i. complex–mediated hypersensitivity
  i. complex–mediated hypersensitivity reaction
  i. conglutinin
  i. cytolysis
  i. deficiency
  i. deficiency disease
  i. deviation
  i. elimination
  i. globulin
  i. hemolysin

immune *(continued)*
-   i. hemolysis
-   i. hemolytic anemia
-   i. human serum globulin
-   humoral secondary i. response
-   i. interferon
-   i.-mediated diseases
-   i. molecule
-   i. opsonin
-   i. paralysis
-   i. polysaccharides
-   i. precipitate
-   i. precipitation reaction
-   primary i. response
-   i. process
-   i. protein
-   i. reaction
-   i. response
-   i. response (Ir) genes
-   i. response (Ir) gene defect
-   secondary i. response
-   i. serum
-   i. serum globulin
-   i. status
-   i. stimulatory complex (IS-COM)
-   i. suppression
-   i. suppressor
-   i. suppressor (Is) genes
-   i. surveillance
-   i. system
-   i. thrombocytopenia
-   i. tolerance

immunity
-   acquired i.
-   acquired specific i.
-   active i.
-   adaptive i.
-   adoptive i.
-   allograft i.
-   antibacterial i.
-   antibody-mediated i.
-   antimicrobial i.
-   antitissue i.
-   antitoxic i.
-   antiviral i.
-   artificial i.

immunity *(continued)*
-   cell-mediated i. (CMI)
-   cellular i.
-   community i.
-   concomitant i.
-   cross i.
-   diminished i.
-   familial i.
-   genetic i.
-   herd i.
-   host i.
-   host protective i.
-   humoral i.
-   infection i.
-   inherent i.
-   inherited i.
-   innate i.
-   intrauterine i.
-   local i.
-   maternal i.
-   Metchnikoff's theory of antimicrobial i.
-   mucosal i.
-   native i.
-   natural i.
-   nonspecific i.
-   passive i.
-   passively acquired i.
-   pertussis i.
-   protective i.
-   smallpox i.
-   species i.
-   specific i.
-   sterile i.
-   T cell–mediated i. (TCMI)
-   tissue i.
-   transference of i.
-   tumor i.
-   *X.* models for studying immunity

immunization
-   active i.
-   adoptive i.
-   antigen dose vs. i.
-   booster i.
-   i. campaigns
-   diphtheria i.
-   genetic i.

immunization *(continued)*
  measles i.
  mumps i.
  i. nonresponders
  passive i.
  pediatric i.
  primary i.
  i. recipient
  repeated i.
  i. responders
  rubella i.
  secondary i.
  tertiary i.
  i. therapy
  toxoid i.
  varicella i.

immunize

immunizing
  median i. dose

immunoabsorption
  quantitative i.

immunoactive hormone

immunoadjuvant
  i. function

immunoadsorbent

immunoadsorption

immunoassay
  enzyme i. (EIA)
  enzyme-linked i.
  fluorescence i. (FIA)
  fluorescent i. (FIA)
  heterogeneous i.
  heterogeneous fluores-
    cence i.
  homogeneous i.
  homogeneous fluores-
    cence i.
  nephelometric inhibition i.
  Northern blot i.
  optical i.
  rapid surface i.
  semiquantitative i.
  sol particle i. (SPIA)
  Southern blot i.

immunoassay *(continued)*
  TDX i.
  Western blot i.

immunobiological

immunobiology

immunoblast

immunoblastic
  i. lymphadenopathy

immunoblot

immunoblotting

immunochemical

immunochemistry

immunocompetence

immunocompetent
  i. host

immunocomplex

immunocompromised

immunoconglutinin

immunocyte
  common i.
  i.-derived amyloidosis

immunocytic
  i. amyloidosis

immunocytoadherence
  i. technique

immunocytochemistry

immunodeficiency
  acquired i.
  antibody i.
  autosomal recessive i.
  autosomal severe com-
    bined i. (SCID)
  cellular i.
  combined i. (CID)
  combined B and T cell i.
  common variable i. (CVID)
  common variable unclassi-
    fiable i.
  congenital i.
  i. diseases

immunodeficiency *(continued)*
   i. with elevated IgM
   i. with hyper-IgM
   inherited i. diseases
   primary i.
   protein i.
   secondary i.
   severe combined i. (SCID)
   i. with short-limbed dwarfism
   i. with thymoma
   X-linked i.
   X-linked severe combined i. (X-linked SCID)

immunodeficient

immunodepression

immunodepressive

immunodetection

immunodeviation

immunodiagnosis

immunodiffusion
   radial i. (RID)
   single radial i. (SRID)

immunodominance

immunodominant
   i. group
   i. region

immunoelectrophoresis (IEP)
   countercurrent i.
   crossed i.
   quantitative i.
   rocket i.

immunoendocrinopathy
   i. syndrome

immunoferritin

immunofiltration

immunofixation (IFIX)

immunofluorescence
   i. assay (IFA)
   direct i.
   indirect i.
   i. microscopy

immunofluorescent
   i. antibody testing
   i. antigen assay
   i. assay (IFA)
   i. techniques

immunogen

immunogenetic

immunogenetics

immunogenic
   i. antigen
   i. determinant
   i. nucleic acid
   i. polypeptide
   i. stimuli

immunogenicity

immunoglobulin (Ig) *(designated* A, D, E, G, and M)
   i.-alpha
   antilymphocyte i.
   i.-beta
   i.-binding factor (IBF)
   cell surface i.
   i. characteristics
   i. classes
   i. concentration
   i. domains
   i. fold
   i. genes
   i. G1 molecule
   i. hinge region
   i. idiotypes
   i. levels
   membrane i.
   membrane-bound i. (mIg)
   i. molecule
   monoclonal i.
   monomeric i.
   oligoclonal i.
   polymeric i.
   secretory i. (sIg)
   secretory i. A
   i. subclasses
   i. superfamily
   i. supergene family (IgSF)
   surface i. (sIg)

immunoglobulin *(continued)*
   i.-synthesizing B lympho-
     cyte
   tailpieces of i's
   thyroid-binding inhibitory
     i's (TBII)
   thyroid-stimulating i's (TSI)
   thyrotropin-binding inhibi-
     tory i's (TBII)
   TSH-binding inhibitory i's
   Xenopus i's

immunoglobulinlike domains

immunoglobulinopathy
   monoclonal i's

immunogold technique

immunohemolytic
   i. anemia

immunohistochemical
   i. staining

immunohistochemistry

immunohistofluorescence

immunoincompetent

immunologic *(also* immunological)
   i. competence
   i. contraceptive methods
   i. deficiency
   i. deficiency theory
   i. dysfunction
   i. ignorance
   i. inertia
   i. injury
   i. memory
   i. paralysis
   primary i. diseases
   i. rejection
   i. relationship
   i. resistance
   sex-linked lymphogenic i.
     disease
   i. studies
   i. surveillance

immunologic *(continued)*
   i. tolerance
   i. unresponsiveness
   i. vasculitis

immunological

immunologically
   i. competent cell
   i. privileged sites

immunologist

immunology
   cellular i.
   neuroendocrine i.
   tumor i.

immunometric assay

immunomicroscopy
   direct i.

immunomodulation

immunomodulator

immunomodulatory
   i. effects

immunopathogenesis

immunopathologic

immunopathology

immunoperoxidase
   i. technique

immunophenotype

immunophilin

immunophysiology

immunopotency

immunopotentiation

immunopotentiator

immunoprecipitation
   i. analysis
   i. techniques

immunoproliferative
   i. small intestine disease

immunoprophylaxis

immunoradiometric
  i. assay (IRMA)

immunoradiometry

immunoreactant
  glucagon i.

immunoreaction

immunoreactive

immunoreactivity
  glucagon-like i.

immunoreceptor
  i. tyrosine-based activation
    motif (ITAM)

immunoregulation

immunoresponsiveness

immunoselection

immunosenescence

immunosorbent

immunostimulant

immunostimulation

immunosuppressant
  i. radiation
  i. reaction

immunosuppression
  i. drugs

immunosuppressive
  i. agent
  i. drugs
  i. therapy

immunosurveillance

immunotherapy
  adoptive i.
  adoptive cellular i.
  passive i.
  tumor i.

immunotoxin

immunotransfusion

impairment
  renal i.

impetigo

implantable matrix

implanted contraceptive

impotence
  drug-induced i.
  endocrinologic i.
  psychogenic i.
  secondary i.

imprinting
  hormonal i.

inactivated
  i. bacteria
  i. serum
  i. toxin
  i. vaccine

inactivation
  complement i.
  heat i.

inactivator
  anaphylatoxin i. (AI)
  C3b i.

inactive X theory

inanition

inapparent
  i. infection
  i. viral infection

inbred
  i. mouse
  i. mouse strain

incidence
  hyperparathyroidism i.

incisura *pl.* incisurae
  i. pancreatis

inclusion
  i. bodies
  cytoplasmic i's
  Guarnieri's i's
  intranuclear i's

incompatibility
  Rh i.

incompatibility *(continued)*
    Rhesus i.

incomplete
    i. agglutinin
    i. androgen insensitivity
    i. antibody
    i. isosexual precocity
    i. testicular feminization

incorporation
    leucine i.
    thymidine i.

incretin

incretion

incubation
    i. period

incubative stage

index *pl.* indexes, indices
    albumin i.
    fever i.
    free thyroxine i.
    free triiodothyronine i.
    maturation i.
    metabolic indices
    opsonic i.
    parasite i.
    penile-brachial blood pres-
        sure i. (PBPI)
    phagocytic i.
    spleen i.
    splenic i.
    splenometric i.
    stimulation i.

Indian tick typhus

indirect
    i. agglutination
    i. antihuman globulin test
    i. contact
    i. Coombs' test
    i. fluorescent antibody
        (IFA) test
    i. hemagglutination
    i. hemagglutination tech-
        nique
    i. immunofluorescence

indirect *(continued)*
    i. immunofluorescence mi-
        croscopy
    i. test of immunofluores-
        cence

individual
    allogeneic i's

indolent
    i. myeloma

induced
    i. phagocytosis

inducer cell

inducible NO synthase (iNOS)

induction
    antibody i.
    lactation i.
    ovulation i.
    i. phase

induration
    laminate i.
    parchment i.

industrial allergy

inertia
    immunologic i.

infant
    i. immunization schedule
    i. mortality rate
    newborn i.
    i. sex reassignment

infantile
    i. cretinism
    i. dwarf
    i. hypothyroidism
    i. (lethal) osteopetrosis
    i. myxedema
    i. paralysis
    i. spinal paralysis

infantilism
    Brissaud's i.
    dysthyroidal i.
    hypophysial i.
    Lévi-Lorain i.
    Lorain's i.

infantilism *(continued)*
    myxedematous i.
    pancreatic i.
    pituitary i.
    regressive i.
    sexual i.
    universal i.

infarction
    myocardial i.

infectible

infection
    adenovirus i.
    agammaglobulinemia i.'s
    airborne i.
    bacterial i.
    chronic i.
    clinical i.
    colonization i.
    congenital cytomegalovi-
        rus i.
    congenital viral i.
    cross i.
    cryptogenic i.
    cytolytic viral i.
    droplet i.
    dust-borne i.
    ectogenous i.
    endogenous i.
    Epstein-Barr latent i.
    exogenous i.
    gastrointestinal i.
    generalized viral i.
    helminth i.'s
    HIV i.
    iatrogenic i.
    i. immunity
    inapparent i.
    inapparent viral i.
    integrated viral i.
    latent i.
    localized i.
    localized viral i.
    mass i.
    mixed i.
    Mycoplasma i.
    nosocomial i.
    opportunistic i.
    pyogenic i.

infection *(continued)*
    resistance to i.
    respiratory tract i.
    secondary i.
    steady-state viral i.
    streptococcal i.
    streptococcal skin i.
    streptococcal upper respir-
        atory i.
    subclinical i.
    systemic i.
    upper respiratory i.
    vector-borne i.
    water-borne i.

infectiosity

infectious
    i. adrenalitis
    i. agent
    i. diarrhea
    i. disease
    i. granuloma
    i. hemolytic anemia
    i. hepatitis
    i. jaundice
    i. material
    i. mononucleosis
    i. nucleic acid
    i. splenomegaly
    i. waste

infectiousness

infective
    i. dose
    i. jaundice
    median i. dose
    i. splenomegaly
    i. thrombosis
    i. thrombus

infectivity

Infektion-Immunität

inferior
    i. border of body of pan-
        creas
    i. border of pancreas
    i. margin of suprarenal
        gland
    i. syndrome of red nucleus
    i. thyroid artery

infertility
    female i.
    idiopathic i.
    lactation-associated i.
    male i.

infiltrate
    inflammatory i.

infiltration
    epituberculous i.
    tuberculous i.

infiltrative
    i. dermopathy
    i. ophthalmopathy

inflammation
    acute i.
    chronic i.
    cytokinine-induced i.
    granulomatous i.
    necrotizing i.
    i. sites
    subacute i.

inflammatory
    acute i. response
    i. CD4 T cells (T_H1 cells)
    i. cell
    i. infiltrate
    i. macrophage
    i. mediators
    i. response
    i. rheumatism
    i. T cells

influenza
    i. A
    Asian i.
    i. A virus
    i. B
    i. B virus
    i. C
    i. C virus
    endemic i.
    Hong Kong i.
    i. hemagglutinin
    Russian i.
    Spanish i.
    i. virus
    i. virus vaccine

influenzal

Influenzavirus
    I. A
    I. B
    I. C

infundibular
    i. body
    i. stalk
    i. stem

infundibulum *pl.* infundibula
    i. of hypophysis
    i. hypothalami
    i. of hypothalamus
    i. lobi posterioris hypophy-
        seos
    i. neurohypophyseos

infusion
    continuous subcutaneous
        insulin i.

ingested allergen

ingestion
    latex bead i.

inguinal adenopathy

inhalation tuberculosis

inhalational
    i. anthrax
    i. challenge
    i. challenge test
    i. provocation

inhaled
    i. allergen
    i. antigen

inherent immunity

inheritance
    pseudoautosomal i.
    recessive i.

inherited
    i. immunity
    i. immunodeficiency dis-
        eases
    i. neutropenia

inhibin

inhibiting
  i. factors
  i. hormones

inhibition
  adrenal steroid i.
  agglutination i.
  allogenic i.
  cold target i.
  contact i.
  hemagglutination i. (HAI, HI)
  migration i.
  ovulation i.
  i. technique

inhibitor
  anaphylatoxin i.
  C1 i.
  C1 esterase i.
  membrane i.
  membrane attack complex i.
  membrane i. of reactive lysis (MIRL)
  protease i.

inhibitory
  i. syndrome

injectable contraceptive

injection
  booster i.
  intracorporeal i.
  secondary i.

injury
  immunologic i.
  spinal cord i.
  tubular cell i.

innate
  i. immune response
  i. immunity
  i. resistance
  i. resistance mechanisms

innocent bystander
  i. b. cell

inocula (*plural of* inoculum)

inoculability

inoculable

inoculate

inoculation
  i. hepatitis
  protective i.
  smallpox i.

inoculum *pl.* inocula

iNOS
  inducible NO synthase

inosinic-cytidylic acid complex

inositol
  i. triphosphate
  i. 1,4,5-triphosphate

insect
  i. bite
  i. sting
  i. venom

insensitivity
  androgen i.
  complete androgen i.
  incomplete androgen i.

insidious rejection

in situ hybridization

insomnia

instability
  vasomotor i.

instructive
  i. model of T cell development
  i. theory of antibody synthesis

insufficiency
  acute adrenocortical i.
  adrenal i.
  adrenocortical i.
  chronic adrenocortical i.
  familial adrenocortical i.
  metabolic i.
  parathyroid i.

insufficiency *(continued)*
   primary adrenal i.
   primary adrenocortical i.
   renal i.
   secondary adrenal i.
   secondary adrenocortical i.
   thyroid i.

insulin
   i. antagonists
   crystalline zinc i.
   i. hypersecretion
   i. hypersensitivity
   i.-induced hypoglycemia
   i. interactions
   intramuscular i.
   Lente i.
   i. levels
   i.-like growth factor
   neutral protamine Hage-
     dorn i. (NPH)
   neutral regular i.
   oral i.
   protamine zinc i.
   i. pump
   i. receptors
   i. receptor substrate-1
   regular i.
   i. release
   i. resistance
   semi-Lente i.
   i. shock
   i. storage
   i. synthesis
   i. therapy
   i. tolerance test

insulin-dependent diabetes mellitus (IDDM)

insulinemia

insulinogenesis

insulinogenic

insulinoma

insulinopathy

insulinopenic

insulitis

insulogenic

insuloma

insusceptibility

intake
   water i.

Intal

integrated viral infection

integration
   neuroendocrine i.

integrin
   β_1 i.
   β_2 i.
   β_3 i.
   leukocyte i's
   macrophage i's

intelligence
   i. quotient (IQ)
   subnormal i.

interaction
   antigen i.
   antigen-antibody i.
   B cell i.
   hormone receptor i.
   host-parasite i's
   hydrophobic i's
   insulin i's
   parasite-host i.
   primary i.
   primary antibody i's
   protein-protein i.
   secondary i.
   secondary antibody i's

interalveolar

intercellular adhesion molecule
   (ICAM) (1 *and* 2)

interception

intercrine

interdigitating
   i. cells

interdigitating *(continued)*
    i. dendritic cells
    i. reticular cell

interference
    methylation i.

interferon (IFN)
    i.-α
    i.-alfa
    alpha i.
    i.-β
    beta i.
    i. beta-2
    chick embryo i.
    epithelial i.
    exogenous i.
    fibroblast i.
    fibroepithelial i.
    i.-γ
    gamma i.
    i.-γ receptor
    immune i.
    i. inducers
    leukocyte i.
    i. receptor
    type I i.
    type II i.

interleukin (IL) *(specific interleukins are designated by an Arabic numeral, as interleukin-1, interleukin-2, IL-1, IL-2)*
    i. receptor
    i. secretion

intermediate
    i. cell
    i. host
    reactive nitrogen i. (RNI)
    reactive oxygen i. (ROI)
    i. thymocyte

intermedin

intermolecular force

internal
    i. image
    i. mammary arteriogram
    i. secretion
    i. secretory system

international insulin unit

intersex
    female i.
    male i.
    true i.

intersexual

intersexuality

interstitial
    i. cells
    i. cell–stimulating hormone
    i. cell tumor
    i. fluid
    i. plasma cell pneumonia
    i. pneumonitis

intervening sequences

intestinal
    i. anthrax
    i. autoimmune disease
    i. flora
    i. myiasis
    i. phase
    i. schistosomiasis
    i. strongyloidiasis

intestine

intolerance
    carbohydrate i.
    heat i.
    hereditary fructose i.
    protein i.

intoxication
    antibody i.
    lead i.
    vitamin D i.
    water i.

intracellular
    i. bacteria
    i. parasite
    i. pathogen
    i. receptor

intracorporeal injection

intracranial tumor

intracrine

intracutaneous
    i. reaction
    i. test

intradermal
    i. reaction
    i. skin test
    i. test

intraepidermal lymphocyte

intraepithelial lymphocyte

intramuscular insulin

intranasal

intranuclear inclusions

intraperitoneal
    i. fetal transfusion
    i. toxemia

intrapituitary
    i. cysts

intrarenal obstruction

intrathoracic
    i. goiter
    i. thyroid

intratubal precipitation

intrauterine
    i. device (IUD)
    i. immunity

intravascular
    i. coagulation
    i. destruction
    i. hemolysis

intravenous
    i. glucose
    i. glucose tolerance test
    i. immune globulin
    i. pyelography
    i. urography

intrinsic
    i. asthma
    i. coagulation mechanism

intrinsic *(continued)*
    i. factor (IF)
    i. factor autoantibodies

intron

inundation fever

invariant chain

invasive
    i. aspergillosis
    i. fibrous thyroiditis
    i. thyroiditis

invasiveness

invermination

inverse anaphylaxis

lnv group antigen

in vitro
    i. v. fertilization (IVF)

in vivo

iod-Basedow

iodide
    i. goiter
    i. oxidation
    i. peroxidase
    plasma inorganic (PI) i.
    renal i. clearance rate
    i. transport

iodination
    organic i.

iodine
    i. deficiency
    i. escape
    excess i.
    i.-induced hyperthyroidism
    Lugol's i.
    i. metabolism
    i. mumps
    protein-bound i.
    radioactive i. uptake

iodogorgoric acid

iodoprotein

iodotherapy

iodothyroglobulin

iodothyronine

iodotyrosine
    i.-coupling defect
    i. dehalogenase defect

ion
    i. channel
    i. exchange
    i. gradient
    i. pump
    i. transport

ionic homeostasis

iopanoate sodium

ipodate sodium

IPV
    poliovirus vaccine inacti-
        vated

IQ
    intelligence quotient
        subnormal IQ

Ir
    immune response
        Ir genes
        Ir gene defect

I region

iridovirus

IRMA
    immunoradiometric assay

iron
    i. storage disease

irradiation
    total lymphoid i. (TLI)

irregularity
    menstrual i.

Is
    immune suppressor
        Is genes

ischemia

ischemic heart disease

ISCOM
    immune stimulatory com-
        plex

island
    blood i.
    i. disease
    i. fever
    i's of Langerhans
    i's of pancreas

islet
    i. amyloid polypeptide
    i. cells
    i. cell adenoma
    i. cell tumor
    i. hormone
    i's of Langerhans
    pancreatic i's
    pancreatic i. cells

isoadrenocorticism

isoagglutination

isoagglutinin

isoandrosterone

isoantibody

isoantigen

isochromosome

isocytolysin

isoelectric focusing

isoenzyme
    Regan i.

isoform

isogeneic
    i. antigen
    i. graft

isogeneric

isogenic
    i. graft

isograft

isohemagglutination

isohemagglutinin

isohemolysin

isohemolysis

isohemolytic

isoimmune
  i. reaction

isoimmunization
  Rh i.

isolated
  i. hypoaldosteronism
  i. IgA deficiency
  i. menarche

isolation
  lymphocyte i.
  protein i.

isoleukoagglutinin

isologous
  i. graft

isolysin

isolysis

isolytic

isomer
  meta i.
  para i.

isophagy

isophil antibody

isophile
  i. antigen

isoplastic
  i. graft

isoprecipitin

isoprenaline

isoprinosine

isosensitization

isosexual precocity
  incomplete i. p.

isosporiasis

isothromboagglutinin

isotope

isotopic
  i. bone scanning
  i. renography

isotransplant

isotransplantation

isotype
  i. detection
  i. distribution
  i. exclusion
  i. function
  secretory i. deficiencies
  i. structure
  i. switch
  i. switching

isotypic
  i. determinants
  i. exclusion
  i. variant
  i. variation

isthmectomy

isthmus *pl.* isthmi
  i. glandulae thyroideae
  i. of thyroid gland

ITAM
  immunoreceptor tyrosine-
    based activation motif

itch
  bakers' i.
  barbers' i.
  Cuban i.
  dew i.
  dhobie i.
  ground i.
  jock i.

Itk

IUD
    intrauterine device

IVF
    in vitro fertilization

IVF-ET
    in vitro fertilization with
      embryo transfer

Ixodes
    I. pacificus
    I. persulcatus
    I. ricinus
    I. scapularis

ixodiasis

ixodism

J
joining
J chain
J gene segments
J region

Jacob-Monod model

jail fever

JAK
Janus family of kinases
JAK3 kinase

Jamestown Canyon virus

Janus
J. family of kinases (JAK)
J. kinase

Japanese
J. encephalitis
J. encephalitis virus
J. flood fever
J. river fever

Jarisch-Herxheimer reaction

jaundice
epidemic j.
homologous serum j.
human serum j.
infectious j.
infective j.
leptospiral j.
spirochetal j.

J chain

JC virus

jejunoileal bypass

Jendrassik's sign

jennerization

Jerne
J. plaque assay
J. plaque technique
J. plaque test

Jeryl Lynn live attenuated
mumps vaccine

J (joining) gene segments

Job's syndrome

jock itch

jodbasedow
j. phenomenon

joining (J)
j. chain
j. gene segments
j. region

joint
coding j.
signal j.

Jones-Mote reaction

JRA
juvenile rheumatoid arthritis

J (joining) region

junction
gap j.

junctional diversity

Junin
J. fever
J. virus

jun oncogene

Jurkat T cell line

juvenile
j. acquired hypothyroidism
j. diabetes mellitus
j. hypothyroidism
j. osteoporosis
j. Paget disease
j. rheumatoid arthritis

juxtaglomerular (JG)
j. cell hyperplasia

K
 potassium
 K antigen
 K cells
 substance K
 K virus

κ
 κ chain

Kahler's disease

kalemia

kaliuresis

kallikrein

Kallmann's syndrome

Kamerun swellings

K antigen

kaolin

Kaposi
 K's sarcoma
 K's sarcoma–associated
 herpesvirus

kappa (κ)
 k. chain
 k. chain marker
 k. light chains

karyotype
 chromosome k.
 XO k.

Katayama
 K. disease
 K. fever

Kayser-Fleischer ring

K cells

κ chain

Kd
 dissociation constant

kD
 kilodalton

Ke (*antigenic marker*)

158

Kearns-Sayre syndrome

Kedani fever

keloidal blastomycosis

Kemerovo virus

Kenny treatment

Kenya tick typhus

keratinization

keratinocyte

keratitis
 anaphylactic k.

keratoconjunctivitis

keratomycosis
 k. nigricans

keratopathy
 hypercalcemic k.

keratosis

Kern

kernicterus

ketoacidosis
 diabetic k.

Keto-Diastix

ketogenesis

ketohydroxyestrin

ketone

ketonemia

ketonuria

ketosis
 k.-prone diabetes mellitus
 k.-resistant diabetes mellitus

ketosteroid
 17-k.

ketotic hypoglycemia

Kew Gardens spotted fever

kidney
- k. disease
- k. failure
- k. function
- myeloma k.
- k. stone
- k. transplantation

killed vaccine

killer
- k. cells
- k. inhibitory receptors (KIR)
- k. T cells

kilodalton (kD)

kinase
- Blk k.
- Bruton's tyrosine k. (Btk)
- calmodulin-dependent multiprotein k.
- DNA-dependent k.
- Fyn k.
- JAK3 k.
- Janus k.
- Janus family of k's (JAK)
- Lck k.
- Lyn k.
- P1 k.
- phosphotyrosine k.
- protein k.
- rhodopsin k.
- Syk k.
- thymidine k.
- tyrosine k.
- ZAP-70 k.

kinetic
- k. diffusion test
- k. technique

kinetochore

kinetoplast

Kingella
- *K. kingae*

kinin
- k. activation
- k. system

Kinkiang fever

KIR
- killer inhibitory receptors

Kirsten murine sarcoma virus

kissing disease

Klebsiella
- *K. friedländeri*
- *K. oxytoca*
- *K. ozaenae*
- *K. pneumoniae*
- *K. pneumoniae ozaenae*
- *K. pneumoniae rhinoscleromatis*
- *K. rhinoscleromatis*
- *K. terrigena*

Kleihauer-Betke test

Kleinschmidt technique

Klinefelter's syndrome

Kluyvera

Km
- kappa chain marker
  - Km allotypes
  - Km antigens

Knies' sign

knockout
- k. animal
- gene k.
- k. mouse

Kober test

Koch
- K's law
- K. phenomenon
- K. postulates

Kocher
- K's sign
- K.-Debré-Sémélaigne syndrome

Koongol virus

Koplik
- K's sign

Koplik *(continued)*
  K's spots

Korean
  K. hemorrhagic fever
  K. hemorrhagic fever virus
  K. hemorrhagic nephroso-
    nephritis

Korin fever

Krabbe disease

K-*ras* oncogene

Ku antibody

Kumba virus

Kumlinge virus

Kunjin virus

Kupffer's cell

kuru

Kussmaul's coma

Kveim
  K. antigen
  K. test

K virus

kwashiorkor

Kyasanur Forest
  K. F. disease
  K. F. disease virus

kyphosis
  dorsal k.

L
    L cells
    L form
    light
        L chain

L+
    limes tod
        L+ dose

L0
    limes nul
        L0 dose

L3T4

La
    La antigen
    La protein

label
    fluorescent l's

labeling
    affinity l. of receptors
    photoaffinity l.
    TdT-dependent dUPT-bio-
        tin nick end l. (TUNEL)

labia (*plural of* labium)

labiomycosis

labium *pl.* labia
    labia majora
    labia minora

laboratory error

lacrimal gland

La Crosse virus

lactate

lactation
    l.-associated infertility
    l. failure
    l. hormone
    l. induction

lactic acidosis

lactoferrin

lactogen
    human placental l. (hPL)
    placental l. function
    l. production

lactogenic
    l. hormone

lactosuria
    postpartum l.

lactotrope
    l. adenoma
    l. cell

lactotroph
    l. adenoma
    l. cell

lactotrophic

lactotrophin

lactotropic
    l. cell

lactotropin

Laënnec's cirrhosis

lagophthalmos

lag period

LAK
    lymphokine-activated killer
        LAK cell

laked

Lalouette's pyramid

lambda (λ)
    l. chain
    l. group light chains
    l. light chains
    l. monoclonal light chains

lambliasis

lambliosis
    lamellar bone

lamina propria

Laminaria

laminarin

laminate induration

Lancereaux-Mathieu disease

Landouzy's disease

Langerhans
L's cell (LC)
L's cell histiocytosis

Landry's paralysis

langerhansian adenoma

Lansing virus

LAP
leukocyte adhesion protein

lapinization

lapinize

La protein

large
l. cleaved cell
l. granular lymphocyte (LGL)
l. granule cells
l. lymphocyte
l. noncleaved cell
l. pre-B cell
l. uncleaved cell

larva pl. larvae
l. currens
cutaneous l. migrans
l. migrans
ocular l. migrans
visceral l. migrans

Laron
L. dwarf
L. dwarfism
L. syndrome
L.-type dwarfism

larva migrans

laryngeal
l. cancer
l. carcinoma
l. diphtheria

laryngeal (continued)
l. tuberculosis

laryngitis
diphtheritic l.
tuberculous l.

laryngophthisis

laryngotracheal diphtheria

larynx

laser
flow cell cytometry l.
YAG-type l.

Lassa
L. fever
L. virus

late
l. benign syphilis
l. latent syphilis
l.-onset osteopetrosis
l. phase reaction
l. pro-B cell
l. rejection
l. syphilis

latency
l. period
l. phase
l. stage

latent
l. allergy
l. cytomegalovirus
l. diabetes
early l. syphilis
l. infection
late l. syphilis
l. period
l. syphilis
l. typhus
l. virus

lateral hermaphroditism

latex
l. agglutination
l. agglutination test
l. bead ingestion
l. fixation

latex *(continued)*
    l. fixation test

LATS
    long-acting thyroid stimula-
        tor
            LATS protector

lattice
    l. formation
    l. hypothesis

laugh
    canine l.
    sardonic l.

Launois' syndrome

Laurell technique

Laurence-Moon-Bardet-Biedl
    syndrome

LAV
    lymphadenopathy virus

law
    Behring's l.
    Godélier's l.
    Golgi's l.
    Koch's l.
    Louis' l.

lawn plate

Lawrence
    L's transfer factor
    L.-type dialyzable transfer
        factor

layer
    mucopolysaccharide-tei-
        choic acid l. (*of Staphylo-
        coccus aureus cell wall*)

lazaretto

lazy
    l. pituitary
    l. leukocyte syndrome

LC
    Langerhans' cell

LCA
    leukocyte common anti-
        gens

LCAT
    lecithin–cholesterol acyl-
        transferase

L cells

L (light) chain

Lck
    Lck kinase

LCL bodies

LCM
    lymphocytic choriomenin-
        gitis
            LCM virus

LCMV
    lymphocytic choriomenin-
        gitis virus

LCMV-LASV complex

LD
    lymphocyte-defined
        LD antigens

LDL
    low-density lipoprotein

LE
    lupus erythematosus
        LE cell
        LE factor

lead
    l. intoxication
    l. poisoning

leader
    l. peptide
    l. sequence

leak
    phosphate l.

LECAM

lecithin–cholesterol acyltrans-
    ferase (LCAT)

lectin
    mannan-binding l. (MBL)
    l. pathway

Lecythophora

Legionella
- *L. bozemanii*
- *L. dumoffii*
- *L. feeleii*
- *L. gormanii*
- *L. jordanis*
- *L. long-beachae*
- *L. micdadei*
- *L. pittsburgensis*
- *L. pneumophila*
- *L. wadsworthii*

legionellosis

legionnaires' disease

Leiner's disease

Leishman's chrome cells

Leishmania
- *L. major*

leishmaniasis

leishmanin
- l. test

length
- amplification fragment l.
- restriction fragment l.

Lente insulin

Lentivirinae

Lentivirus

lentivirus

Leon virus

lepra reaction

leprechaunism

lepromatous leprosy

lepromin
- l. reaction
- l. test

leprosy
- lepromatous l.
- tuberculoid l.

leptin

Leptospira

leptospiral jaundice

leptospirosis
- anicteric l.
- benign l.
- l. icterohaemorrhagica

leptospiruria

leptothricosis

leptotrichosis

Lesch-Nyhan syndrome

lesion
- Councilman's l.
- granulomatous l.
- macular l.
- parenchymal l.
- renal vascular l.
- ulcerative l.
- vascular l's

lesser pancreas

lethal
- l. gene

lethargy

leucine
- l. incorporation
- l.-induced hypoglycemia
- oral l. test
- l. test

leu-enkephalin

leukemia
- acute lymphoblastic l.
  (ALL)
- acute lymphocytic l. (ALL)
- l. cells
- chronic lymphocytic l.
  (CLL)
- hairy cell l.
- l. inhibitory factor
- lymphatic l.
- non-T, non-B acute lym-
  phoblastic l.
- pre-B cell l.

leukemia *(continued)*
  l. virus
  virus-induced l.

leukemic reticuloendotheliosis

leukemogenesis

leukin

leukoagglutinin

leukocidin

leukocyte
  l. adherence inhibition
    technique
  l. adhesion deficiency
  l. adhesion protein (LAP)
  l. agglutinin
  agranular l.
  l. common antigens (LCA)
  l. count
  l. culture antigens
  l. diapedesis
  l. extravasation
  l. function–associated anti-
    gen (LFA) (1–3)
  l. inhibitory factor (LIF)
  l. integrins
  l. interferon
  neutrophilic polymorpho-
    nuclear l's
  passenger l.
  polymorphonuclear l.
  polymorphonuclear neutro-
    philic l.
  l. recruitment
  l. typing serum

leukocytic
  l. pyrogen

leukocytoclastic
  l. angiitis
  l. vasculitis

leukocytolysin

leukocytophagy

leukocytosis

leukocytotoxicity

leukodystrophy
  metachromatic l.

leukoencephalopathy

leukokinin

leukolysin

leukopenia

leukophagocytosis

leukoprecipitin

leukotactic factor

leukotaxin

leukothrombin

leukotoxic

leukotoxicity

leukotoxin

leukotriene

leukovirus

leu-M1 antigen

level
  androgen plasma l's
  calcium l.
  electrolyte l's
  glucose l.
  immunoglobulin l's
  insulin l's
  phosphorus plasma l.
  plasma calcitonin l's
  thyroid-stimulating hor-
    mone l.
  thyroxine (T_4) l.

Lévi
  L.-Lorain dwarf
  L.-Lorain dwarfism
  L.-Lorain infantilism

Levinthal-Coles-Lillie bodies

levodopa

levothyroxine sodium

Lewis
  L. antigen

Lewis *(continued)*
    L's phenomenon

Leydig cell
    L. c. agenesis
    L. c. failure
    L. c. hypoplasia
    L. c. tumor

Lf
    limes flocculating
        Lf dose
        Lf unit

LFA
    leukocyte function–associ-
        ated antigen
            LFA-1
            LFA-2
    lymphocyte function–asso-
        ciated antigen
            LFA-1
            LFA-2
            LFA-3

L form

LH
    luteinizing hormone

LHRH
    luteinizing hormone–
        releasing hormone

Liacopoulos phenomenon

libido

library
    phage display l.

lichen
    l. amyloidosis
    cutaneous l. amyloidosis

Liddle sign

LIF
    leukocyte inhibitory factor

lifelong obesity

ligand
    altered peptide l's
    l. assay
    c-kit l.

ligand *(continued)*
    Fas l.
    heterogeneous l. assay

ligase

light
    l. cells
    ultraviolet l. (UV)

light (L) chain
    light chain disease
    kappa (κ) light chains
    lambda (λ) light chains
    lambda (λ) group light
        chains
    lambda (λ) monoclonal
        light chains
    light chain nephropathy
    light chain–related amyloi-
        dosis
    surrogate light chains

ligneous
    l. struma
    l. thyroiditis

limbic encephalitis

Liley chart

limes
    l. flocculating
    l. nul
    l. nul dose
    l. reacting
    l. tod
    l. zero dose

limit
    permissible exposure l.

limiting dilution assay

line
    adrenal l.
    cell l's
    cloned T cell l.
    embryonic stem cell l's
    Jurkat T cell l.
    Pastia's l's
    precipitin l.
    Sergent's white adrenal l.
    T cell l's

line *(continued)*
    white adrenal l.

lineage
    hematopoietic l.

linear
    l. determinants
    l. epitope

lingual
    l. goiter
    l. thyroid

linguatuliasis

linguatulosis

linkage
    l. disequilibrium

linked recognition

liothyronine
    l. euthyroidism
    l. I 125
    l. toxicosis

lipase
    lipoprotein l. (LPL)

lipemia
    carbohydrate-induced l.
    diabetic l.
    endogenous l.

lipid
    l. A
    l.-lowering drugs
    l. mediators
    l. metabolism
    serum l.

lipoadenoma

lipoatrophy

lipocortin

lipodystrophy

lipoid adrenal hyperplasia

lipolysis

lipolytic hormones

lipoma

lipomodulin

lipopolysaccharide (LPS)
    l.-binding protein

lipoprotein
    high-density l. (HDL)
    l. lipase (LPL)
    low-density l. (LDL)
    very-low-density l. (VLDL)

liposome

lipotroph

lipotropic hormone (LPH)

lipotropin
    β-l.

lipovaccine

lipoxin

lipoxygenase
    l. pathway

Lipschütz bodies

listerellosis

Listeria
    L. monocytogenes

listeriosis

lithiasis
    renal l.

live
    l. attenuated vaccine
    natural l. vaccine
    l. vaccine

liver
    bronze l.
    l. damage
    l. disease
    l. dysfunction
    l. failure
    l. transplantation

living
    l. nonrelated donor transplantation
    l. related donor transplantation

living *(continued)*
l. unrelated donor transplantation

LMEF
lymphocyte migration–enhancing factor

LMF
lymphocyte mitogenic factor

LMIF
lymphocyte migration–inhibiting factor

LNPF
lymph node permeability factor

loaiasis

lobe
anterior l.
anterior l. of hypophysis
anterior l. of pituitary gland
posterior l.
pyramidal l.
pyramidal l. of thyroid gland
l. of thyroid gland

lobectomy
thyroid l.

Loboa

Lobo's disease

lobomycosis

lobule
l. of pancreas
thymic l.
l's of thyroid gland

lobulus *pl.* lobuli
lobuli glandulae thyroideae

lobus *pl.* lobi
l. anterior hypophyseos
l. glandulae thyroideae
l. glandularis hypophyseos

lobus *(continued)*
l. pyramidalis glandulae thyroideae

local
l. anaphylaxis
l. hormone
l. immunity
l. mediator

localization
microorganism l.
l. procedures

localized
l. fungus
l. infection
l. myeloma
l. viral infection

locus
cim l.
H-2 l.
minor lymphocyte stimulating loci
minor lymphocyte stimulatory loci
Mls loci
MLS loci

loiasis

Lone Star fever

long
l.-acting antiestrogen
l.-acting thyroid stimulator (LATS)
l.-incubation hepatitis
l. terminal redundancy
l. terminal repeat (LTR)
l. terminal repeat segments
l. terminal repeat sequences

longitudinal growth

loop
amplification l.
positive feedback l.

Lorain
L's disease

Lorain *(continued)*
  L's infantilism
  L.-Lévi dwarf
  L.-Lévi dwarfism
  L.-Lévi syndrome

loss
  age-related bone l.
  bone l.

Lostorfer
  L's bodies
  L's corpuscles

Louis' law

Louis-Bar's syndrome

louping ill virus

louse-borne typhus

low
  l.-density lipoprotein (LDL)
  l.-dose dexamethasone suppression test
  l.-dose tolerance
  l.-frequency antigens
  l.-incidence antigens
  l. T$_3$ (triiodothyronine) syndrome
  l.-turnover osteomalacia
  l.-zone tolerance

LPH
  lipotropic hormone
    β-LPH

LPL
  lipoprotein lipase

LPS
  lipopolysaccharide

Lr
  limes reacting
    Lr dose

L-selectin

LT
  lymphotoxin

LTF
  lymphocyte-transforming
    factor

LTR
  long terminal repeat

L-tryptophan

lues

luetic

Lugol
  L's iodine
  L's iodine stain
  L's solution

luliberin

lumbricosis

lumen *pl.* lumina, lumens
  residual l.

lumina (*plural of* lumen)

luminescence

lung
  farmer's l.
  l. disease
  l. failure
  l. transplantation

lupus
  l. band test
  cutaneous l. erythematosus
  discoid l. erythematosus
  l. erythematosus
  l. erythematosus–like syndrome
  systemic l. erythematosus (SLE)

luteal hormone

luteal
  l. hormone
  l. phase dysfunction

luteinization

luteinizing
  l. hormone (LH)
  l. hormone–releasing hormone (LHRH)

luteolysis

luteotropic
  l. hormone

luteotropin

lutropin

Lutz-Splendore-Almeida disease

Ly
  Ly 6
  Ly 6 molecule
  Ly 49
  Ly antigens

17,20-lyase deficiency

Lyb antigens

Lyme
  L. arthritis
  L. borreliosis
  L. carditis
  L. disease
  L. disease vaccine (recom-
    binant OspA)
  L. meningitis

LYMErix

lymph
  afferent l. vessels
  l. cell
  efferent l. vessels
  l. follicles
  l. node
  l. node permeability factor
    (LNPF)
  l. vessels

lymphadenitis
  regional l.
  tuberculoid l.
  tuberculous l.

lymphadenoid
  l. goiter

lymphadenopathy
  angioimmunoblastic l.
  angioimmunoblastic l. with
    dysproteinemia (AILD)
  l.-associated virus
  immunoblastic l.

lymphadenopathy *(continued)*
  l. syndrome
  tuberculous l.
  l. virus (LAV)

lymphapheresis

lymphatic
  l. leukemia
  l. spaces
  l. system
  l. vessels

lymphatolytic
  l. serum

lymphoblast
  B l.

lymphoblastic

lymphocerastism

Lymphocryptovirus

lymphocytapheresis

lymphocyte
  activated l.
  activated B l.
  l.-activating factor
  l. activation
  amplifier T l.
  l. antigen receptors
  antigen-specific B l's
  antigen-specific T l's
  l.-associated virus
  atypical (reactive) l's
  B l.
  l. blastogenic factor (BF)
  bystander B l's
  l. circulation
  l. count
  cytolytic T l.
  cytotoxic T l. (CTL)
  l.-defined (LD)
  l.-defined (LD) antigens
  l. function–associated anti-
    gen (LFA)
  l. function–associated anti-
    gen-3 (LFA-3)
  helper T l's

lymphocyte *(continued)*
  immature B l.
  l. immune globulin
  immunoglobulin-synthesiz-
    ing B l.
  l.-inherited deficiencies
  intraepidermal l.
  intraepithelial l.
  l. isolation
  large l.
  large granular l.
  l.-limiting dilution assay
  mature B l.
  l.-mediated reaction
  l. migration–enhancing fac-
    tor (LMEF)
  l. migration–inhibiting fac-
    tor (LMIF)
  l. mitogenic factor (LMF)
  naive l's
  natural killer l.
  peripheral blood l.
  plasmacytoid l.
  pre-B l.
  l. product
  l. proliferation
  l. proliferation assay
  l. proliferation test
  l.-promoting factor
  l. purification
  l. receptors
  l. recirculation
  l. repertoire
  sensitized l.
  sensitized T l.
  l. series
  small l.
  suppressor l.
  l. surface antigen
  l. surface marker
  l. surface receptor
  T l.
  thymus-dependent l.
  thymus-independent l.
  l. tolerance
  l. transformation
  l.-transforming factor (LTF)

lymphocyte *(continued)*
  tumor-infiltrating l. (TIL)
  variable l.

lymphocytic
  l. choriomeningitis (LCM)
  l. choriomeningitis virus
    (LCMV)
  l. hypophysitis
  l. series
  l. thyroiditis

lymphocytoblast

lymphocytoma

lymphocytopenia

lymphocytopheresis

lymphocytopoiesis

lymphocytopoietic

lymphocytorrhexis

lymphocytosis
  acute infectious l.
  relative l.

lymphocytotic

lymphocytotoxicity

lymphocytotoxin

lymphogranuloma
  l. inguinale
  l. venereum
  l. venereum skin test

lymphogranulomatosis
  l. inguinalis

lymphohistiocytic

lymphohistiocytosis
  erythrophagocytic l.
  hemophagocytic l.

lymphohistioplasmacytic

lymphoid
  l. cells
  l. follicles
  l. hypertrophy
  l. organs

lymphoid *(continued)*
l. progenitor
secondary l. tissue
l. stem cell
l. system
l. thyroiditis
l. tissue

lymphokentric

lymphokine
l.-activated killer (LAK)
l.-activated killer cell (LAK cell)

lympholysis
cell-mediated l. (CML)

lympholytic

lymphoma
B cell l.
Burkitt's l.
cutaneous l.
cutaneous T cell l.
follicular center cell l.
Hodgkin's l.
Mediterranean l.
non-Hodgkin's l.
T cell l.
thyroid l.
virus-induced l.

lymphopathia
l. venerea

lymphopenia

lymphopenic
l. dysgammaglobulinemia
l. immunologic deficiency

lymphoplasmapheresis

lymphopoiesis

lymphopoietic

lymphopoietin-1

lymphoproliferative
l. disease
l. disorder
l. syndrome

lymphoreticular
l. system
l. tissue
l. tissue graft

lymphoreticulosis
benign l.

lymphorrhoid

lymphosarcoma

lymphotactin

lymphotaxis

lymphotoxin (LT)

lymphotropic
l. papovavirus

Lyn kinase

Lyon hypothesis

lypressin

lysate
staphylococcal bacterio-phage l.

lyse

lysin
beta l.

lysine vasopressin

lysinogen

lysis
bystander l.
hot-cold l.
reactive l.

lysogen

lysogenesis

lysogenic
l. bacterium

lysogenicity

lysogeny

lysosomal enzyme

lysozyme
hen egg-white l. (HEL)

lysozyme *(continued)*
    partridge l.
    turkey l.
    phagocyte l.

lyssa
    l. bodies

Lyssavirus

lyssic

lyssoid

lysylbradykinin

Lyt
    Lyt antigens
    Lyt marker

lytic
    l. pathway
    l. virus

M

M
- M antigen
- M cells
- M component
- M protein
- M-25 virus

μ
- μ heavy chain
- μ heavy chain disease

MAb
- monoclonal antibody

MAC
- membrane attack complex
- *Mycobacterium avium* complex
  - MAC disease

Mac-1
- Mac-1 antigen
- glycoprotein Mac-1

McArdle's disease

McCune-Albright syndrome

Machado
- M. reaction
- M. test
- M.-Guerreiro reaction
- M.-Guerreiro test

Machupo virus

macroadenoma

macrofollicular
- m. adenoma

macrogenitosomia
- m. praecox

macroglobulin
- alpha m.
- alpha$_2$-m.

macroglobulinemia
- Waldenström's m.

macrolymphocyte

macromastia

macromonocyte

macronodular hyperplasia

macro-orchidism

macrophage
- activated m.
- m.-activating factor
- m. activation
- m. aggregating factor
- alveolar m's
- armed m's
- m. chemoattractant and activating factor/protein (MCAF)
- m. chemotactic factor
- m. colony-stimulating factor (M-CSF)
- m. cytokines
- dermal m.
- fixed m.
- free m.
- m. growth factor
- inflammatory m.
- m. inhibitory factor
- m. integrins
- m. intracellular pathogens
- m. migration inhibitory factor
- m. pinocytotic activity
- m. progenitors
- m. recruitment
- resident m.
- surface m.
- m. system
- thymic m.
- tingible body m.
- tumor-associated m.

macrophagocyte

macroprolactinoma

macrosomatia
- m. adiposa congenita

macrosomia
- fetal m.
- neonatal m.

macrotechnique
- Rantz and Randall m.

macrovascular disease

macula *pl.* maculae
    m. gonorrhoeica
    Saenger's m.

macular
    m. lesion

maculopapular

mad

MadCAM-1
    mucosal addressin cell adhesion molecule

madness
    myxedema m.

Madonna fingers

Madura foot

maduromycosis

maedi/visna virus

MAF
    macrophage-activating factor

MAGE-1 gene (melanoma antigen gene)

magnesium

magnicellular
    m. neurons
    m. nuclei

Majocchi's granuloma

major
    m. agglutinin
    m. basic protein (MBP)
    m. histocompatibility antigens
    m. histocompatibility complex (MHC)

Makonde virus

mal
    m. morado

malabsorption
    m. syndrome

malaise

malaria

malarial
    m. pigment
    m. stippling

male
    m. climacteric
    m. feminization
    m. homosexuality
    m. hypogonadism
    m. infertility
    m. intersex
    m. pattern baldness
    m. pseudohermaphrodism
    m. pseudohermaphrodite
    m. pseudohermaphroditism
    m. puberty
    m. reproduction
    m. sex hormone

malic enzyme

malignancy

malignant
    m. hypertension
    m. melanoma
    m. pheochromocytoma
    m. Swiss-type agammaglobulinemia
    m. tumor

mallein
    m. test

malnutrition
    m.-related diabetes mellitus

MALT
    mucosa-associated lymphoid tissue
    mucosal-associated lymphoid tissue

Malta fever

M-aminobenzene sulphate

mammalian
    m. adenoviruses

mammalian *(continued)*
    m. type C retroviruses

mammatroph

mammogen

mammoplasia
    benign infantile m.

mammosomatotrope

mammosomatotroph
    m. adenoma

mammotroph

mammotrophic

mammotropic

mammotropin

management
    dietary m.
    psychological m.
    waste m.

Manchurian typhus

Mancini test

manifestation
    gastrointestinal m's
    headache m. of pituitary
        tumor
    XYY clinical m's

manipulation
    endocrine m.
    hormonal m.

Mann's sign

mannan-binding lectin (MBL)

mannose
    m.-binding protein
    m. receptor

Manson
    M's disease
    M's hemoptysis
    M's schistosomiasis

mansonelliasis

mansonellosis

M antigen

mantle zone

Mantoux test

MAO
    monoamine oxidase
    MAO inhibitor

maple syrup urine disease

marasmus

marble bone disease

Marburg
    M. disease
    M. hemorrhagic fever
    M. virus
    M. virus disease

Marfan
    M's sign
    M's syndrome

margin
    inferior m. of suprarenal
        gland
    medial m. of adrenal gland
    medial m. of suprarenal
        gland
    superior m. of adrenal
        gland
    superior m. of suprarenal
        gland

marginal zone

margination

margo *pl.* margines
    m. anterior corporis pan-
        creatis
    m. inferior corporis pan-
        creatis
    m. medialis glandulae su-
        prarenalis
    m. posterior corporis pan-
        creatis
    m. superior corporis pan-
        creatis
    m. superior glandulae su-
        prarenalis

Marie
    M's disease

Marie *(continued)*
   M's sign

marijuana

marker
   allotypic m's
   alpha chain m. (Am)
   Am m.
   CD m.
   cell m.
   cell-surface m.
   gamma chain m. (Gm)
   genetic m's
   lymphocyte surface m.
   Lyt m.
   surface m.
   thymocyte-specific sur-
     face m.
   tumor m's

Maroteaux-Lamy syndrome

marrow
   bone m.

Marseilles fever

Marsh's disease

MART
   MART-1

masculine

masculinity

masculinization

masculinize

masculinizing

masked
   m. hyperthyroidism
   m. virus

masking
   m. of antigens

mas oncogene

mass
   m. action hypothesis
   m. infection
   sellar m.
   skeletal m.

Mastadenovirus

mastalgia

mast cell

mastitis

mastocytosis
   cutaneous m.

matching
   cross m.
   tissue m.

material
   cross-reacting m. (CRM)
   infectious m.

maternal
   m. age
   m. androgen
   m. antibody
   m. behavior
   m. deprivation syndrome
   m. diabetes
   m. homologous antibodies
   m. immunity

matrix
   m. GLA protein
   implantable m.
   noncollagen organic m.
   nuclear m.
   organic m.
   m. protein

maturation
   affinity m.
   m. index

maturational arrest

mature
   m. B cells
   m. T cells
   m. thymocyte

maturity
   m.-onset diabetes mellitus
   m.-onset diabetes of youth

Maurer
   M's clefts

Maurer *(continued)*
    M's dots
    M's spots
    M's stippling

Mauriac syndrome

maximum tolerated dose

Mayaro virus

MBL
    mannan-binding lectin

MBP
    major basic protein
    myelin basic protein

MCAF
    macrophage chemoattrac-
        tant and activating factor

M cells

MCF
    macrophage chemotactic
        factor

Mcg

M component

MCP
    membrane cofactor protein
    MCP-1
        monocyte chemotactic
            protein-1

M-CSF
    macrophage colony-stimu-
        lating factor

MDP
    muramyldipeptide

MEA
    multiple endocrine aden-
        omatosis
        familial MEA
        type I MEA
        type IIA MEA
        type IIB MEA

Mean's sign

measles
    atypical m.
    black m.
    Edmonston strain of m.
    German m.
    hemorrhagic m.
    m. immunization
    m.-like viruses
    Moraten strain of m.
    m., mumps, and rubella vi-
        rus vaccine live
    m. and mumps virus vac-
        cine live
    m. and rubella virus vac-
        cine live
    Schwartz strain of m.
    three-day m.
    m. vaccine
    m. vaccination
    m. virus
    m. virus vaccine live

measurement
    antibody m.
    skinfold m.
    virulence m.

mechanical vector

mechanism
    antimicrobial m.
    body temperature m.
    collision-coupling m.
    host defense m's
    innate resistance m's
    intrinsic coagulation m.
    rejection m's
    rejection effector m's
    renal countercurrent m's

Mechnikov *(variant of* Metchnikoff)

medial
    m. border of adrenal gland
    m. border of suprarenal
        gland
    m. margin of adrenal gland
    m. margin of suprarenal
        gland

median
  m. eminence
  m. strumectomy
  m. tissue culture infective
    dose

mediastinum

mediate contact

mediator
  m. cell
  inflammatory m's
  lipid m's
  local m.
  paracrine m's
  preformed m.
  soluble m.
  soluble protein m.

medical thyroidectomy

Medin's disease

Mediterranean
  M. fever
  M. lymphoma

medium
  contrast m.
  culture m.
  radiographic contrast me-
    dia
  Yssel's m.

medroxyprogesterone

medulla *pl.* medullae
  adrenal m.
  m. of adrenal gland
  m. glandulae suprarenalis
  ovarian m.
  suprarenal m.
  m. of suprarenal gland

medullary
  m. cancer
  m. carcinoma of thyroid
    gland
  m. chromaffinoma
  m. paraganglioma
  m. thyroid carcinoma

medulloadrenal

megacolon
  myxedema m.

megakaryocyte

megakaryocytic thrombocytopenic purpura

megasoma

meiosis

Meissner's plexus

melanin

melanocyte
  m.-stimulating hormone

melanoderma
  parasitic m.

melanoma
  m. antigen
  m. antigen gene
  malignant m.

melanophage

melanophore-stimulating hormone

melanotroph

melanotropin

melasma

melatonin

melioidosis

mellituria

membrane
  accidental m.
  apical plasma m.
  m. attack complex (MAC)
  m. attack complex inhibitor
  capillary basement m.
  cell m.
  m. cofactor protein (MCP)
  extraembryonic m's
  false m.

membrane *(continued)*
    glomerular basement m.
    m. immunoglobulin
    m. inhibitor
    m. inhibitor of reactive ly-
      sis (MIRL)
    mucous m.
    plasma m.
    presynaptic m.
    m. receptor
    m. transplant regulation
    tubular basement m.
    Volkmann's m.

membranous
    m. cells
    m. glomerulonephritis

memory
    m. B cells
    m. cells
    cytotoxic m.
    immunologic m.
    m. response
    T cell m.
    m. T cells

MEN
    multiple endocrine neopla-
      sia
        MEN 1
        MEN 2A
        MEN 2B

menarche
    delayed m.
    isolated m.
    premature m.

mendelian segregation

Mengo virus

meningeal
    m. anthrax
    m. plague

meningitis *pl.* meningitides
    aseptic m.
    eosinophilic m.
    Lyme m.
    plague m.

meningococcal polysaccharide
    vaccine

meningococcemia

meningococcin

meningococcosis

meningococcus

meningoencephalitis
    amebic m.
    eosinophilic m.
    primary amebic m.
    toxoplasmic m.

meningorecurrence

meningovascular
    m. neurosyphilis

menopausal
    m. ovary
    m. syndrome

menopause

menotropins

menses

menstrual
    m. cycle
    m. extraction
    m. irregularity

menstruation

6-mercaptopurine

merozoite

merthiolate

mesenchyma
    feminizing m.
    gonadal m.
    ovarian m.
    sex m.

mesenchyme

mesodermal

mesothelium

mesovarian fold

messenger
  anchored m's
  biochemical m.
  first m.
  peptide m's
  m. RNA (mRNA)
  second m.

metabolic
  m. acidosis
  m. clearance rate (MCR)
  m. control
  m. defects
  m. disorder
  m. indices
  m. inhibition test
  m. insufficiency
  m. myopathy

metabolism
  anaerobic m.
  androgen m.
  bone m.
  calcium m.
  carbohydrate m.
  estrogen m.
  hormone m.
  iodine m.
  lipid m.
  nucleic acid m.
  phosphate m.
  phosphorus m.
  protein m.
  purine m.
  pyrimidine m.
  water m.

metabolite
  arachidonic acid m's

metachromatic leukodystrophy

metagonimiasis

metainfective

meta isomer

metanephrine

metaplasia

metaraminol

metastasis

metastatic
  m. cancer
  m. disease
  m. orchitis
  osteoblastic m. disease
  m. tuberculous abscess

metazoa

metazoan disease

Metchnikoff (*spelled also* Mech-nikov)
  M's cellular immunity the-ory
  M's theory of antimicrobial immunity

met-enkephalin

methacholine challenge

methacrylate

method
  absorption m.
  double diffusion m.
  growth inhibition m.
  histochemical antibody m's
  immunologic contraceptive m's
  mucus m.
  Ouchterlony double diffu-sion m.
  separation m's
  symptothermal m. of natu-ral family planning
  m's for thyroid activity

methotrexate

methylation
  m. interference

α-methyldopa

methyltestosterone

methyltransferase
  phenylethanolamine *N*-m. (PNMT)

metyrapone test

Meuse fever

Mexican typhus

MG agglutinin

MGF
　　macrophage growth factor

MHA-TP
　　microhemagglutination as-
　　say–*Treponema pallidum*
　　(MHA-TP)

MHC
　　major histocompatibility
　　　complex
　　　　MHC class I molecules
　　　　MHC class IB genes/
　　　　　molecules
　　　　MHC class II compart-
　　　　　ment (MIIC)
　　　　MHC class II molecules
　　　　MHC class II transacti-
　　　　　vator (CIITA)
　　　　MHC class III genes
　　　　MHC congenic
　　　　MHC haplotype
　　　　MHC molecule
　　　　MHC mutant
　　　　MHC recombinant
　　　　MHC restricted
　　　　MHC restriction
　　　　Xenopus MHC

μ heavy chain disease

micelles

microabsorption

microadenectomy

microadenoma
　　prolactin-secreting m.

microadenomectomy

microbe

microbial
　　m. agents
　　m. antigens
　　m. test antigen
　　m. virulence factors

microbicidal activity

microcytotoxicity
　　m. assay

microencephaly

microenvironment
　　favorable m.
　　unfavorable m.

microfilaremia

microfilaria

microfollicular
　　m. adenoma

microgenitalism

microglia

microglial nodules

microglobulin
　　β_2-m.
　　beta$_2$-m.

micrograft

microhemagglutination assay–
　　Treponema pallidum (MHA-
　　TP)

micro-indirect immunofluores-
　　cence assay

micronodular dysplasia

microorganism
　　m. dissemination
　　m. localization
　　nonpathogenic m.
　　pathogenic m.
　　m. persistence

microphage

microphagocyte

microphallus

microplasia

microplate

Micropolyspora
　　M. faeni

microprecipitation
  m. test

microprolactinoma

microscope
  confocal fluorescent m.
  darkfield m.
  electron m.
  epi-illumination fluores-
    cence m.
  fluorescent m.
  transmitted light m.

microscopy
  darkfield m.
  fluorescent m.
  immunofluorescence m.

microsoma

microsomia

microsporidia

microsporidial

microsporidiosis

microsporosis
  m. nigra

Microsporum
  M. audouinii
  M. canis
  M. cookei
  M. felineum
  M. ferrugineum
  M. fulvum
  M. gallinae
  M. gypseum
  M. lanosum
  M. nanum
  M. persicolor
  M. vanbreuseghemii

microvascular disease

microxycyte

microxyphil

midcycle ovulation

middle
  m.-age spread

middle *(continued)*
  m. binders

midget

MIF
  migration-inhibiting factor
  migration inhibition factor
  migration inhibitory factor
    MIF test
  MSH-inhibitory factor

mIg
  membrane-bound immuno-
    globulin

migration
  m.-inhibiting factor
  m. inhibition
  m. inhibition factor
  m. inhibitory factor
  m. inhibitory factor test
  monocyte m.

MIIC
  class II MHC compartment

mild hypothyroidism

miliary
  m. tubercle
  m. tuberculosis

milk
  m.-alkali syndrome
  m. let-down reflex

milker
  m's nodes
  m's node virus
  m's nodules

milkpox

milzbrand

mimicry
  molecular m.

mineral
  m. balance
  m. salts

mineralization
  bone m.

mineralization *(continued)*
    m. of bones

mineralocorticoid
    urinary m.

miners' anemia

minor
    m. agglutinin
    m. H antigens
    m. histocompatibility antigens
    m. lymphocyte stimulating antigen
    m. lymphocyte stimulating gene
    m. lymphocyte stimulating loci
    m. lymphocyte stimulatory antigen
    m. lymphocyte stimulatory gene
    m. lymphocyte stimulatory loci

miracidium

Mirchamp's sign

MIRL
    membrane inhibitor of reactive lysis

MIT
    monoiodotyrosine

mite
    house dust m.
    m.-borne typhus

mitochondria

mitochondrial antibodies

mitogen
    B cell m's
    pokeweed m. (PWM)
    polyclonal m.

mitogenesis

mitogenic
    m. factor

mitosis

Mitsuda
    M. antigen
    M. reaction
    M. test

mixed
    m. agglutination reaction
    m.-cell adenoma
    m. chancre
    m. connective tissue disease
    m. gland
    m. gonadal dysgenesis
    m. hypoglycemia
    m. infection
    m. leukocyte reaction
    m. lymphocyte culture (MLC)
    m. lymphocyte culture assay
    m. lymphocyte culture test
    m. lymphocyte reaction
    m. somatotroph-lactotroph adenoma
    m. sore
    m. vaccine

MLC
    mixed lymphocyte culture
        MLC antigens
        MLC assay

Mls
    minor lymphocyte stimulating
        Mls antigen
        Mls gene
        Mls loci
    minor lymphocyte stimulatory

MLS
    minor lymphocyte stimulating
        MLS antigen
        MLS gene
        MLS loci
    minor lymphocyte stimulatory

MMR
measles, mumps, and ru-
bella virus vaccine live

MMTV
mouse mammary tumor vi-
rus
murine mammary tumor vi-
rus

MM virus

mobility
electrophoretic m.

mobilization in hypercalcemia

Möbius' sign (*spelled also* Moebius)

model
affinity m.
determinant selection m.
instructive m. of T cell development
Jacob-Monod m.
selection m.
stochastic m.
X. models for studying immunity

modeling
skeletal m.

modification
behavior m.
molecular m.
posttranslational m.

modified
m. antigen
m. smallpox

modifier
biological response m's

Modoc virus

modulation
antigenic m.

Moebius (*variant of* Möbius)

molecular
m. genetics

molecular (*continued*)
m. mimicry
m. modification
m. pathogenesis
m. probe hybridization
m. weight

molecule
accessory m's
adhesion m's
allogeneic MHC m's
CD m.
cell adhesion m. (CAM)
cell interaction (CI) m's
CI m's
class I MHC m's
class IB MHC m's
class II MHC m's
class III MHC m's
cytotoxic effector m's
DM m.
DO m.
effector m's
endothelial leukocyte adhesion m. (ELAM)
extracellular matrix m.
glycan-bearing cell adhe-
sion m.-1 (GlyCAM-1)
immune m.
immunoglobulin m.
immunoglobulin G1 m.
intercellular adhesion m.
(ICAM) (1 *and* 2)
Ly 6 m.
MHC (major histocompati-
bility complex) m's
mucosal addressin cell adhesion m.
surface m's
vascular cell adhesion m.
(VCAM)
vascular cell adhesion m. 1
(VCAM-1)
very late activation m's

Molisch
M's reaction
M's test

Molluscipoxvirus

molluscum contagiosum virus

Moloney
- M. reaction
- M. test
- M. virus

Monilia

monilial granuloma

moniliasis

moniliosis

monitoring
- rejection m.

monkeypox
- m. virus

monoamine oxidase (MAO)
- m. o. inhibitor (MAOI)

monoblast

monoclonal
- m. antibody (MAb)
- benign m. gammopathy
- m. gammopathies
- m. gammopathy type
- m. hypergammaglobuline-mias
- m. immunoglobulin
- m. immunoglobulin deposition disease
- m. immunoglobulinopa-thies
- m. populations
- m. protein

monocyte
- m. chemoattractants
- m. chemotactic factor
- m. chemotactic protein-1
- m. count
- m. function
- m. migration
- m. progenitors
- m. series
- surface m.

monocytic
- m. pyrogen

monocytic *(continued)*
- m. series

monocytoid

monocytolysis

monogen

monoinfection

monoiodotyrosine (MIT)

monokine

monomer

monomeric immunoglobulin

monomorphic epitope

mononeuropathy
- diabetic m.

mononuclear
- m. cell
- m. phagocyte
- m. phagocyte system (MPS)

mononucleosis
- cytomegalovirus m.
- infectious m.
- posttransfusion m.

monophage

monorecidive chancre

MonoSlide

monospecific antisera

monospecificity

Monospot test

Monosticon Dri-Dot

monovalent
- m. serum

mons pubis

Montana myotic leukoencepha-litis virus

Montenegro
- M. reaction

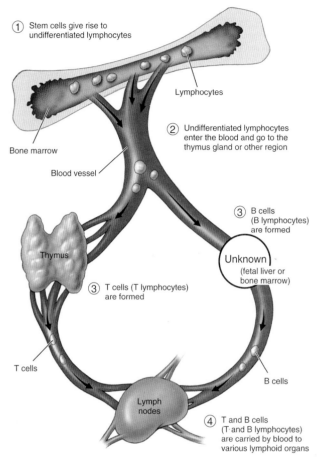

① Stem cells give rise to
undifferentiated lymphocytes

Lymphocytes

② Undifferentiated lymphocytes
enter the blood and go to the
thymus gland or other region

Bone marrow

Blood vessel

③ B cells
(B lymphocytes)
are formed

Thymus

Unknown
(fetal liver or
bone marrow)

③ T cells (T lymphocytes)
are formed

T cells

B cells

Lymph
nodes

④ T and B cells
(T and B lymphocytes)
are carried by blood to
various lymphoid organs

Formation of lymphocytes (T and B cells). (*1*) Stem cells give rise to undifferentiated lymphocytes in the bone marrow. (*2*) Undifferentiated lymphocytes leave the bone marrow by way of the blood. (*3*) Some lymphocytes travel to the thymus gland, where they mature and are transformed into T lymphocytes, or T cells. Some lymphocytes go to another part of the body, probably the fetal liver or bone marrow. Here they mature and become B lymphocytes, or B cells. (*4*) T and B cells travel to other lymphoid tissue, such as lymph nodes, where they live, work, and reproduce. (From Herlihy, B, Maebius, NK: The Human Body in Health and Illness. Philadelphia, W.B. Saunders Company, 2000.)

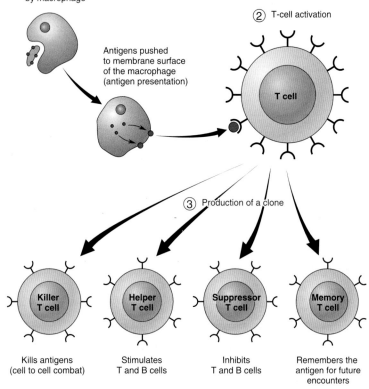

Cell-mediated immunity: T cell function. (*1*) The macrophage ingests the antigen (pathogen). The macrophage processes the antigen and pushes the antigen to its surface (antigen presentation). (*2*) The T cell is activated. (*3*) A clone is produced. The clone includes the four subgroups of the activated T cell: killer T cells, helper T cells, suppressor T cells, and memory T cells. (From Herlihy, B, Maebius, NK: The Human Body in Health and Illness. Philadelphia, W.B. Saunders Company, 2000.)

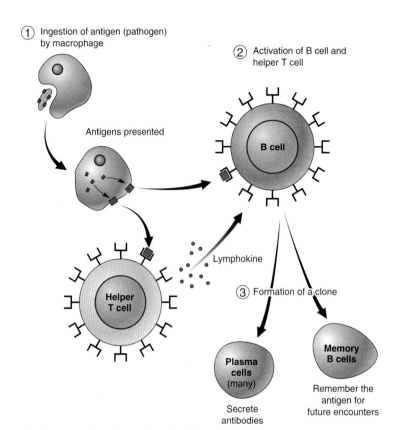

Antibody-mediated immunity: B cell function. (*1*) The macrophage ingests the antigen (pathogen). The macrophage processes the antigen and pushes it to the macrophage surface (antigen presentation). (*2*) Both B and helper T cells are activated. The helper T cell secretes a lymphokine, which further stimulates the B cell. (*3*) A clone is produced. The clone includes the two subgroups of the B cell: plasma cells and memory B cells. The function of each cell is identified. (From Herlihy, B, Maebius, NK: The Human Body in Health and Illness. Philadelphia, W.B. Saunders Company, 2000.)

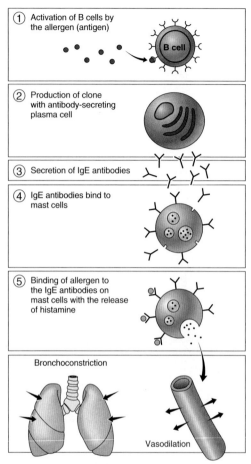

Immediate-reaction allergy (immediate hypersensitivity reaction). (*1*) An allergen (antigen) binds to the receptor on a B cell; this event activates the B cell. (*2*) The activated B cell produces a clone, including plasma cells. (*3*) The plasma cells secrete IgE antibodies. (*4*) The IgE antibodies bind mast cells. (*5*) When additional allergen is introduced, the allergen binds to the antibody on the mast cells. This process rebinds to the antibody on the mast cells. This process releases a dangerous amount of histamine into the blood. The lowest panel illustrates the effects of histamine. Histamine causes a narrowing of the respiratory passages. This narrowing, in turn, decreases the amount of air that can be inhaled and causes severe wheezing. Histamine also causes widespread dilation of the blood vessels and a severe drop in blood pressure. (From Herlihy, B, Maebius, NK: The Human Body in Health and Illness. Philadelphia, W.B. Saunders Company, 2000.)

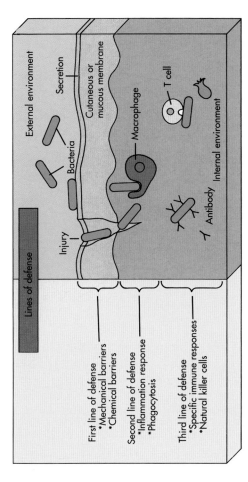

Lines of defense. Immune function, that is, defense of the internal environment against foreign cells, proteins, and viruses, includes three layers of protection. The first line of defense is a set of barriers between the internal and external environment; the second line of defense involves the nonspecific inflammatory response (including phagocytosis); and the third line of defense includes the specific immune responses and the nonspecific defense offered by NK cells. Of course, tumor cells that arise in the body are already past the first two lines of defense and must be attacked by the third line of defense. This diagram is a simplification of the complex function of the immune system; in reality, there is a great deal of crossover of mechanisms between these "lines of defense." (From Thibodeau, GA, Patton, KT: Anthony's Textbook of Anatomy & Physiology, 16th ed. St. Louis, Mosby, Inc., 1999.)

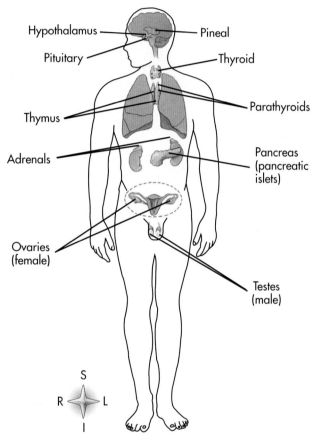

Locations of the major endocrine glands. (From Thibodeau, GA, Patton, KT: Anthony's Textbook of Anatomy & Physiology, 16th ed. St. Louis, Mosby, Inc., 1999.)

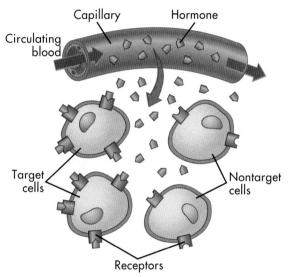

The target cell concept. A hormone acts only on cells that have receptors specific to that hormone because the shape of the receptor determines which hormone can react with it. This is an example of the lock-and-key model of biochemical reactions. (From Thibodeau, GA, Patton, KT: Anthony's Textbook of Anatomy & Physiology, 16th ed. St. Louis, Mosby, Inc., 1999.)

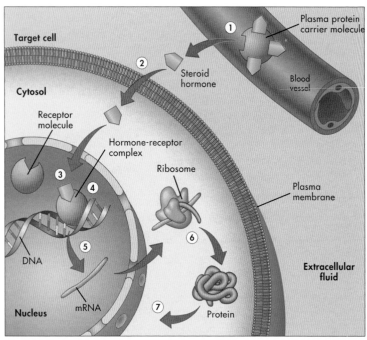

Steroid hormone mechanism. According to the mobile-receptor hypothesis, lipid-soluble steroid hormone molecules detach from a carrier protein (*1*) and pass through the plasma membrane (*2*). The hormone molecules then pass into the nucleus, where they bind with a mobile receptor to form a hormone-receptor complex (*3*). This complex then binds to a specific site on a DNA molecule (*4*), triggering transcription of the genetic information encoded there (*5*). The resulting mRNA molecule moves to the cytosol, where it associates with a ribosome, initiating synthesis of a new protein (*6*). This new protein—usually an enzyme or channel protein—produces specific effects in the target cell (*7*). (From Thibodeau, GA, Patton, KT: Anthony's Textbook of Anatomy & Physiology, 16th ed. St. Louis, Mosby, Inc., 1999.)

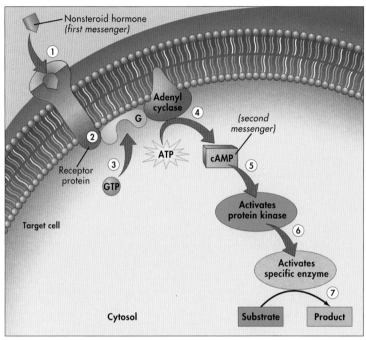

Example of a second-messenger mechanism. A nonsteroid hormone (*first messenger*) binds to a fixed receptor in the plasma membrane of the target cell (*1*). The hormone-receptor complex activates the G protein (*2*). The activated G protein reacts with GTP, which in turn activates the membrane-bound enzyme adenyl cyclase (*3*). Adenyl cyclase removes phosphate from ATP, converting it to cAMP (*second messenger*) (*4*). cAMP activates or inactivates protein kinases (*5*). Protein kinases activate specific cellular systems (*6*). These activated enzymes then influence specific cellular reactions, thus producing the target cell's response to the hormone (*7*). (From Thibodeau, GA, Patton, KT: Anthony's Textbook of Anatomy & Physiology, 16th ed. St. Louis, Mosby, Inc., 1999.)

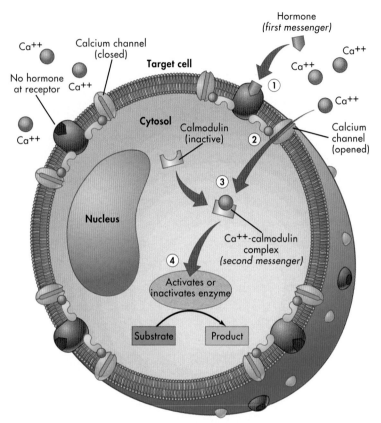

Calcium-calmodulin as a second messenger. In this example of a second-messenger mechanism, a nonsteroid hormone (*first messenger*) first binds to a fixed receptor in the plasma membrane (*1*), which activates membrane-bound proteins (G protein and PIP2) that trigger the opening of calcium channels (*2*). Calcium ions, which are normally at a higher concentration in the extracellular fluid, diffuse into the cell and bind to a calmodulin molecule (*3*). The Ca^{++}-calmodulin complex thus formed is a second messenger that binds to an enzyme to produce an allosteric effect that promotes or inhibits the enzyme's regulatory effect in the target cell (*4*). (From Thibodeau, GA, Patton, KT: Anthony's Textbook of Anatomy & Physiology, 16th ed. St. Louis, Mosby, Inc., 1999.)

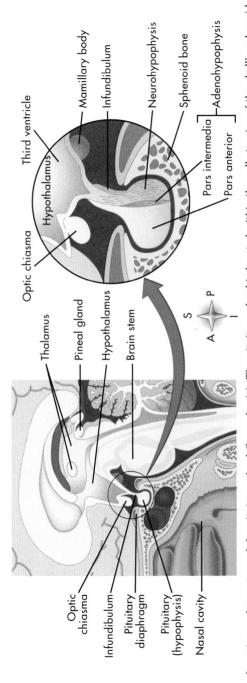

Location and structure of the pituitary gland (hypophysis). The pituitary gland is located within the sella turcica of the skull's sphenoid bone and is connected to the hypothalamus by a stalklike infundibulum. The infundibulum passes through a gap in the portion of the dura mater that covers the pituitary (the pituitary diaphragm). The *inset* shows that the pituitary is divided into an anterior portion, the adenohypophysis, and a posterior portion, the neurohypophysis. The adenohypophysis is further subdivided into the pars anterior and the pars intermedia. The pars intermedia is almost absent in the adult pituitary. (From Thibodeau, GA, Patton, KT: Anthony's Textbook of Anatomy & Physiology, 16th ed. St. Louis, Mosby, Inc., 1999.)

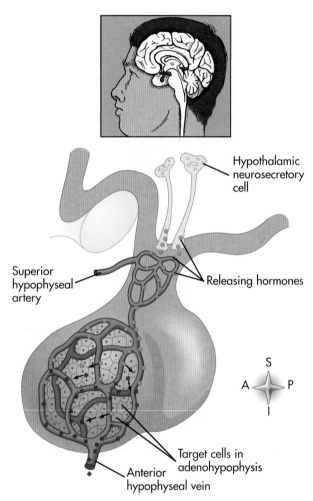

Hypophyseal portal system. Neurons in the hypothalamus secrete releasing hormones into veins that carry the releasing hormones directly to the vessels of the adenohypophysis, thus bypassing the normal circulatory route. (From Thibodeau, GA, Patton, KT: Anthony's Textbook of Anatomy & Physiology, 16th ed. St. Louis, Mosby, Inc., 1999.)

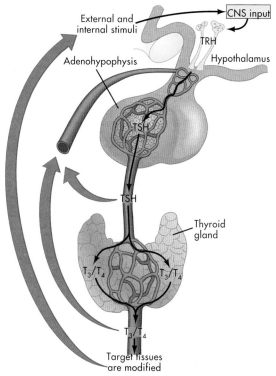

Negative feedback control by the hypothalamus. In this example, the secretion of thyroid hormone (T_3 and T_4) is regulated by a number of negative feedback loops. A long negative feedback loop (*thin line*) allows the CNS to influence hypothalamic secretion of thyrotropin-releasing hormone (*TRH*) by nervous feedback from the targets of T_3/T_4 (as well as from other nerve inputs). The secretion of TRH by the hypothalamus and thyroid-stimulating hormone (*TSH*) by the adenohypophysis is also influenced by shorter feedback loops (*thicker lines*), allowing great precision in the control of this system. (From Thibodeau, GA, Patton, KT: Anthony's Textbook of Anatomy & Physiology, 16th ed. St. Louis, Mosby, Inc., 1999.)

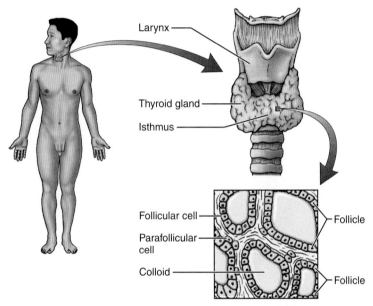

Larynx

Thyroid gland

Isthmus

Follicular cell

Parafollicular cell

Colloid

Follicle

Follicle

Thyroid gland. Location in the anterior neck, and the thyroid follicle. (From Herlihy, B, Maebius, NK: The Human Body in Health and Illness. Philadelphia, W.B. Saunders Company, 2000.)

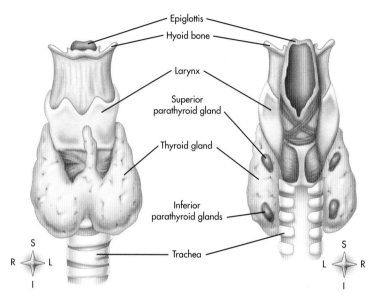

Thyroid and parathyroid glands. Note the relationships of the thyroid and parathyroid glands to each other, to the larynx, and to the trachea. (From Thibodeau, GA, Patton, KT: Anthony's Textbook of Anatomy & Physiology, 16th ed. St. Louis, Mosby, Inc., 1999.)

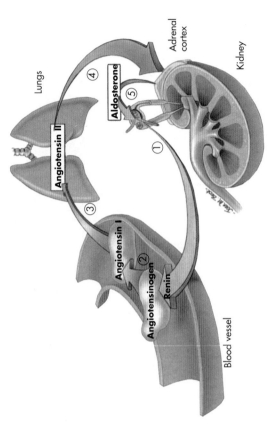

Renin-angiotensin mechanism for regulating aldosterone secretion. (*1*) When incoming blood pressure in the kidneys drops below a certain level, the juxtaglomerular apparatus secretes renin into the blood. (*2*) Renin causes angiotensinogen, a normal constituent of the blood, to be converted into angiotensin I. (*3*) Angiotensin I circulates to the lungs, where converting enzymes in the capillaries split the molecule, forming angiotensin II. (*4*) Angiotensin II circulates to the adrenal cortex, where it stimulates the secretion of aldosterone. (*5*) Aldosterone causes increased reabsorption, which causes increased water retention. As water is retained, the blood volume increases. The increased volume of blood creates higher blood pressure—which then causes the renin-angiotensin mechanism to stop. (From Thibodeau, GA, Patton, KT: Anthony's Textbook of Anatomy & Physiology, 16th ed. St. Louis, Mosby, Inc., 1999.)

Montenegro *(continued)*
    M. test

moon
    m. face
    m. facies
    m.-shaped face

Mooser bodies

Moraten
    M. measles virus vaccine
    M. strain *(of measles)*

Moraxella
    M. *(Branhamella) catar-*
        rhalis
    M. *(Moraxella) lacunata*

morbidity

morbilli

Morbillivirus

morbillous

Morganella
    M. morganii

morphine injector's septicemia

morphogenetic protein

morphologic correlation

morphological
    m. sex

Morquio syndrome

Morris syndrome

mortality

morula

morular cell

mosaicism
    chromosomal m.
    XO/XX m.
    XY/XXY m.

Moscow typhus

Mossman fever

mosquito

motheaten mutant mouse

motif
    antigen receptor activa-
        tion m. (ARAM)
    antigen recognition activa-
        tion m.
    immunoreceptor tyrosine-
        based activation m.
        (ITAM)
    sequence m.

motilin

motility

Mott cell

mountain tick fever

mouse
    athymic m.
    Biozzi m.
    congenic mice
    gene knockout m.
    inbred m.
    knockout m.
    m. mammary tumor virus
        (MMTV)
    motheaten mutant m.
    New Zealand black
        (NZB) m.
    nude m.
    NZB (New Zealand
        black) m.
    SCID (severe combined im-
        munodeficiency) m.
    syngeneic m.
    transgenic m.
    m. unit

mouth
    purse-string m.

M protein

MPS
    mononuclear phagocyte
        system

mRNA
    messenger RNA
        precursor mRNA (pre-
            mRNA)

MSA
　　multiplication-stimulating
　　activity

MSH
　　melanocyte-stimulating
　　hormone
　　　α MSH
　　　β MSH
　　　MSH-inhibitory factor
　　　(MIF)

MS-1 hepatitis

MS-2 hepatitis

MTD
　　maximum tolerated dose

mu
　　m. chain disease
　　m. heavy chain
　　m. heavy chain disease

MUC-1
　　mucin-1

Mucambo virus

Much's granules

mu chain disease

mucin
　　m.-1

mucinlike vascular addressins

mucinous
　　m. adenocarcinoma
　　m. carcinoma

mucocutaneous candidiasis

mucopolysaccharide
　　m.-teichoic acid
　　m.-teichoic acid layer (of
　　　Staphylococcus aureus cell
　　　wall)

mucopolysaccharidosis

Mucor
　　M. circinelloides
　　M. racemosissimus

mucormycosis
　　cerebral m.
　　rhinocerebral m.

mucosa
　　m.-associated lymphoid tis-
　　　sue (MALT)
　　buccal m.
　　respiratory m.
　　vaginal m.

mucosal
　　m. addressin cell adhesion
　　　molecule (MadCAM)
　　m.-associated lymphoid tis-
　　　sue (MALT)
　　m. disease virus
　　m. immune system
　　m. immunity
　　m. neuroma syndrome
　　m. surfaces
　　m. tissues

mucous
　　m. carcinoma
　　m. edema
　　m. membrane
　　m. patch

mucus
　　endocervical m.
　　m. method

mud fever

mu heavy chain disease

mulberry cell

müllerian
　　m. agenesis
　　m. ducts
　　m. duct cysts
　　m. duct inhibitory factor
　　m. inhibiting factor
　　m. inhibiting substance
　　m. regression factor
　　m. tract

multicolony stimulating factor
　　mCSF

multicontaminated

multiglandular

multi-infection

multilaminar vesicle

multilineage colony-stimulating factor

multinodular
m. goiter
m. toxic goiter

multinucleated cell

multiple
m. adenoma
m. endocrine adenomatosis (MEA)
m. endocrine deficiency syndrome
m. endocrine neoplasia (MEN) (types I, II, IIA, IIB, III)
m. glandular deficiency syndrome
m. hormone
m. hormone–secreting tumor
m. myeloma
m. organ failure
m. plasmacytoma of bone
m.-puncture test
m. sclerosis
m. stem cell (MSC)
m. system atrophy

multiplication
adenovirus m.
m.-stimulating activity

multipotent

multipotential stem cell

multisensitivity

multivalency

multivalent
m. antigen

multivesicular body

mumps
m. immunization

mumps *(continued)*
iodine m.
m. skin test
m. skin test antigen
m. vaccine
m. virus
m. virus vaccine live

muramyldipeptide
MDP

murine
m. hybridoma
m. mammary tumor virus (MMTV)
m. typhus

muromonab-CD3

Murray Valley encephalitis virus

muscle
m. atrophy
m. autoimmune disease
skeletal m.
smooth m.
striated m.
vascular smooth m.

muscular dystrophy
Duchenne m. d.

musculoskeletal system

mustard
phosphoramide m.

mutagenesis

mutant
MHC m.

mutation
clear plaque m.
nude m.
oncogenic m's
unc m.

M-25 virus

Mx protein

myalgia
epidemic m.

myasthenia gravis

myasthenic syndrome

mycethemia

mycetogenic

mycetogenous

mycetoma
    actinomycotic m.
    eumycotic m.

mycobacterial
    m. adjuvant

mycobacteriosis

Mycobacterium
    M. abscessus
    M. africanum
    M. aquae
    M. avium complex disease
    M. avium-intracellulare
    M. balnei
    M. borstelense
    M. bovis
    M. brunense
    M. buruli
    M. chelonae
    M. flavescens
    M. fortuitum
    M. gastri
    M. giae
    M. gordonae
    M. habana
    M. haemophilum
    M. intracellulare
    M. kansasii
    M. leprae
    M. lepraemurium
    M. littorale
    M. luciflavum
    M. malmoense
    M. marianum
    M. marinum
    M. microti
    M. minetti
    M. moelleri
    M. nonchromogenicum
    M. paraffinicum

Mycobacterium (continued)
    M. paratuberculosis
    M. phlei
    M. platypoecilus
    M. ranae
    M. scrofulaceum
    M. simiae
    M. smegmatis
    M. susceptibility
    M. szulgai
    M. terrae
    M. triviale
    M. tuberculosis
    M. tuberculosis
    M. tuberculosis var. *avium*
    M. tuberculosis var. *bovis*
    M. tuberculosis var. *hominis*
    M. tuberculosis var. *muris*
    M. ulcerans
    M. vaccae
    M. xenopi

Mycocentrospora
    M. acerina

mycohemia

mycology

mycophage

Mycoplasma
    M. gallisepticum
    M. hemagglutination inhibi-
        tion test
    M. hominis
    M. infection
    M. laidlawii
    M. mycoides
    M. pneumoniae
    M. replication
    M. serology
    M. vaccine

mycoplasma
    bacteria vs. m's

mycoplasmosis

mycosis
    m. fungoides
    Gilchrist's m.

mycosis *(continued)*
    Posadas' m.

mycotic

myc proto-oncogene

myelin
    m. basic protein (MBP)
    m. sheath

myelinolysis
    central pontine m.

myelitis

myelocytoma

myeloid
    m. cells
    m. progenitors

myelolipoma

myeloma
    m. cell
    m. clone
    indolent m.
    m. kidney
    localized m.
    multiple m.
    plasma cell m.
    m. protein (M protein)
    solitary m.

myelomatoid

myelomatosis

myelopathy
    chronic progressive m.
    diabetic m.
    HTLV-1–associated m.

myeloperoxidase
    m. deficiency

myelophage

myelopoiesis

myeloproliferative disease

myelosarcoma

myelosarcomatosis

myiasis
    creeping m.
    cutaneous m.
    cutaneous blowfly m.
    dermal m.
    intestinal m.
    m. linearis
    nasal m.
    traumatic m.

myiosis

myocardial infarction

myocarditis
    experimental autoim-
        mune m.

myocardium

myoma
    submucous m.

myopathy
    metabolic m.
    thyrotoxic m.

myophosphorylase deficiency
    glycogenosis

myosin

myositis
    m. ossificans progressiva
    trichinous m.

myotonia dystrophica

myotonic dystrophy

Myrothecium

myxedema
    circumscribed m.
    m. coma
    congenital m.
    m. heart
    m. ileus
    infantile m.
    m. madness
    m. megacolon
    nodular m.
    operative m.

myxedema *(continued)*
    pituitary m.
    pretibial m.
    primary m.
    secondary m.

myxedematoid

myxedematous
    m. cretinism
    m. infantilism

myxomatosis

myxovirus

N
  N protein
  N region

Na
  sodium

naegleriasis

nail
  Plummer's n.

Nairovirus

naive
  n. B cells
  n. cell
  n. lymphocytes
  n. T cells

naked virus

Nakiwogo virus

nanism
  pituitary n.

nanoid

nanosoma

nanosomia

nanous

nanukayami
  n. disease
  n. fever

nanus

NAP-2

narcosis
  carbon dioxide n.
  chronic carbon dioxide n.
  chronic CO_2 n.

narcotic
  n. analgesics
  n. opiates

nasal
  n. administration
  n. diphtheria
  n. myiasis

nasopharyngeal
  n. carcinoma
  n. diphtheria

National Commission for Clinical Laboratory Standards (NCCLS)

National Hemophilia Foundation

National Marrow Donor Program

native immunity

natural
  n. antibodies
  n. autoantibodies
  n. family planning
  n. immunity
  n. killer (NK)
  n. killer cells
  n. killer lymphocytes
  n. live vaccine
  n. resistance
  n. selection theory
  n. suppressor cells
  n. tolerance

nausea

NBT
  nitroblue tetrazolium
    NBT test

NCF
  neutrophil chemotactic factor

necatoriasis

necrobiosis lipoidica diabeticorum

necrosis *pl.* necroses
  avascular n.
  caseation n.
  fibrinoid n.
  focal n.
  postpartum pituitary n.
  septic n.
  syphilitic n.

necrosis *(continued)*
    tissue n.

necrotizing
    n. angiitis
    n. vasculitis

nef gene

negative
    n. anergy
    n. cooperativity
    n. phase
    n. selection
    n. staining

negatively regulated steroid response element

Negishi virus

Negri bodies

Neisser-Wechsberg phenomenon

Neisseria
    N. flavescens
    N. gonorrhoeae
    N. lactamica
    N. meningitidis
    N. mucosa
    N. subflava

Nelson's syndrome

nemathelminthiasis

nematization

nematode

nematodiasis

nematosis

neoantigen

neoarsphenamine

neogenesis
    T_3 (triiodothyronine) n.

neomembrane

neomycin
    n. resistance (*neor*) gene

neonatal
    n. bursectomy
    n. hyperparathyroidism
    n. hypoadrenocorticism
    n. hypoglycemia
    n. macrosomia
    n. septicemia
    n. thymectomy

neonatally-induced tolerance

neonate

neoplasia
    multiple endocrine n.
        (MEN) (*types I, II, IIA, IIB, III*)

neoplasm
    sex cord n.

neoplastic
    n. disease

neor (neomycin resistance)
    gene

neostigmine

nephelometric
    n. endpoint
    n. inhibition immunoassay

nephelometry

nephritic syndrome

nephritis
    Heymann's n.

nephritogenic

nephrocalcinosis

nephrogenic diabetes insipidus

nephrolithiasis

nephron

nephropathia
    n. epidemica

nephropathy
    analgesic n.
    autoimmune n.
    light chain n.

nephroplasty

nephrosis

nephrosonephritis
   hemorrhagic n.
   Korean hemorrhagic n.

nephrotic syndrome

nephrotoxic

nerve
   n. endings
   n. growth factor
   n. recordings
   nonmyelinated n.
   vagus n.

nervosa
   bulimia n.

nervousness

nervous system
   adrenergic n. s.
   aminergic n. s.
   autonomic n. s.
   central n. s.
   enteric n. s.
   peptidergic n. s.
   sympathetic n. s.

nesidiectomy

nesidioblast

nesidioblastoma

nesidioblastosis

network
   artificial neural n. (ANN)
   n. hypothesis
   idiotype–anti-idiotype n.
   idiotypic n.
   n. theory

Neudoerfl virus

neu oncogene

neural stalk

neuritis
   allergic n.
   cranial nerve n.
   experimental allergic n.

neuritis *(continued)*
   postfebrile n.

neuroamebiasis

neuroblast

neuroblastoma
   adrenal n.

neuroborreliosis

neurocysticercosis

neuroendocrine
   n. cells
   n. disease
   n. immunology
   n. integration
   n. system
   n. transducer

neuroendocrinology

neurofibromatosis

neurogenic hypogonadism

neuroglycopenia

neurohormonal
   n. cells

neurohormone

neurohumor

neurohypophysial
   n. hormones

neurohypophysis
   fetal n.

neuroimmunologic

neuroimmunology

neuroimmunomodulation

neuroleptic

neurologic
   n. cretinism
   n. sequelae

neurological disorders

neurolysin

neuromuscular disorders

neuron
    facilitator n.
    magnicellular n's
    peptidergic n.
    tuberohypophyseal n.

neuropathy
    autonomic n.
    diabetic n.
    diabetic cardiovascular n.
    peripheral n.
    sensory n.

neuropeptide
    n. Y

neurophysin

neuroprobasia

neuropsychiatric disease

neuroschistosomiasis

neurosecretion

neurosecretory
    n. cell
    n. fibers
    n. granule (NSG)

neurosteroid

neurosyphilis
    asymptomatic n.
    meningovascular n.
    parenchymatous n.
    paretic n.

neurotensin

neurotensinoma

neurotoxic cytokine

neurotoxin

neurotransmitter
    false n.

neurotripsy

neurotrophin

neurotropic virus

neurovaccine

neurovariola

neurovirus

neutral
    n. protamine Hagedorn in-
      sulin (NPH)
    n. regular insulin

neutralization
    antibody-mediated n.
    n. test
    toxin n.
    viral n.

neutralize

neutralizing antibody

neutron activation analysis

neutropenia
    acquired n.
    autoimmune n.
    inherited n.

neutrophil
    n. chemotactic factor
      (NCF)
    circulating n's
    n. count
    n. cytochrome deficiency
    n. dysfunction syndrome
    n. extravasation
    n. factor in cytokine ac-
      tions
    n. progenitors

neutrophilic polymorphonuclear leukocytes

newborn
    n. hemolytic disease
    n. infant
    n. pneumonitis virus

Newcastle
    N. disease
    N. disease virus

New Zealand black mouse

Nezelof syndrome

NFAT
  nuclear factor of activated
    T cells

NFIL-2A

N-formylmethionine

NGF
  nerve growth factor
    NGF β

niacin

nickel
  n. sensitivity

Nickerson-Kveim test

Nicolas-Favre disease

nicotine

nicotinic acid

NIDDM
  non–insulin-dependent dia-
    betes mellitus

Niemann-Pick disease

night sweat

nine-mile fever

Nipah virus

nitric oxide

nitroblue
  n. tetrazolium (NBT)
  n. tetrazolium dye reduc-
    tion
  n. tetrazolium test

nitrogen
  n. balance
  blood urea n. (BUN)

NK
  natural killer
    NK cells

N-nucleotides

Nocardia
  N. asteroides

Nocardia (continued)
  N. brasiliensis
  N. caviae
  N. coeliaca
  N. farcinica
  N. lutea
  N. madurae
  N. otitidis-caviarum

nocardiasis

Nocardiopsis

nocardiosis

nocturnal
  n. hemoglobinuria
  n. penile tumescence (NPT)

node
  Dürck's n's
  Heberden's n's
  iliac n's
  lymph n.
  milker's n's
  n's of Ranvier

nodular
  n. adrenal hyperplasia
  n. goiter
  n. myxedema
  n. sclerosis

nodule
  cold n.
  Fraenkel's n's
  hot n.
  microglial n's
  milker's n's
  rheumatic n's
  secondary n.
  thyroid n's
  typhoid n.
  typhus n's
  warm n.
  Wohlbach's n's

non-A–E hepatitis

nonamer

nonan

non-A, non-B hepatitis

non-A, non-B hepatitis virus

nonantigenic

non–beta cell tumor

noncleaved cell

noncollagen organic matrix

nondiabetic
n. glycosuria

nondisjunction

nonenveloped virus

nonenzymatic glycosylation

nonfunctional
n. adenoma
n. tumor

nonfunctioning
n. adenoma
n. tumor

nongoitrous
n. autoimmune thyroiditis

non-Hodgkin's lymphoma

nonhormonal therapy

nonhyperglycemic glycosuria

nonicteric

nonidentity

nonimmune precipitation

nonimmunogenic
n. polypeptide

noninfectious

non–insulin-dependent diabetes mellitus (NIDDM)

nonketotic hyperosmolar coma

nonlinear coupling

nonmyelinated nerve

non-oncogenic virus

non–organ-specific autoimmunity

nonosmotic pathway

nonparalytic poliomyelitis

nonpathogenic
n. autoantibodies
n. microorganism

nonphagocytic cell

nonpituitary
n. sellar mass

nonproductive rearrangement

nonreceptor hormone–binding protein

nonreplicative vaccine

nonresponder
immunization n's

nonseasonal
n. allergic rhinitis
n. hay fever
n. rhinitis

nonsecreting
n. adenoma

nonsecretory
n. adenoma

nonself

nonspecific
n. immunity
n. staining

nonsteroidal
n. antiinflammatory drug
n. contraceptive

nonsuppressible
n. insulinlike activity
n. insulinlike protein

nonsusceptibility

nonsymptomatic

non-T, non-B acute lymphoblastic leukemia

nontoxic goiter

nonvenereal syphilis

nonviral oncogene

Noonan's syndrome

Noon pollen unit

noradrenaline

noradrenergic
    n. pathway

norepinephrine (NE)

norethindrone

normal
    n. dwarf
    n. flora
    n. gigantism
    n. serum
    n. variation

normetanephrine

normocalcemia

normocrinic

normocytic normochromic anemia

normoglycemia

normoglycemic
    n. glycosuria

North American blastomycosis

North Asian tick typhus

Northern
    N. blot
    N. blot hybridization
    N. blot immunoassay
    N. blotting
    N. RNA transfer
    N. transfer

North Queensland tick typhus

Norwalk virus

Norwegian scabies

nosematosis

nosocomial
    n. infection

nosomycosis

nosoparasite

nosophyte

NO synthase
    inducible NO s. (iNOS)

notch
    pancreatic n.

notoedric

not-self

N protein

NPT
    nocturnal penile tumescence

NRC
    Nuclear Regulatory Commission

N region
    N r. diversification

NSG
    neurosecretory granule

nSRE
    negatively regulated steroid response element

nuclear
    n. antigens
    n. factor of activated T cells
    n. matrix
    n. proteins

Nuclear Regulatory Commission (NRC)

nuclei (*plural of* nucleus)

nucleic acid
    immunogenic n. a.
    infectious n. a.
    n. a. metabolism

nucleocapsid
    n. core factor

nucleoid

nucleophagocytosis

nucleoside phosphorylase deficiency

nucleosome

nucleotide
    N-n's

nucleus *pl.* nuclei
    droplet nuclei
    magnicellular n.
    paraventricular n. (PVN)
    SC n.
    subventricular n.
    suprachiasmatic (SC) n.
    supraoptic n. (SON)
    unstable n.

nude
    n. mouse
    n. mutation

null
    n. cells
    n.-cell adenoma

number
    triangulation n.

numerical classification

nurse cell

nutrition

nutritional gynecomastia

nux vomica

Nyando virus

nyctohemeral

NZB (New Zealand black) mouse

O
O agglutination
O agglutinin
O antigen (*of Salmonella typhi*)

OAF
osteoclast-activating factor

O agglutination

O agglutinin

Oakley
O.-Fulthorpe technique
O.-Fulthorpe test

O antigen

obesity
adult-onset o.
android o.
central o.
endogenous o.
exogenous o.
experimental o.
gynoid o.
hyperinsulinar o.
hypogonadal o.
hypothyroid o.
lifelong o.
peripheral o.
secondary o.
o. treatment

obstruction
intrarenal o.

obstructive sleep apnea syndrome

OC
oral contraceptive

occlusion hypothesis

octan

octopamine

ocular larva migrans

oculocraniosomatic
o. disease

oculocraniosomatic *(continued)*
o. muscular disease

oculomotor paresis

oesophagostomiasis

oestriasis

off-rate constants

OGTT
oral glucose tolerance test

Ohara's disease

OKT3 monoclonal antibody

oligo-adenylate synthetase

oligoclonal immunoglobulin

oligomenorrhea

oligonucleotide
o. probe hybridization

olympian brow

olympic brow

omental
o. eminence of body of pancreas
o. tuber of body of pancreas

Omsk
O. hemorrhagic fever
O. hemorrhagic fever virus

onchocerciasis

onchocercoma

onchocercosis

oncocytic adenoma

oncocytoma

oncofetal
o. antigen
o. proteins

oncogene
c-kit o.
o. cloning
dominant negative o.

201

oncogene *(continued)*
   erb-B o.
   jun o.
   K-*ras* o.
   mas o.
   neu o.
   nonviral o.
   proto-o.
   ras o.
   src o.
   viral o.

oncogenesis

oncogenic
   o. mutations
   o. viruses

oncologist

oncology

oncosphere

oncostatin M

oncovirus

on-rate constants

onychomycosis
   dermatophytic o.

o'nyong-nyong
   o. virus

oocyst

oocyte
   Xenopus o's

oogenesis

oophorectomy

oophoritis
   autoimmune o.

open tuberculosis

operative myxedema

ophthalmia
   sympathetic o.

ophthalmology

ophthalmopathy
   dysthyroid o.

ophthalmopathy *(continued)*
   Graves' o.
   infiltrative o.

opiate
   endogenous o.
   narcotic o's

Opie paradox

opioid
   adrenomedullary o.

opisthorchiasis

opisthorchosis

opportunistic
   o. fungus
   o. infection
   o. pathogen
   o. tumor

opsonic
   o. activity
   o. adherence
   o. index

opsonin
   immune o.

opsonization
   HIV o.

opsonize

opsonizing antibody

opsonocytophagic
   o. test

opsonophagocytosis

opsonophilia

opsonophilic

optic
   o. atrophy
   o. chiasm

optical immunoassay

optimal proportions

OPV
   poliovirus vaccine live oral

oral
   o. candidiasis

oral *(continued)*
    o. contraceptive (OC)
    o. glucose
    o. glucose tolerance test
    (OGTT)
    o. insulin
    o. leucine test
    o. tolerance

orangeophil

orbitopathy
    dysthyroid o.
    Graves' o.

Orbivirus

orbivirus

orchiectomy

orchiopexy

orchitis
    metastatic o.
    o. variolosa
    viral o.

organ
    central lymphoid o's
    circumventricular o's
    generative lymphoid o's
    o. growth
    lymphoid o's
    peripheral lymphoid o's
    periventricular o's
    o. of shock
    shock o.
    subcommissural o. (SCO)
    subfornical o. (SFO)
    target o.
    o. transplantation
    transplanted o.

organa *(plural of* organum)

organic matrix
    noncollagen o. m.

organification defect

organism
    pleuropneumonia-like o's
    unicellular o.

organization
    thymocyte o.

organotherapy

organotropism

organ-specific
    o.-s. antigen
    o.-s. autoantibodies
    o.-s. autoimmune disease
    o.-s. autoimmunity
    o.-s. disease

organum *pl.* organa
    o. subcommissurale
    o. subfornicale
    o. vasculosum of the lamina terminalis (OVLT)

orgasm

Oriental
    O. hemoptysis
    O. lung fluke disease
    O. ringworm
    O. schistosomiasis
    O. spotted fever

orificial tuberculosis

origin
    tumor o.

original antigenic sin phenomenon

Orimune

ornithine carbamyl transferase

ornithosis

oropharyngeal
    o. reflex
    o. tularemia

oropharynx

Oropouche virus

orosomucoid

Oroya fever

orphan
    o. receptor sequence

orphan *(continued)*
    o. viruses

orthoglycemic
    o. glycosuria

Orthohepadnavirus

Orthomyxoviridae

orthomyxovirus

orthophosphate

Orthopoxvirus

orthopoxvirus

Orthoreovirus

orthostatic hypotension

orthotopic
    o. transplantation

Orungo virus

osmolality
    serum o.
    urine o.

osmolarity

osmole
    idiogenic o.

osmoreceptor

osmotic
    o. diuresis
    o. homeostasis
    o. pathway
    o. regulation
    o. stimuli
    o. threshold

O-specific polysaccharide

ossification
    dystrophic o.
    eutrophic o.
    extraskeletal o.

osteitis
    o. deformans
    o. fibrosa cystica

osteoarthritis
    hypertrophic o.

osteoarthropathy
    pulmonary o.

osteoarthrosis

osteoblast

osteoblastic metastatic disease

osteocalcin

osteoclast
    o.-activating factor (OAF)

osteocyte

osteodystrophy
    Albright hereditary o.
    (AHO)
    renal o.
    uremic o.

osteoectasia

osteogenesis
    o. imperfecta tarda

osteohydatidosis

osteomalacia
    anticonvulsant-induced o.
    axial o.
    biochemically recogniza-
      ble o.
    hyperphosphatemic o.
    low-turnover o.
    tumor o.

osteomyelitis
    typhoid o.
    o. variolosa

osteonecrosis

osteonectin

osteopenia

osteopetrosis
    early-onset nonlethal o.
    infantile (lethal) o.
    late-onset o.

osteophyte
    vertebral o.

osteopontin

osteoporosis
    age-related o.
    juvenile o.
    postmenopausal o.
    primary o.
    o. prophylaxis
    secondary o.
    senile o.

osteoporotic
    o. pain

otiobiosis

otitis media

otobiosis

otodectic

Ouchterlony
    O. double diffusion method
    O. gel-diffusion assay
    O. quantitative precipitin
      reaction
    O. technique
    O. test

Oudin
    O. technique
    O. test

outlet
    relaxed vaginal o.
    vaginal o.

ovalbumin

ovarian
    o. agenesis
    o. amenorrhea
    o. androgen
    o. cortex
    o. cyst
    o. follicles
    o. growth factor
    o. hilar cells
    o. hilum
    o. hormones
    o. medulla
    o. mesenchyma
    o. premature failure
    o. steroid

ovarian *(continued)*
    o. stroma
    o. tumor
    o. tunica
    o. vein
    o. wedge resection

ovariectomy

ovariotestis

ovary
    aging o.
    gonodotropin-resistant o.
    menopausal o.
    polycystic o.
    postmenopausal o.
    prunelike o.

overactivity

overfeeding

overlap syndrome

overnutrition
    relative o.

oviduct

OVLT
    organum vasculosum of
      the lamina terminalis

ovotestis

ovulation
    o. induction
    o. inhibition
    midcycle o.

ovum

oxalate

oxidation
    iodide o.

oxosteroid

ox-warble disease

oxygen
    o.-derived product
    singlet o.

oxyntomodulin

oxyphil
 o. cells
 o. cell tumor

oxyphilic
 o. adenoma
 o. cells
 o. granular cell adenoma

oxytocin
 o. synthesis

oxyuria

oxyuriasis

oxyuriosis

Oz
 O. allotype
 O. antigen
 O. factor

Ozzard's filariasis

P
P antigen
factor P
properdin
substance P

P1
P1 bacteriophage recombi-
nation system
P1 kinase

p24
p. protein (*in HIV infection*)

p150,95

pachycephalia

pachycephalic

pachycephalous

pachycephaly

PADGEM (CD62P)

Paecilomyces

paecilomycosis

PAF
platelet-activating factor
PAF-acether

PAGE
polyacrylamide gel electrophoresis
SDS-PAGE

Paget disease
juvenile P. d.

Pahvant Valley
P. V. fever
P. V. plague

pain
osteoporotic p.

painless thyroiditis

paint
antiseptic p.

pair
hormone p's

palatine
p. tonsil

palmitic acid

palmoplantar sign

palpitation

PALS
periarteriolar lymphatic
sheath

panagglutinable

panagglutination

panagglutinin

pancreas *pl.* pancreata
endocrine p.
fetal p.
lesser p.
p. transplantation
Willis' p.
Winslow's p.

pancreata (*plural of* pancreas)

pancreatectomy

pancreatic
p. calcitoninoma
p. cholera
p. cholera syndrome
p. clear cells
p. duct
p. gland
p. infantilism
p. islets
p. islet cells
p. notch
p. oncofetal antigen (POA)
p. polypeptide (PP)
p. polypeptide–producing
tumor
p. tumor

pancreatitis

pancreatography

pancreozymin

panel-reactive antibody (PRA)

panencephalitis
  subacute sclerosing p.
    (SSP)

panhypogammaglobulinemia

panhypogonadism

panhypopituitarism
  prepubertal p.

panimmunity

panning

pan–T-cell antigens

P antigen (*of adenovirus*)

Panton-Valentine leukocidin
  toxoid

PAP
  peroxidase-antiperoxidase
    PAP technique

papain
  p. allergy
  p. antibody cleavage
  p.-treated erythrocyte

paper
  Whatman p.

papilla *pl.* papillae
  vaginal papillae

papillary
  p. adenocarcinoma
  p. carcinoma of thyroid
    gland
  p. cystadenoma
  p. cystadenoma of thyroid
  p. cystic adenoma
  p. thyroid carcinoma

papilledema

papillitis

papilloma

Papillomavirus

papillomavirus
  human p.

Papovaviridae

papovavirus
  lymphotropic p.

pappataci fever
  p. f. virus

papule

para-aminosalicylic acid

paracalcitol

paracholera

paracoccidioidal granuloma

Paracoccidioides

paracoccidioidomycosis

paracortex

paracortical
  p. area
  p. region of lymph node

paracrine
  p. action
  p. control
  p. growth factor
  p. mediators
  p. secretion

paradox
  Opie p.

paradysentery

parafollicular
  p. areas
  p. cells

parafrenal glands

paraganglia

paraganglioma
  medullary p.

paraganglion *pl.* paraganglia

paragonimiasis

paragonimosis

Paragonimus westermani

parahormone

parahypophysis

parainfectious

parainfluenza virus

para isomer

parallergic
    p. reaction

parallergy

paralysis *pl.* paralyses
    diphtheric p.
    diphtheritic p.
    immune p.
    immunologic p.
    infantile p.
    infantile spinal p.
    Landry's p.
    parotitic p.
    periodic p., thyrotoxic
    postdiphtheritic p.
    serum p.
    tick p.

paralytic
    p. disease
    p. hydrophobia
    p. poliomyelitis
    p. rabies

paramagnetic beads

paramphistomiasis

Paramyxoviridae

Paramyxovirinae

Paramyxovirus

paramyxovirus
    avian p. 1

paraneoplastic syndrome

paranephric

paranephritis

paranephroma

paraparesis
    tropical spastic p.

parapertussis

parapestis

paraplegia
    tropical spastic p.

paraprotein

paraproteinemia

parasite
    extracellular p.
    p.-host interaction
    p. index
    intracellular p.

parasitemia

parasitic
    p. hemoptysis
    p. melanoderma
    p. worm

parasitism

parasitosis

parastruma

parasympathetic
    p. nervous system

parathormone

parathyrin

parathyrinoma

parathyroid
    p. adenoma
    p. adenoma of thymus
    p. arteries
    p. bodies
    p. cancer
    p. carcinoma
    p. glands
    p. hormone (PTH)
    p. hormone–like peptide
    p. hormone–like protein
    p. hormone–related pep-
      tide
    p. hormone–related pro-
      tein (PTHRP)
    p. hormone resistance
    p. hyperplasia
    p. insufficiency

parathyroid *(continued)*
   p. metastatic disease
   p. poisoning
   p. secretory proteins
   p. tissue

parathyroidal

parathyroidectomize

parathyroidectomy

parathyroidlike polypeptide

parathyroidoma

parathyroprival

parathyroprivia

parathyroprivic

parathyroprivous

parathyrotrophic

parathyrotropic

paratope

paratuberculosis

paratuberculous

paratyphoid
   p. fever

paravaccinia
   p. virus

paraventricular nucleus (PVN)

parchment induration

parenchyma

parenchymal
   p. lesion

parenchymatous
   p. goiter
   p. neurosyphilis

parenteral

parenteric fever

paresis
   oculomotor p.

paretic neurosyphilis

Parinaud syndrome

Parkinson's disease

parkinsonian
   p. gait
   p. tremor

parotid gland
   accessory p. g.

parotin

parotitic paralysis

parotitis
   epidemic p.
   postoperative p.
   staphylococcal p.

paroxysm

paroxysmal
   p. cold hemoglobinuria
   (PCH)
   p. nocturnal hemoglobinuria (PNH)

Parry's disease

pars *pl.* partes
   p. distalis
   p. distalis adenohypophy-
   seos
   p. distalis lobi anterioris
   hypophyseos
   p. endocrina pancreatis
   p. infundibularis adenohy-
   pophyseos
   p. intermedia
   p. intermedia adenohypo-
   physeos
   p. intermedia lobi anterioris hypophyseos
   p. tuberalis
   p. tuberalis adenohypophy-
   seos
   p. tuberalis lobi anterioris
   hypophyseos

part
   endocrine p. of pancreas

partes (*plural of* pars)

partial
　p. agglutinin
　p. agonist peptides
　p. antigen
　p. identity
　p. thromboplastin time
　　(PTT)

particle
　p. agglutination
　beta p's
　Dane p.
　sol p.
　viral p.
　virus p.

particulate antigen

parturition

parvicellular neurons

parvoviral

Parvoviridae

Parvovirinae

Parvovirus

parvovirus
　human p. B19
　human p. RA-1

Paschen
　P's bodies
　P's corpuscles
　P's granules

passenger
　p. cells
　p. leukocyte
　p. leukocyte hypothesis

passive
　p. agglutination
　p. anaphylaxis
　p. antibody
　p. cutaneous anaphylaxis
　　(PCA)
　p. cutaneous anaphylaxis
　　reaction

passive *(continued)*
　p. cutaneous anaphylaxis
　　test
　p. cutaneous Arthus reac-
　　tion
　p. hemagglutination
　p. hemagglutination tech-
　　nique
　p. hemolysis
　p. immunity
　p. immunization
　p. immunotherapy
　p. latex agglutination
　p. protection test
　p. transfer
　p. transfer of cellular resis-
　　tance
　p. transfer test
　p. tumor
　p. vaccination

passively acquired immunity

Pasteur's theory

Pasteurella
　P. multocida
　P. pneumotropica
　P. septica

pasteurellosis

pasteurization

Pastia
　P's lines
　P's sign

patch
　mucous p.
　Peyer's p's
　p. skin test
　p. test

paternity testing

pathergia

pathergic

pathergy

pathogen
　extracellular p.

pathogen *(continued)*
    p.-generated autoanti-
        bodies
    intracellular p.
    macrophage intracellular
        p's
    opportunistic p.
    successful p.
    p. types

pathogenesis
    molecular p.
    pertussis p.

pathogenic
    p. microorganism
    p. staphylococcus

pathogenicity
    balanced p.

pathologic
    p. glycosuria
    p. gynecomastia

pathology

pathophysiology

pathway
    adrenergic p's
    alternative p.
    alternative complement p.
    cholinergic p's
    classic p.
    classical p.
    classical complement p.
    complement p's
    default p.
    dopaminergic p's
    glycolytic p.
    lectin p.
    lipoxygenase p.
    lytic p.
    nonosmotic p.
    noradrenergic p.
    osmotic p.
    peptidergic p.
    polyol p.
    prohormone p.
    properdin p.

pathway *(continued)*
    serotoninergic p's
    tuberoinfundibular p.

pattern

Paul-Bunnell test

P1 bacteriophage recombina-
    tion system

PBPC
    peripheral blood progeni-
        tor cells

PBPI
    penile-brachial blood pres-
        sure index

PC
    phosphatidylcholine

PCA
    passive cutaneous anaphy-
        laxis
            PCA test

PCEC
    purified chick embryo cell
        vaccine

PCH
    paroxysmal cold hemoglo-
        binuria

PCNA
    proliferating cell nuclear
        antigen

PCOS
    polycystic ovary syndrome

PCR
    polymerase chain reaction

PDGF
    platelet-derived growth fac-
        tor

pea soup stool

PECAM (CD31)

pediatric immunization

pediculosis
    p. capitis

pediculosis *(continued)*
   p. vestimentorum

PEG
   polyethylene glycol

pellet
   testosterone p's

Pellizzi's syndrome

Pelodera dermatitis

Pemberton's sign

pemphigoid
   bullous p.

pemphigus vulgaris

Pendred's syndrome

penicillin
   p. allergy
   p. hypersensitivity
   p. resistance

penicilliosis

penicilloyl polylysine

Penicillium
   P. chrysogenum
   P. citreoviride
   P. citrinum
   P. claviforme
   P. crustaceum
   P. cyclopium
   P. expansum
   P. glaucum
   P. griseofulvum
   P. leucopus
   P. melinii
   P. notatum
   P. patulum
   P. purpurogenum
   P. rubrum
   P. uticale
   P. viridicatum

penile
   p. arteriography
   p.-brachial blood pressure
     index (PBPI)
   p. erection
   p. prosthesis

pentadecacatechol

pentamer

pentastomiasis

pentosuria
   chronic essential p.
   essential p.

pentraxin

peplomer

peplos

pepsin
   p. antibody cleavage
   p. proteolysis

peptic ulcer

peptidase
   signal p.

peptide
   agonist p.
   p. agonist
   p. anchor residues
   antagonist p.
   p. antagonist
   p. antigen
   antigenic p's
   atrial p's
   atrial natriuretic p.
   p.-binding region
   brain natriuretic p. (BNP)
   C p.
   calcitonin gene–related p.
   p. chain
   corticotropin-like interme-
     diate lobe p.
   gastric inhibitory p. (GIP)
   gastrin-releasing p.
   p. growth factors
   HIV mutant p's
   p. hormones
   p. hormone cascade
   leader p.
   p. messengers
   parathyroid hormone–
     like p.
   parathyroid hormone–
     related p.

peptide *(continued)*
    partial agonist p's
    placental p. hormone
    serum p.
    signal p.
    p. stability
    p. transport
    vasoactive intestinal p. (VIP)

peptidergic
    p. nervous system
    p. neuron
    p. pathway

Peptococcus
    P. anaerobius
    P. asaccharolyticus
    P. constellatus
    P. magnus

Peptostreptococcus
    P. anaerobius
    P. lanceolatus
    P. micros
    P. parvulus
    P. productus

perceptual abnormalities

perchlorate discharge test

perennial rhinitis

perforation

perforin

performance
    athletic p.

periarteriolar lymphatic sheath
    (PALS)

periarteritis nodosa

pericarditis
    amebic p.

peri-islet

perimenopause

perinatal

perineal
    p. region

period
    convalescence p.

period *(continued)*
    incubation p.
    lag p.
    latency p.
    latent p.
    prodromal p.

peripatetic

peripheral
    p. blood lymphocyte
    p. blood mononuclear cells
    p. blood progenitor cells
      (PBPC)
    p. blood stem cells
    p. lymphoid organs
    p. lymphoid tissue
    p. neuropathy
    p. obesity
    p. tolerance
    p. vascular disease

peripolesis

peristrumitis

peristrumous

perithyroiditis

peritonitis
    fungal p.

perivascular goiter

periventricular organs

permeability
    solute p.
    vascular p.

permissible exposure limit

pernicious anemia

peroxidase

peroxidase-antiperoxidase
    (PAP)
    p.-a. technique

peroxide
    hydrogen p.

persistence
    microorganism p.

persistent
    p. estrus syndrome

persistent *(continued)*
    p. hyposthenuria
    p. müllerian duct syndrome

pertechnetate uptake

pertussis
    acellular p. vaccine
    p. antitoxin
    p. cough
    p. immune globulin
    p. immunity
    p.-like syndrome
    p. pathogenesis
    p. syndrome
    p. toxin
    p. vaccine

pertussoid

Peruvian wart

pest

pesticemia

pestiferous

pestilence

pestilential

pestis
    p. ambulans
    p. bubonica
    p. fulminans
    p. major
    p. minor
    p. siderans

petechia *pl.* petechiae

Peutz-Jeghers syndrome

Peyer's patches

PFC
    plaque-forming cell

Pfeiffer
    P's disease
    P's glandular fever
    P's phenomenon

PG
    prostaglandin

Pgp-1 (CD44)

pH
    p. gradient
    urine p.

PHA
    phytohemagglutinin

phaeohyphomycosis

phaeosporotrichosis

phage
    p. cross
    p. display
    p. display library

phagedenic chancroid

phagocytable

phagocyte
    blood p.
    p. chemoattractants
    p. lysozyme
    mononuclear p.
    p. recruitment
    tissue p.

phagocytic
    p. amebocyte
    p. capacity
    p. cell
    p. cell deficiencies
    p. dysfunction disorders
    p. index
    p. Langerhans cell

phagocytin

phagocytize

phagocytolysis

phagocytolytic

phagocytose

phagocytosis
    deficient p.
    induced p.
    spontaneous p.
    surface p.

phagocytotic
    p. vesicle

phagological

phagolysis

phagolysosome

phagolytic

phagosome

pharmacoendocrinology

pharyngeal
   p. diphtheria
   p. plague
   p. pouch
   p. pouch syndrome
   p. tonsil

pharyngitis
   aphthous p.
   diphtheritic p.
   p. herpetica
   plague p.
   streptococcal p.
   vesicular p.

pharyngoconjunctival
   p. fever
   p. fever virus

pharyngoconjunctivitis

pharyngotyphoid

pharynx

phase
   activation p.
   cephalic p.
   cognitive p.
   effector p. of immune re-
     sponse
   gastric p.
   induction p.
   intestinal p.
   latency p.
   negative p.
   positive p.
   proliferative p.

phenol

phenomenon *pl.* phenomena
   Arthus p.
   Becker's p.
   Bordet-Gengou p.
   capping p.

phenomenon *(continued)*
   cartilage sulfation p.
   Chase-Sulzberger p.
   Dale p.
   Danysz's p.
   dawn p.
   Debré's p.
   Denys-Leclef p.
   d'Herelle's p.
   first-set p.
   Gengou p.
   Hektoen p.
   Houssay p.
   jodbasedow p.
   Koch p.
   Lewis' p.
   Liacopoulos p.
   Neisser-Wechsberg p.
   original antigenic sin p.
   Pfeiffer's p.
   prozone p.
   Raynaud p.
   second-set p.
   Somogyi p.
   Staub-Traugott p.
   Sulzberger-Chase p.
   Twort-d'Herelle p.

phenothiazine

phenotype

phenotypic sex

phenoxybenzamine

phentermine

phentolamine
   p. test

phenylalanine hydroxylase

phenylbutazone

phenylethanolamine *N*-methyl-
   transferase (PNMT)

phenylketonuria (PKU)

phenytoin

pheochrome
   p. body
   p. cells

pheochromoblast

pheochromoblastoma

pheochromocyte

pheochromocytoma
    adrenal p.
    familial p.
    familial medullary thyroid
        carcinoma–p. syndrome
    malignant p.

pheromone

Phialophora

Philip's glands

Philippine hemorrhagic fever

phlebosclerosis

phlebotomus fever
    p. f. virus

Phlebovirus

Phleum

phlogocyte

phlogocytosis

Phocas' disease

Phoma

phorbol ester
    p. e. response element

phosphatase

phosphate
    p.-buffered saline
    p. deficiency syndrome
    p. leak
    p. metabolism
    plasma p.
    SHP p.
    tubular reabsorption of p.
        (TRP)
    urinary p.

phosphatidylcholine (PC)
    p.-specific phospholipase

phosphatidylinositol (PI)
    p. 4,5-bisphosphate
    p. 4-phosphate
    p. turnover

1-phosphatidylinositol phos-
    phodiesterase

phosphatidylinositol phospholi-
    pase C

phosphodiesterase

phosphoinositide

phospholipase
    p. A_2
    p. C
    p. D
    phosphatidylcholine-speci-
        fic p.
    phosphatidylinositol p. C

phospholipid

phosphoprotein

phosphoramide mustard

phosphorescence

phosphoribosyltransferase
    hypoxanthine-guanine p.

phosphorus
    p. distribution
    p. excretion
    p. metabolism
    p. plasma level

phosphorylase
    purine nucleoside p. (PNP)

phosphorylation
    amplification via p.
    rhodopsin p.

phosphorylcholine

phosphotungstic acid
    p. a. negative staining

phosphotyrosine kinase

photoaffinity labeling

photoallergen

photoallergic

photoallergy

photocoagulation

photoinactivation

photomicrograph

photon absorptiometry

photosensitivity
p. reaction

phototherapy

PHP
pseudohypoparathyroidism

phthisis

phycomycetosis

phycomycetous

phycomycosis
subcutaneous p.

phylactic

phylaxis

physalopteriasis

physical
p. activity
p. allergy

physicochemical assay

physiologic
p. antisepsis
p. dwarf
p. hypogammaglobulinemia

physiological
p. antiestrogen
p. gynecomastia

phytoanaphylactogen

phytohemagglutinin (PHA)

phytomitogen

phytoprecipitin

phytosensitinogen

phytosis

PI
phosphatidylinositol

pian
hemorrhagic p.

Picchini's syndrome

Pichinde virus

pickwickian syndrome

Picornaviridae

picornavirus

piece
secretory p.

piedra
black p.
white p.

Piedraia

PIF
prolactin-inhibiting factor

pig
transgenic p.

pigment
malarial p.

pigmentation

pilus *pl.* pili

pineal
p. body
p. cell
p. choriocarcinoma
p. gland
p. syndrome
p. tumor

pinealectomy

pinealism

pinealoblastoma

pinealocyte

pinealocytoma

pinealoma
ectopic p.

pinealopathy

pineoblastoma

pineocytoma

pinocytic activity

pinocytosis

pinta
    p. fever

pinus

pipestem fibrosis

piroplasmosis

Pirquet
    P. reaction
    P. test

Piry virus

pit
    coated p's

pituicyte

pituitarism

pituitary
    p. adamantinoma
    p. adenoma
    p. adiposity
    p.-adrenal suppression
    p. ameloblastoma
    p. amenorrhea
    anterior p.
    p. apoplexy
    p. basophilism
    p. body
    p. cachexia
    p. diabetes insipidus
    p. diverticulum
    p. dwarf
    p. dwarfism
    p. failure
    p. gigantism
    p. gland
    p. hormone
    p. hypogonadism
    p. hypothyroidism
    p. infantilism

pituitary *(continued)*
    p. isolation syndrome
    lazy p.
    p. myxedema
    p. nanism
    p. portal system
    posterior p.
    p. reserve
    p. stalk
    p.-thyroid axis
    p. tumor
    p. vesicle

pituitectomy

pityriasis
    p. nigra

P-K
    Prausnitz-Küstner
        P-K antibodies
        P-K reaction
        P-K test

p58/p70 killer inhibitory receptor

P1 kinase

PKU
    phenylketonuria

Pl(A1) antigen

placebo

placenta

placental
    p. growth hormone
    p. hormones
    human p. lactogen (hPL)
    p. lactogen function
    p. sulfatase
    p. sulfatase deficiency
    p. transfer antibody

plague
    ambulatory p.
    black p.
    bubonic p.
    glandular p.
    hemorrhagic p.
    meningeal p.
    p. meningitis

plague *(continued)*
    Pahvant Valley p.
    pharyngeal p.
    p. pharyngitis
    pneumonic p.
    pulmonic p.
    p. septicemia
    septicemic p.
    siderating p.
    sylvatic p.
    p. vaccine

plakins

plaque
    p. assay
    bacteriophage p.
    calcium p's
    p.-forming cell (PFC)
    p.-forming unit
    p. reduction test
    p. technique

plasma
    p. catecholamine
    hypotonic p.
    p. inorganic (PI) iodide
    p. phosphate
    p. protein
    p. renin
    p. renin activity (PRA)

plasmablast

plasma cell
    p. c. disorders
    p. c. dyscrasias
    p. c. myeloma
    p. c. tumor

plasmacyte
    p. series

plasmacytic
    p. series

plasmacytoid
    p. lymphocyte

plasmacytoma
    multiple p. of bone

plasmapheresis
    p. method

plasmid

plasmin

plasminogen
    p. activator

plasmocyte

plasmocytoma

Plasmodium

plasmoma

plasticity

plate
    lawn p.

platelet
    p.-activating factor (PAF)
    p. agglutination
    p. agglutinin
    p. antigen
    p. count
    p.-derived growth factor
      (PDGF)
    p. factor (1–4)
    p. group
    p. immunofluorescence test

Platyhelminthes

Plesiomonas
    P. shigelloides

pleura

pleuritis

pleurodynia
    epidemic p.

pleuropneumonia-like orga-
nisms

plexus
    Auerbach's p.

plot
    variability p.
    Wu and Kabat p's

PLT
   primed lymphocyte typing

Plummer
   P's disease
   P's nail
   P's sign

plunging goiter

pluriglandular
   p. adenomatosis

plurihormonal
   p. adenoma

pluripotent
   p. stem cell

PMN
   polymorphonuclear
   polymorphonuclear neutro-
      phil

PMS
   premenstrual syndrome

pneumococcal
   p. pneumonia
   p. polysaccharide
   p. vaccine polyvalent

pneumococcemia

pneumococcosis

Pneumococcus

pneumococcus polysaccharide

Pneumocystis
   P. carinii
   P. carinii pneumonia

pneumomelanosis

pneumomycosis

pneumonia
   amebic p.
   atypical p.
   caseous p.
   cheesy p.
   interstitial plasma cell p.
   pneumococcal p.
   Pneumocystis carinii p.

pneumonia *(continued)*
   primary atypical p.
   woolsorter's p.

pneumonic plague

pneumonitis
   Ascaris p.
   histosensitive p.
   hypersensitive p.
   hypersensitivity p.
   interstitial p.

Pneumovax 23

Pneumovirinae

Pneumovirus

PNH
   paroxysmal nocturnal he-
      moglobinuria

PNMT
   phenylethanolamine *N*-
      methyltransferase

PNP
   purine nucleoside phos-
      phorylase
         PNP deficiency

P-nucleotides

POA
   pancreatic oncofetal anti-
      gen

Poa

pocket
   Rathke's p.

POEMS
   plasma cell dyscrasia with
      polyneuropathy, organo-
      megaly, endocrinopathy,
      M protein, and skin
      changes
         POEMS syndrome

pogoniasis

point
   p. of dilution

point *(continued)*
  equivalence p.

poisoning
  food p.
  lead p.
  parathyroid p.

poison ivy
  p. i. extract

poison oak
  p. o. extract

poison sumac

Poisson distribution

pokeweed mitogen (PWM)

pol gene *(of HIV)*

poliencephalitis

poliencephalomyelitis

polio
  p. vaccine
  p. virus

poliocidal

polioclastic

polioencephalomyelitis

poliomyelencephalitis

poliomyeliticidal

poliomyelitis
  abortive p.
  acute anterior p.
  acute lateral p.
  anterior p.
  ascending p.
  bulbar p.
  cerebral p.
  endemic p.
  epidemic p.
  p.-like diseases
  nonparalytic p.
  paralytic p.
  postinoculation p.
  posttonsillectomy p.
  postvaccinal p.

poliomyelitis *(continued)*
  spinal paralytic p.
  p. vaccine
  p. virus

poliomyeloencephalitis

polioviral

poliovirus
  p. vaccine
  p. vaccine inactivated (IPV)
  p. vaccine live oral (OPV)
  p. vaccine live oral trivalent (TOPV)

pollen
  p. allergen
  p. allergy
  p. antigen
  p. extract

pollenogenic

pollenosis

pollinosis

polyacrylamide gel electrophoresis (PAGE)

polyadenopathy

polyadenosis

polyadenous

polyadenylation

polyarteritis
  p. nodosa

polyarthritis
  epidemic p.
  p. rheumatica acuta

poly-C9 (complement component)

polyclonal
  p. activation
  p. activator
  p. antibody
  p. gammopathy
  p. hypergammaglobulinemia

polyclonal *(continued)*
    p. mitogen

polycystic
    p. ovary
    p. ovary syndrome (PCOS)

polycythemia

polydipsia

polyendocrine
    p. adenomatosis
    p. autoimmune diseases

polyendocrinoma

polyendocrinopathy

polyester
    sucrose p.

polyethylene glycol

polygenic

polyglandular
    p. autoimmune diseases
    p. autoimmune syndromes

polyhedral theca lutein-like cell

poly-Ig receptor

polyinfection

polylysine

polymer
    polypeptide p.

polymerase
    p. chain reaction (PCR)
    p. chain reaction technique

polymeric immunoglobulin

polymicrobial

polymicrobic

polymorphic
    p. gene

polymorphism
    amplification fragment
        length p. (AFLP)
    ethnic p.

polymorphism *(continued)*
    restriction fragment
        length p.

polymorphocyte

polymorphonuclear (PMN)
    p. granulocyte
    p. leukocyte
    p. neutrophil (PMN)
    p. neutrophilic leukocyte

polymyositis
    trichinous p.

polyneuritis
    acute idiopathic p.
    idiopathic p.

polyneuropathy
    symmetrical peripheral p.

polynucleotide

polyol pathway

Polyomavirus

polyomavirus

polyp
    colonic p.
    endocervical p.
    endometrial p.

polypeptide
    gastric inhibitory p.
    glucose-dependent insu-
        linotropic p.
    p. growth factors
    p. hormone
    immunogenic p.
    islet amyloid p.
    nonimmunogenic p.
    pancreatic p. (PP)
    parathyroidlike p.
    p. polymer
    p. structures
    vasoactive intestinal p.
        (VIP)

polyperforin

polyphosphoinositide

polypoid adenocarcinoma

polysaccharide
  bacterial p.
  capsular p.
  p. complex
  core p.
  immune p's
  O-specific p.
  pneumococcal p.
  pneumococcus p.
  specific p's
  p. vaccine

polyserositis

polyspecificity

polyuria
  hypokalemic p.

polyvalent
  p. allergy
  p. attenuated vaccine
  p. serum
  p. vaccine

POMC
  pro-opiomelanocortin
    POMC gene

Pomona fever

Pompe's disease

Pongola virus

Pontiac fever

pool
  sympathetic nerve ending
    storage p's

pooled serums

population
  monoclonal p's
  p. study

poradenitis
  p. nostras
  subacute inguinal p.
  p. venerea

poradenolymphitis

pore-forming protein

pork trichina skin test

porocephaliasis

porocephalosis

Porphyromonas
  P. asaccharolytica

portal
  p. circulation
  p. veins of hypophysis

Porter
  P.-Silber chromogen
  P.-Silber reaction

Posadas
  P's disease
  P's mycosis
  P.-Wernicke disease

positive
  p. anergy
  p. cooperativity
  p. cooperativity of ovarian
    steroid hormones
  p. feedback loop
  p. phase
  p. selection

postablative hypothyroidism

postabsorptive hypoglycemia

postbranchial bodies

postcapillary high endothelial
  venule

postcardiotomy syndrome

postcoital contraception

postdiphtheritic
  p. paralysis

posterior
  p. lobe
  p. pituitary
  p. pituitary gland
  p. pituitary hormones
  p. surface of adrenal gland

posterior *(continued)*
    p. surface of body of pancreas
    p. surface of suprarenal gland

postfebrile neuritis

posthypoglycemic coma

postinoculation poliomyelitis

postmenopausal
    p. hypercalcemia
    p. osteoporosis
    p. ovary

postmenopause

post–myocardial infarction syndrome

postnatal

postoccipital lobe

postoperative parotitis

postpartum
    p. lactosuria
    p. pituitary necrosis
    p. thyroiditis
    p. thyroiditis syndrome

postperfusion syndrome

postpolio sequela

postpoliomyelitis
    p. sequela
    p. syndrome

postprandial hypoglycemia

postprimary tuberculosis

postradioiodine hypothyroidism

poststreptococcal glomerulonephritis

postsynaptic membrane

posttonsillectomy poliomyelitis

posttranscriptional processing

posttransfusion
    p. hepatitis
    p. mononucleosis
    p. syndrome

posttranslational
    p. modification
    p. processing

postulate
    Koch p's
    Witebsky's p's

postvaccinal
    p. poliomyelitis

postvaccinial

postvenereal

postzone

potassemia

potassium
    p. citrate
    p. depletion
    p. deprivation
    p. iodide
    p. perchlorate
    p. supplementation
    total body p.

potential
    p. abnormality of glucose tolerance
    action p.
    zeta p.

potomania
    beer p.

pouch
    craniobuccal p.
    craniopharyngeal p.
    pharyngeal p.
    Rathke's p.

Powassan virus

pox
    p. virus

Poxviridae

poxvirus

PP
    pancreatic polypeptide
        PP cells

PPD
    purified protein derivative
        PPD skin test

PPHP
    pseudopseudohypopara-
        thyroidism

p24 protein (*in HIV infection*)

PRA
    panel-reactive antibody
    plasma renin activity

practice
    safety p's

Prader-Willi syndrome

Pr antigen

Prausnitz
    P.-Küstner (P-K) antibodies
    P.-Küstner (P-K) reaction
    P.-Küstner (P-K) test

PRE
    progesterone response ele-
        ment

prealbumin
    T_4-binding p. (TBPA)

prebacillary

pre-B cell
    large p.-B c.
    p.-B c. leukemia
    p.-B c. proliferation
    p.-B c. receptor
    small p.-B c.

pre-B lymphocyte

precipitate
    immune p.

precipitation
    aluminum p.
    group p.
    immune p. reaction

precipitation (*continued*)
    intratubal p.
    nonimmune p.
    p. reaction
    p. test

precipitin
    p. line
    p. reaction
    rheumatoid arthritis p.
    p. test
    p. test ring variations

precipitinogen

precipitogen

preclinical diabetes

precocious
    central p. puberty
    constitutional p. puberty
    contrasexual p. puberty
    factitious p. puberty
    familial p. puberty
    gonadotropin-dependent p.
        puberty
    heterosexual p. puberty
    idiopathic p. puberty
    incomplete p. puberty
    isosexual p. puberty
    neurogenic p. puberty
    p. pseudopuberty
    p. puberty
    true p. puberty

precocity
    contrasexual p.
    incomplete isosexual p.
    sexual p.

precursor
    p. cell
    p. mRNA (pre-mRNA)
    p. substance

prediabetes

prediction
    adult stature p.
    rejection p.

prednisone

preeclampsia

preeruptive stage

pre-existing antibody

preformed mediator

pregnancy
p. cell
ectopic p.
p. gland
p.-induced hypertension
p. serum

pregnane

pregnanediol

pregnanetriol

pregnant
p. mare serum gonadotro-
pin

pregnene

pregneninolone

pregnenolone

prehormone

prehyoid glands

prehypophyseal

prehypophysial

prehypophysis

premature
p. adrenarche
p. menarche
p. thelarche

prematurity

premenopause

premenstrual
p. syndrome (PMS)
p. tension syndrome

premonocyte

pre-mRNA
precursor mRNA

premunition

premunitive

prenatal
p. hormone

Pre-Pen

preprohormone

preproinsulin

preprotein

prepubertal panhypopituitarism

presentation
antigen p.

pressor substance

pressure
blood p.

presynaptic membrane

pre-T cell

prethyroid

prethyroideal

prethyroidean

pretibial
p. fever
p. myxedema

pre-T lymphocyte

pretuberculosis

pretuberculous proteinuria

prevention
atherosclerosis p.
rejection p.

previous abnormality of glucose tolerance

Prevnar

Prevotella
P. bivia
P. buccae
P. corporis
P. denticola
P. disiens
P. heparinolytica

Prevotella (continued)
    P. intermedia
    P. melaninogenica
    P. oralis
    P. oris

prezone

PRF
    prolactin-releasing factor

prick test

primary
    p. adrenal insufficiency
    p. adrenocortical nodular
      dysplasia
    p. aldosteronism
    p. amebic meningoenceph-
      alitis
    p. amenorrhea
    p. amyloidosis
    p. antibody interactions
    p. antibody repertoire
    p. antibody response
    p. atypical pneumonia
    p. bubo
    p. complex
    p. complication
    p. focus
    p. follicles
    p. hemochromatosis
    p. hyperaldosteronism
    p. hyperparathyroidism
    p. hypogonadism
    p. hypothyroidism
    p. immune response
    p. immunization
    p. immunodeficiency
    p. immunoglobulin defi-
      ciency
    p. inoculation complex
    p. inoculation tuberculosis
    p. interaction
    p. lymphoid tissues
    p. myxedema
    p. osteoporosis
    p. response
    p. sex characters
    p. syphilis

primary *(continued)*
    p. tuberculosis
    p. tuberculous complex

prime

primed
    p. lymphocyte typing (PLT)

priming

primitive stem cell

primordial dwarf

primordial dwarfism

principal cells

prion
    p. disease
    p. protein (PrP)

PRIST
    paper radioimmunosorbent
      test

private
    p. antigens
    p. specificity

PRL
    prolactin

proactivator
    C3 p. (C3PA)

probacteriophage

pro-B cell
    early p.-B c.
    late p.-B c.
    p.-B c. proliferation

probe
    DNA p.

procainamide hydrochloride

procedure
    localization p's

proceptivity

process
    immune p.
    selection p.
    uncinate p. of pancreas

processing
   antigen p. (APC)
   posttranscriptional p.
   posttranslational p.
   receptor p.

processus *pl.* processus
   p. uncinatus pancreatis

prodromal
   p. period
   p. stage

prodrome

product
   advanced glycation end p's
   bacterial p's
   lymphocyte p.
   soybean p's

production
   antibody p.
   estradiol p.
   lactogen p.
   somatic mutation theory of
      antibody p.

productive tuberculosis

proestrogen

professional antigen-presenting
   cell

profile
   antigenic p.

profiling
   renin-sodium p.

progastrin

progenitor
   basophil p's
   p. cell
   lymphoid p.
   macrophage p's
   monocyte p's
   myeloid p's
   neutrophil p's

progeria

progestagen

progestational
   p. agent
   p. hormone

progesterone
   p. antagonist
   p. breakthrough bleeding
   p. receptor
   p. response element (PRE)

progestin

progestogen

proglottid

progoitrin

programmed cell death

progressive
   p. coccidioidomycosis
   p. disseminated histoplas-
      mosis
   p. muscular atrophy
   p. systemic sclerosis
   p. vaccinia

ProHIBiT

prohormone
   p. pathway

proinflammatory

proinsulin

prolactin (PRL)
   p. cell
   p. cell adenoma
   p.-inhibiting factor (PIF)
   p.-inhibiting hormone
   p. receptor system
   p.-releasing factor (PRF)
   p.-releasing hormone
   p.-secreting adenoma
   p.-secreting microadenoma
   p.-secreting tumor

prolactinoma

prolactoliberin

prolactostatin

prolan

prolapse
    uterine p.

proliferating
    p. B cells
    p. cell nuclear antigen
        (PCNA)

proliferation
    antigen-induced p.
    cell p.
    lymphocyte p.
    pre-B cell p.
    pro-B cell p.

proliferative
    p. inhibitory factor
    p. phase
    p. retinopathy

prolymphocyte

promonocyte

promoter
    chicken ovalbumin up-
        stream p. (COUP)

prontosil

pronuclear stage tubal transfer
    PROST

pro-opiomelanocortin (POMC)

proparathyroid
    p. hormone

properdin (P)
    p. deficiency
    p. pathway
    p. system

prophage

prophylactic gonadectomy

prophylaxis

Propionibacterium
    P. acnes
    P. granulosum
    P. propionicum

proplasmacyte

proportion
    optimal p's
    segmental p's

proptosis

prosecretin

PROST
    pronuclear stage tubal
        transfer

prostacyclin

prostaglandin (PG)
    p. D_2
    p. E_1
    p. E_2
    p. $F_{2\alpha}$
    p. G_2
    p. H_2
    p. I_2
    p. synthetase

prostate
    p. cancer
    p. gland
    p.-specific antigen (PSA)
    p. tumor

prostatectomy
    transurethral p.

prostatic

prosthesis
    penile p.

prostration
    heat p.

protamine zinc insulin

protease
    p. activity
    p. inhibitor
    serine p.

proteasome (CD59)

protectin

protection test

protective
    p. antibody

protective *(continued)*
    p. immunity
    p. inoculation

protector
    LATS p.

protein
    p. A
    ABC p's
    acute phase p's
    acute phase plasma p's
    amyloid p.
    p. antigen
    AP-1 p.
    ATP-binding cassette p.
    B7 p.
    bactericidal permeability
      increasing p. (BPI)
    Bence Jones p.
    binding p.
    B-lineage specific activa-
      tor p. (BSAP)
    p.-bound iodine
    p.-bound iodine test
    carrier p.
    cationic p's
    C4 binding p.
    complement control p.
      (CCP)
    C-reactive p.
    cyclic adenosine mono-
      phosphate response ele-
      ment–binding p. (CREB)
    cytoplasmic p's
    DNA-binding p.
    DNA-dependent p. kinase
    docking p.
    E1A p.
    encephalitogenic p.
    endogenous p. antigen
    eosinophil cationic p.
    exogenous p. antigen
    Fas p.
    fetal p.
    folding of p's
    G p.
    p. G
    heat shock p.
    H1 histone p.

protein *(continued)*
    HIV p's
    p. hormone
    IGF-binding p. (IGFBP)
    immune p.
    p. immunodeficiency
    p. intolerance
    p. isolation
    p. kinase
    p. kinase A
    p. kinase C
    La p.
    leukocyte adhesion p.
      (LAP)
    lipopolysaccharide-bind-
      ing p.
    M p.
    macrophage chemoattrac-
      tant and activating factor/
      p.
    major basic p. (MBP)
    mannose-binding p.
    matrix p.
    matrix GLA p.
    membrane cofactor p.
      (MCP)
    p. metabolism
    monoclonal p.
    monocyte chemotactic p.-1
    Mx p.
    myelin basic p. (MBP)
    myeloma p. (M protein)
    N p.
    nonreceptor hormone-
      binding p.
    nonsuppressible insulin-
      like p.
    nuclear p's
    oncofetal p's
    p24 p. *(in HIV infection)*
    parathyroid hormone–
      like p.
    parathyroid hormone–re-
      lated p. (PTHRP)
    parathyroid secretory p's
    plasma p.
    pore-forming p.
    prion p. (PrP)
    p.-p. interaction

protein *(continued)*
    proteolipid p.
    p. purification
    ras p.
    rev p.
    S p.
    serum p.
    serum amyloid p.
    staphylococcal p. A
    surfactant p. A
    surfactant p. D
    p. synthesis
    tat p.
    thymus-dependent p. antigen
    tolerogenic p. antigen
    translation inhibitory p.
    transport p's
    van Dyke p.
    viral p's
    zeta-associated p. (ZAP)
    zeta-associated p.-70 (ZAP-70)

proteinase

proteinemia
    Bence Jones p.

protein-glutamine γ-glutamyl-transferase

protein kinase
    p. k. A
    B cell progenitor p. k.
    p. k. C
    cAMP-dependent p. k.
    cyclic AMP–dependent p. k.
    DNA-dependent p. k.

protein-tyrosine kinase

proteinuria
    Bence Jones p.
    pretuberculous p.

proteoglycan
    bone p's

proteolipid
    p. protein

proteolysis

proteolytic enzyme

Proteus
    P. mirabilis
    P. vulgaris

prothoracicotropic hormone

prothrombin time (PT)

prothymocyte

protirelin

protobiology

protocol

proto-oncogene
    myc p.-o.

protothecosis

protozoa (*plural of* protozoon)

protozoan

protozoiasis

protozoon *pl.* protozoa

protozoophage

protozoosis

protransglutaminase

Providencia
    P. alcalifaciens
    P. rettgeri
    P. stuartii

provirus
    HIV p.

provisional cortex

provocation
    bronchial p.
    inhalational p.
    p. test
    p. typhoid

provocative
    p. diet
    p. test

prozonal

prozone
  p. effect
  p. phenomenon
  p. reaction

PrP
  prion protein

prunelike ovary

PSA
  prostate-specific antigen

P-selectin (CD62P)

pseudoagglutination

pseudoaldosteronism

pseudoallele

pseudoallergic reaction

pseudallescheriasis

pseudoanaphylactic

pseudoanaphylaxis

pseudoautosomal inheritance

pseudobasedow

pseudocapsule

pseudochancre
  p. redux

pseudocholecystitis

pseudocowpox
  p. virus

pseudo–Cushing's syndrome

pseudocyst
  adrenal p.

pseudodiabetes
  uremic p. mellitus

pseudodiphtheria

pseudogene

pseudogout

pseudo–Graefe's sign

pseudogynecomastia

pseudohermaphrodism
  female p.
  male p.

pseudohermaphrodite
  female p.
  male p.

pseudohermaphroditism
  female p.
  male p.

pseudohypoaldosteronism

pseudohyponatremia

pseudohypoparathyroidism
  (PHP)

pseudohypothyroidism

pseudomembrane

pseudomembranous

Pseudomonas
  P. acidovorans
  P. alcaligenes
  P. cepacia
  P. fluorescens
  P. paucimobilis
  P. pseudoalcaligenes
  P. putida
  P. stutzeri

pseudomucinous cyst adenoma

pseudopoliomyelitis

pseudoprecocious puberty

pseudoprimary
  p. aldosteronism
  p. hyperaldosteronism

pseudopseudohypoparathy-
roidism (PPHP)

pseudopuberty
  precocious p.

pseudorabies virus

pseudoreaction

pseudorheumatism

pseudoscarlatina

pseudoscrotum

pseudosubstrate site

pseudotuberculous thyroiditis

pseudo–Turner syndrome

pseudotyphus

pseudovaginal
    p. perineoscrotal hypospadias

psittacosis

psoriatic arthropathy

psoroptic

psychic distress

psychoendocrinology

psychogenic
    p. amenorrhea
    p. impotence
    p. water drinking

psychological
    p. factors
    p. management

psychoneuroendocrinology

psychoneuroimmunology

psychosexual
    p. differentiation

psychosis

psychosocial
    p. deprivation syndrome
    p. dwarfism
    p. factors

psychotherapy

PT
    prothrombin time

PTH
    parathyroid hormone
        PTH fragments
        PTH resistance

PTHRP
    parathyroid hormone–related protein

PTT
    partial thromboplastin time

pubarche

puberal

pubertal
    p. growth spurt

pubertas
    p. praecox

puberty
    central precocious p.
    constitutional precocious p.
    contrasexual precocious p.
    delayed p.
    factitious precocious p.
    familial precocious p.
    gonadotropin-dependent precocious p.
    heterosexual precocious p.
    idiopathic p.
    idiopathic precocious p.
    incomplete precocious p.
    isosexual precocious p.
    male p.
    neurogenic precocious p.
    precocious p.
    pseudoprecocious p.
    true precocious p.

pubescence

pubescent

pubic hair

public
    p. antigens
    P. Health Service
    p. specificity

pudendal ulcer

pulmonary
　　p. amebiasis
　　p. anthrax
　　p. ascariasis
　　p. aspergillosis
　　p. distomiasis
　　p. edema
　　p. hypersensitivity disease
　　p. osteoarthropathy
　　p. schistosomiasis
　　p. strongyloidiasis
　　p. tuberculosis
　　p. tularemia

pulmonic
　　p. plague
　　p. tularemia

pulp
　　red p.
　　white p.

pump
　　insulin p.
　　ion p.

punctuation
　　Schüffner's p.

puncture
　　Bernard's p.
　　p. diabetes
　　diabetic p.

pure
　　p. antiestrogen
　　p. dwarf
　　p. gonadal dysgenesis
　　p. theca cell tumor

purge

purification
　　lymphocyte p.
　　protein p.

purified
　　p. chick embryo cell vac-
　　　cine (PCEC)
　　p. protein derivative (PPD)
　　p. protein derivative (PPD)
　　　skin test

purine
　　p. analogue
　　p. metabolism
　　p. nucleoside phosphory-
　　　lase (PNP)
　　p. nucleoside phosphory-
　　　lase (PNP) deficiency

puromycin

purpura
　　autoimmune p.
　　autoimmune thrombo-
　　　cytic p.
　　Henoch-Schönlein p.
　　Schönlein-Henoch p.
　　thrombocytopenic p.

purse-string mouth

Purtilo's syndrome

pus

pustule
　　malignant p.

Puumala virus

PVN
　　paraventricular nucleus

PWM
　　pokeweed mitogen

pyelography
　　intravenous p.

pyelonephritis

pygmy

pyknodysostosis

pyknotic bodies

pyocyanosis

pyoderma

pyogenic
　　p. bacterium
　　p. infection

pyramid
　　Lalouette's p.
　　p. of thyroid

pyramidal
    p. lobe
    p. lobe of thyroid gland

pyrimidine
    p. analogue
    p. metabolism

pyrogen
    endogenous p.

pyrogen *(continued)*
    exogenous p's
    granulocytic p.
    leukocytic p.
    monocytic p.

pyroglobulin

pyroglobulinemia

Q fever

Qa
    Q. antigen
    Q. genes

quantitative
    q. determination
    q. hypothesis
    q. immunoelectrophoresis
    q. immunoabsorption

Quaranfil virus

quarantine

Queensland tick typhus

Quellung reaction

quenching
    fluorescence q.

quiescent

Quinacrine sterilization

quintan
    q. fever

quotient
    intelligence q. (IQ)

RA
    rheumatoid arthritis
    rheumatoid serum agglutin-
      ator
        RA cell

RabAvert

rabbit
    r. fever
    r. myxoma virus
    r. syphilis

rabid

rabies
    dumb r.
    furious r.
    r. immune globulin
    r.-like viruses
    paralytic r.
    r. vaccine
    r. vaccine adsorbed (RVA)
    r. virus

rabiform

Rabson-Mendenhall syndrome

radial immunodiffusion (RID)
    r. i. test

radiation
    r. bone marrow chimeras
    r. chimera
    immunosuppressant r.
    r. therapy
    r. thyroiditis

radiculopathy

radioactive
    r. antiglobulin test
    r. iodine uptake (RAIU)

radioallergosorbent
    r. test (RAST)

radiodensitometry

radioenzymatic assay

radiography
    dual energy r.

radiographic contrast media

radioimmunoassay (RIA)
    competitive r.
    direct r.
    sandwich r.
    solid phase r.

radioimmunodiffusion

radioimmunoelectrophoresis

radioimmunoprecipitation
    r. assay (RIPA)

radioimmunosorbent
    r. test (RIST)

radioiodide
    r. uptake

radioiodine
    r. uptake
    r. uptake test

radioisotope

radioreceptor assay

RAG
    recombination activating
      gene
        RAG-1
        RAG-2
        RAG mutations
        RAG rescue

ragocyte

ragpicker's disease

ragsorter's disease

ragweed
    r. allergen

raillietiniasis

RAIU
    radioactive iodine uptake

Raji
    R. cell
    R. cell assay

Ralstonia
    R. pickettii

Ramon flocculation test

range
host r.

Ranke
R. complex
R's stages

RANTES chemokine

Rantz and Randall macrotechnique

Ranvier
nodes of R.

RAP
rheumatoid arthritis precipitin

rapamycin

rapid
r. latex agglutination
r. plasma reagin (RPR) card test
r. slide test
r. surface immunoassay

ras oncogene

ras protein

rash

RAST
radioallergosorbent test

rat
r.-bite disease
r.-bite fever

rate
androgen production r's
basal metabolic r. (BMR)
r. constant
erythrocyte sedimentation r. (ESR)
infant mortality r.
metabolic clearance r. (MCR)
renal iodide clearance r.
transcription r.

Rathke
R's cleft cysts
R's cysts

Rathke *(continued)*
R's pocket
R's pouch
R's pouch tumor
R's tumor

ratio
stimulation r. (SR)
waist/hip r.
weight/height r.

Rauscher virus

Raynaud
R. disease
R. phenomenon

RBC
red blood cell

RCA
regulator of complement activation

reabsorption
calcium r.
sodium r.
tubular r. of phosphate (TRP)

reactant
acute phase r's

reacting dose

reaction
alarm r.
allergic r.
allogeneic mixed leukocyte r.
allograft r.
anamnestic r.
anaphylactic r.
anaphylactoid r.
antibody-mediated cytotoxic hypersensitivity r.
antibody-mediated hypersensitivity r.
antigen-antibody r.
antiglobulin r.
antitissue r.
aromatase r.
Arthus r.
Arthus-type r.

reaction *(continued)*
  Bordet-Gengou r.
  cell-mediated hypersensi-
    tivity r.
  r. center
  chromaffin r.
  cockade r.
  complement fixation r.
  conglutination r.
  cross r.
  cutaneous r.
  cytotoxic r.
  cytotoxic hypersensitivi-
    ty r.
  Dale r.
  delayed hypersensitivity r.
  downgrading r.
  equivalence zone r.
  Fernandez r.
  fight-or-flight r.
  foreign body r.
  graft-versus-host (GVH) r.
  granulomatous r.
  group r.
  hemagglutination r.
  hemagglutination inhibi-
    tion r.
  Henle's r.
  Herxheimer's r.
  homograft r.
  host r's
  hypersensitivity r. *(types I–
    IV)*
  r. of identity
  immediate hypersensitivi-
    ty r.
  immune r.
  immune complex–medi-
    ated hypersensitivity r.
  immune precipitation r.
  immunosuppressant r.
  intracutaneous r.
  intradermal r.
  isoimmune r.
  Jarisch-Herxheimer r.
  Jones-Mote r.
  late phase r.
  lepra r.
  lepromin r.

reaction *(continued)*
  Machado r.
  Machado-Guerreiro r.
  Mitsuda r.
  mixed agglutination r.
  mixed leukocyte r.
  mixed lymphocyte r.
  Molisch's r.
  Moloney r.
  Montenegro r.
  r. of nonidentity
  Ouchterlony quantitative
    precipitin r.
  parallergic r.
  r. of partial identity
  passive cutaneous anaphy-
    laxis r.
  passive cutaneous Ar-
    thus r.
  photosensitivity r.
  Pirquet r.
  P-K (Prausnitz-Küstner) r.
  polymerase chain r. (PCR)
  Porter-Silber r.
  Prausnitz-Küstner (P-K) r.
  precipitation r.
  precipitin r.
  prozone r.
  pseudoallergic r.
  Quellung r.
  reversal r.
  reverse passive Arthus r.
  reverse transcriptase
    polymerase chain r.
    (RT-PCR)
  Schultz-Dale r.
  second-set r.
  serologic r.
  serum r.
  serum sickness–like r.
  Shwartzman r.
  skin r.
  stress r.
  sympathetic stress r.
  T cell–mediated hypersen-
    sitivity r.
  toxin-antitoxin r.
  transfusion r.
  tuberculin skin test r.

reaction *(continued)*
    type I hypersensitivity r.
    type II hypersensitivity r.
    type III hypersensitivity r.
    type IV hypersensitivity r.
    upgrading r.
    von Pirquet r.
    water repletion r.
    wheal and erythema r.
    wheal and flare r.
    white-graft r.
    Widal r.

reactivate

reactivation
    r. of serum
    r. tuberculosis

reactive
    r. arthritis
    r. hypoglycemia
    r. lysis
    r. nitrogen intermediate (RNI)
    r. oxygen intermediate (ROI)

reactivity
    Arthus-type r.

reactogenic

reagent
    antihuman globulin r.
    binding r.
    contaminated r.

reagin
    r. antibody
    r. screen test
    syphilitic r.

reaginic
    r. antibody

rearranged gene segments

rearrangement
    chromosomal r.
    nonproductive r.

reassignment
    infant sex r.
    sex r.

rebound hyperglycemia

Rebuck
    R. skin window technique
    R. test

recall antigen

receptivity

receptor
    α-adrenergic r's
    acetylcholine r's
    adrenergic r's
    r. affinity
    alpha r's
    alpha beta T cell r's
    androgen r.
    antigen r.
    r. autoantibodies
    β-adrenergic r's
    beta r's
    C r.
    CC-CCKR-5 cell surface r.
    CD2 r.
    cellular r.
    chemokine r.
    cholinergic r's
    complement r. (CR)
    crystalline fragment r.
    cytokine r.
    desensitization r's
    r.-destroying enzyme
    dopaminergic r's
    Duffy r.
    r. editing
    r.-effector system
    estrogen r.
    r. family hematopoietins
    Fc r.
    fya r.
    gamma delta T r's
    glucocorticoid r.
    H r.
    homing r.
    hormone r.
    IgE r's
    insulin r's
    interferon r.
    interferon-γ r.

receptor *(continued)*
    interleukin r.
    intracellular r.
    killer inhibitory r's (KIR)
    lymphocyte r's
    lymphocyte antigen r's
    lymphocyte surface r.
    mannose r.
    r.-mediated endocytosis
    membrane r.
    p58/p70 killer inhibitory r.
    poly-Ig r.
    pre-B cell r.
    progesterone r.
    r. processing
    r. repertoire
    scavenger r.
    sheep blood cell r.
    sheep red blood cell r.
    r. signals
    spare r.
    r. specificity
    steroid r.
    r.-steroid complex
    steroid hormone r.
    T cell r.
    T cell antigen r.
    transferrin r.
    transmembrane r.
    tumor complement r.
    variable T cell r.
    vitronectin r.
    volume r's

recessive
    r. gene
    r. inheritance
    r. lethal gene
    r. trait

recipient
    immunization r.
    universal r.

recirculation
    lymphocyte r.
    r. of lymphocytes

recognition
    allogeneic r.
    antigen r.

recognition *(continued)*
    linked r.
    r. sequence
    signal r.
    signal r. particle complex

recombinant
    recombination activating
        gene (RAG)
    r. DNA
    hGH-r.
    r. human erythropoietin
    r. inbred strains
    MHC r.
    r. vaccine

recombinase

recombination
    homologous r.
    r. activating genes
    r. signal sequences
    somatic r.
    switch r.

recombinational germline theory

Recombivax HB

recording
    nerve r's

recrudescent typhus

recruitment
    r. factor
    leukocyte r.
    macrophage r.
    phagocyte r.

recurrent
    r. fever
    r. idiotype

red
    r. blood cell
    r. blood cell destruction
    r. cell antigen
    r. cell autoantibody
    r. pulp

reductase
    5α-r.

redundancy
  long terminal r.

Reed-Sternberg cell

refeeding gynecomastia

reflex
  suckling r.

refractory
  r. anemia

Refsum disease

Regan isoenzyme

regeneration
  tissue r.

regimen
  vaccine r.

region
  C (constant) r.
  complement-determining r.
    (CDR) (1–3)
  constant r.
  D (diversity) r.
  Fab r.
  Fc r.
  framework r's
  hinge r.
  homology r's
  HV r.
  hypervariable r's
  I r.
  immunodominant r.
  immunoglobulin hinge r.
  J (joining) r.
  N r.
  N r. diversification
  paracortical r. of lymph
    node
  peptide-binding r.
  perineal r.
  regulatory r.
  switch r's
  thymus-dependent r.
  thymus-independent r.
  transcriptional activation r.
  V (variable) r.

regional
  r. adenopathy
  r. ileitis
  r. lymphadenitis

regressive infantilism

regular insulin

regulation
  appetite r.
  complement r.
  corticotropin-releasing fac-
    tor r.
  membrane transplant r.
  osmotic r.
  transcriptional r.
  volume r.

regulator
  r. of complement activation
    (RCA)

regulatory
  r. region

rehabilitation gynecomastia

Reifenstein's syndrome

reinfection
  r. tuberculosis

reinoculation

Reissner fiber

Reiter
  R's arthritis
  R. antigen
  R's syndrome

rejection
  acute r.
  acute cellular r.
  acute early r.
  acute late r.
  cellular r.
  chronic r.
  r. effector mechanisms
  first-set r.
  graft r.
  homogeneous r.
  homograft r.

rejection *(continued)*
    hyperacute r.
    immunologic r.
    insidious r.
    late r.
    r. mechanisms
    r. monitoring
    r. prediction
    r. prevention
    second-set r.
    second-set graft r.
    skin graft r.
    r. treatment
    vascular r.

relapsing fever

relationship
    immunologic r.

relative
    r. lymphocytosis
    r. overnutrition
    r. risk

relaxin

release
    adrenaline r.
    catecholamine r.
    cytotoxic cytokine r.
    insulin r.

releasing
    r. factors
    r. hormones

remnant
    chylomicron r's

remodeling
    skeletal r.

removal
    spleen r.

renal
    r. adenoma
    r.-adrenal axis
    r. blood flow
    r. calculi
    r. colic
    r. countercurrent mechanisms

renal *(continued)*
    r. diabetes
    r. disease
    r. failure
    r. glycosuria
    r. hypercalciuria
    r. hypertension
    r. impairment
    r. insufficiency
    r. iodide clearance rate
    r. lithiasis
    r. osteodystrophy
    r. parenchymal disease
    r. stone
    r. surface of adrenal gland
    r. surface of suprarenal gland
    r. tubular acidosis
    r. tubular disorders
    r. vascular lesion
    r. vein renin

renin
    r.-angiotensin-aldosterone system
    r.-angiotensin system
    plasma r.
    plasma r. activity (PRA)
    r.-secreting tumor
    r. secretion
    r.-sodium profiling
    r. substrate
    renal vein r.

renography
    isotopic r.

renovascular hypertension

reorientation
    cytoskeletal r.

Reoviridae

repeat
    long terminal r. (LTR)
    short consensus r. (SCR)

reovirus

repeated immunization

repertoire
    antibody r.

repertoire *(continued)*
    lymphocyte r.
    primary antibody r.
    receptor r.

replacement therapy
    androgen r. t.

replicability

replication
    HIV r.
    Mycoplasma r.
    virus r.

replicative vaccine

reporter genes

reproduction
    female r.
    male r.
    sexual r.

reproductive
    r. cycle
    r. system
    r. tract

RES
    reticuloendothelial system

resection
    ovarian wedge r.

resectoscope

reserve
    ACTH r.
    adrenal r.
    adrenocortical r.
    adrenocorticotropic hor-
      mone r.
    pituitary r.
    thyroid r.

reservoir
    r. host
    r. of infection

resident macrophages

residual lumen

resistance
    acquired r.

resistance *(continued)*
    androgen r.
    antibiotic r.
    cellular r.
    complete androgen r.
    drug r.
    HIV drug r.
    hormone r.
    host r.
    incomplete androgen r.
    innate r. mechanisms
    insulin r.
    natural r.
    parathyroid hormone
      (PTH) r.
    passive transfer of cellu-
      lar r.
    penicillin r.
    immunologic r.
    vitamin D r.

resorption
    bone r.
    subperiosteal r. of the mid-
      dle phalanx

respiratory
    r. burst
    r. disease
    r. distress syndrome
    r. mucosa
    r. syncytial viruses (RSV)
    r. system
    r. tract
    r. tract infection
    upper r. infection
    r. viruses

responder
    high r.
    immunization r's

response
    acute phase r.
    adaptive immune r.
    adrenal r.
    amnestic antibody r.
    anamnestic r.
    antibody r.
    autoimmune r.

response *(continued)*
    booster r.
    cell-mediated secondary
        immune r.
    HIV immune r.
    hormone r. elements
    humoral immune r.
    humoral secondary immu-
        ne r.
    immune r.
    inflammatory r.
    innate immune r.
    memory r.
    primary r.
    primary antibody r.
    primary immune r.
    secondary r.
    secondary antibody r.
    secondary immune r.
    skin test r.
    tertiary r.
    triple r. *(of Lewis)*
    vascular r.
    vasopressin r.
    wheal and flare r.

rest
    adrenal r.
    suprarenal r's

resting
    r. macrophages
    r. wandering cell

restricted
    MHC r.

restriction
    class I r.
    class II r.
    dietary r's
    r. endonucleases
    genetic r.
    MHC r.

restriction fragment
    r. f. length
    r. f. length polymorphism

reticular
    r. cell

reticular *(continued)*
    r. dysgenesis
    r. zone

reticulate body

reticulin
    r. M

reticulocyte

reticuloendothelial
    r. blockade
    r. cell
    r. system (RES)

reticuloendotheliosis
    leukemic r.

reticuloendothelium

reticulohistiocytary

reticulum
    endoplasmic r.
    sarcoplasmic r.

retinal
    r. cerebellar hemangioblas-
        tomatosis

retinitis

retinopathy
    diabetic r.
    proliferative r.

retroauricular

retrogenic antigens

retrosternal thyroid

retrovascular goiter

Retroviridae

retrovirus
    BLV-HTLV r's
    mammalian type C r's

rev gene

rev protein

revaccination
    smallpox r.

reversal
  r. reaction
  sex r.

reverse
  r. anaphylaxis
  r. Arthus reaction
  r. genetics
  r. passive agglutination
  r. passive Arthus reaction
  r. passive hemagglutination
  r. T$_3$ (triiodothyronine)
  r. transcriptase
  r. transcriptase activity
  r. transcriptase polymerase
    chain reaction (RT-PCR)
  r. triiodothyronine (T$_3$)

reversion
  antigenic r.

Reye's syndrome

RF
  rheumatoid factor

Rh
  Rhesus
    Rh antibodies
    Rh antigen
    Rh blood group anti-
      gen
    Rh disease
    Rh factor
    Rh incompatibility
    Rh isoimmunization
    Rh sensitization
    Rh$_0$(D) immune globu-
      lin

rhabditic dermatitis

Rhabdoviridae

rhabdovirus

rhagiocrine cell

rheophoresis

Rhesus (Rh)
  R. factor
  R. incompatibility

rheumatic
  r. fever
  r. heart disease (RHD)
  r. nodules

rheumatism
  articular r., acute
  cerebral r.
  desert r.
  gonorrheal r.
  r. of the heart
  inflammatory r.

rheumatogenic group A streptococci

rheumatoid
  r. arthritis (RA)
  r. factor (RF)
  r. serum agglutinator

rhinallergosis

rhinitis
  allergic r.
  anaphylactic r.
  atopic r.
  nonseasonal r.
  nonseasonal allergic r.
  perennial r.
  seasonal r.
  seasonal allergic r.

rhinocerebral
  r. mucormycosis
  r. zygomycosis

Rhinocladiella
  R. aquaspersa

rhinoentomophthoromycosis

rhinofacial zygomycosis

rhinophycomycosis

rhinorrhea

rhinosporidiosis

Rhinosporidium seeberi

rhinoviral

Rhinovirus

rhinovirus

Rhizomucor

Rhizopus

rhodamine
r. dye

Rhodesian trypanosomiasis

Rhodococcus
R. bronchialis
R. equi

rhodopsin
r. desensitization
r. kinase
r. phosphorylation
r. signal transduction

Rhodotorula

rhythm
circadian r.
ultradian r.

RIA
radioimmunosorbent assay
radioimmunoassay

Ribas-Torres disease

ribonucleic acid (RNA)

ribonucleoprotein

ribovirus

rice-field fever

rice-water stools

ricin

rickettsemia

rickets

Rickettsia
R. akamushi
R. akari
R. australis
R. burnetii
R. canis
R. conorii
R. diaporica

Rickettsia (continued)
R. felis
R. honei
R. japonica
R. mooseri
R. muricola
R. nipponica
R. orientalis
R. pediculi
R. prowazekii
R. quintana
R. rickettsii
R. sennetsu
R. sibirica
R. tsutsugamushi
R. typhi
R. typhi (mooseri)
R. wolhynica

rickettsial disease

rickettsialpox

rickettsiosis

RID
radial immunodiffusion
RID test

Riedel
R. disease
R. struma
R. thyroiditis

Riesman's sign

Rift Valley fever virus

Riley-Day syndrome

ring
r. chromosome
Kayser-Fleischer r.
vaginal r's
Waldeyer's r.

ringworm
r. of the beard
black-dot r.
r. of the body
r. of the face
r. of the foot
gray-patch r.
r. of the groin

ringworm *(continued)*
    r. of the hand
    honeycomb r.
    r. of the nails
    Oriental r.
    r. of the scalp
    Tokelau r.

Rio Bravo virus

RIPA
    radioimmunoprecipitation
      assay

risk
    relative r.

RIST
    radioimmunosorbent test

risus
    r. caninus
    r. sardonicus

river blindness

RNA
    ribonucleic acid
      ambisense RNA
      complementary RNA
      DNA-like RNA
      double-stranded RNA
      heteronuclear RNA
      messenger RNA
      negative-sense RNA
      RNA oncogenic virus
      positive-sense RNA
      RNA splicing
      RNA virus
      virus-specific RNA

RNI
    reactive nitrogen interme-
      diate

RNP
    ribonucleoprotein
      RNP antigen

Ro antigen

Rochalimaea
    R. quintana

Rocio virus

rocket
    r. electrophoresis
    r. immunoelectrophoresis

Rocky Mountain
    R. M. spotted fever
    R. M. spotted fever vaccine

rod cell

ROI
    reactive oxygen intermedi-
      ate

rope sign

rose
    r. fever
    r. spots

Roseolovirus

rosette
    E r.
    EAC r.

rosetting

Rose-Waaler test

Rosewater's syndrome

Ross's bodies

Ross River virus

Rotavirus

RotaShield

rotaviral

rotavirus
    r. vaccine live oral

rotazyme

rouleaux
    r. formation

Rous sarcoma virus

route
    venereal r.

RRE sequence

rT3
    reverse triiodothyronine

rubella
  r. immunization
  r. and mumps virus vac-
    cine live
  r. syndrome
  r. vaccine
  r. virus
  r. virus vaccine live

rubeola
  r. vaccine

Rubivirus

Rubner's test

Rubrascan
  (for passive latex agglutina-
    tion test)

Rubulavirus

rudimentary
  r. testis
  r. testis syndrome

ruga *pl.* rugae
  vaginal rugae

rule
  12/23 r.

rupture
  defense r.

Russell
  R. dwarf
  R. dwarfism
  R. syndrome
  R.-Silver dwarfism
  R.-Silver syndrome

Russian
  R. influenza
  R. spring-summer encepha-
    litis virus

RVA
  rabies vaccine adsorbed

S

    S cells
    S gene
    S protein
    S value

Sabia virus

Sabin
    S. poliovirus vaccine
    S.-type vaccine
    S. vaccine
    S.-Feldman dye test

sac
    yolk s.

saccharimeter test

Saccharomyces
    S. cerevisiae
    S. fragilis

Saccharomycopsis

Saenger's macula

safety practices

St. Louis encephalitis
    St. L. e. virus

saline
    s. agglutinin
    s. antibody
    hypotonic s.
    phosphate-buffered s.
    s. suppression test

saliva

salivary
    s. gland disease
    s. gland system
    s. gland virus

Salk
    S.-type poliovirus vaccine
    S.-type vaccine
    S. vaccine

Salmonella
    S. abortus equi
    S. abortus ovis

Salmonella (continued)
    S. agona
    S. arizonae
    S. bongor
    S. brandenburg
    S. choleraesuis
    S. choleraesuis var. *kuzendorf*
    S. choleraesuis var. *typhisuis*
    S. dublin
    S. enteritidis
    S. enteritidis serotype *abortus equi*
    S. enteritidis serotype *abortus ovis*
    S. enteritidis serotype *agona*
    S. enteritidis serotype *dublin*
    S. enteritidis serotype *gallinarum*
    S. enteritidis serotype *heidelberg*
    S. enteritidis serotype *hirschfeldii*
    S. enteritidis serotype *infantis*
    S. enteritidis serotype *newport*
    S. enteritidis serotype *paratyphi A*
    S. enteritidis serotype *pullorum*
    S. enteritidis serotype *schottmuelleri*
    S. enteritidis serotype *sendai*
    S. enteritidis serotype *typhimurium*
    S. gallinarum
    S. heidelberg
    S. hirschfeldii
    S. houtenae
    S. infantis
    S. morgani
    S. newport
    S. paratyphi
    S. paratyphi A
    S. paratyphi B
    S. paratyphi C
    S. pullorum
    S. salamae

Salmonella (continued)
  S. schottmuelleri
  S. sendai
  S. suipestifer
  S. typhi
  S. typhi endotoxin
  S. typhimurium
  S. typhisuis
  S. typhosa

salmonella
  s. arthritis

salmonellosis

salt
  s. agglutination
  mineral s.'s

salvarsan

sandfly
  s. fever
  s. fever viruses
  s. fever-Naples virus
  s. fever-Sicilian virus

Sandhoff disease

Sandström
  S's bodies
  S's glands

sandwich
  s. assay
  s. ELISA
  s. radioimmunoassay
  s. test

sandworm disease

Sanfilippo syndrome

San Joaquin Valley disease

São Paulo typhus

sapronosis

sarcocystosis

sarcoidosis

sarcolemma

sarcoma
  Kaposi's s.

sarcoplasm

sarcoplasmic reticulum

sarcoptic

sarcoptidosis

sarcosporidiasis

sarcosporidiosis

sardonic
  s. laugh

satellite virus

satiation
  thirst s.

SC
  secretory component
  sickle cell
    SC disease
  suprachiasmatic
    SC nucleus

scabetic

scabies
  crusted s.
  Norwegian s.

scabietic

scale
  Gaffky s.

scan
  bone s.
  computed tomography s.
  CT s.
  thyroid s.

scanning
  bone s.
  duplex s.
  fluorescent s.
  isotopic bone s.

scarification test

scarlatina
  s. anginosa

scarlatinal

scarlatiniform

scarlatinoid

scarlet fever

SCAT
  sheep cell agglutination
    test

Scatchard analysis

scavenger
  s. cell
  s. receptor

scedosporiosis

Scedosporium

S cells

schedule
  infant immunization s.
  tuberculin testing s.

Scheie syndrome

Schick
  S. skin test
  S. test

Schilder's disease

Schistosoma mansoni

schistosome

schistosomiasis
  cutaneous s.
  eastern s.
  genitourinary s.
  s. haematobia
  hepatic s.
  s. intercalatum
  intestinal s.
  s. japonica
  Manson's s.
  s. mansoni
  Oriental s.
  pulmonary s.
  urinary s.
  vesical s.
  visceral s.

schistosomule

schistosomulum

Schizophyllum

schizophrenia

Schlepper

Schmidt
  S's syndrome

Schönlein-Henoch purpura

Schottmüller
  S's disease
  S's fever

Schrön-Much granules

Schüffner
  S's dots
  S's granules
  S's punctuation
  S's stippling

Schultz
  S.-Dale reaction
  S.-Dale technique

Schwartz
  S. leukemia virus
  S. measles virus vaccine
  S. strain (*of measles*)

SCID
  severe combined immuno-
    deficiency, severe com-
    bined immunodeficiency
    disease
      autosomal SCID
      SCID mouse
      X-linked SCID

scintigraphy

scintillation
  crystal s.

scintiscanning
  external s.

Sclavo's serum

scleredema adultorum

sclerodactyly

scleroderma

sclerosing thyroiditis

sclerosis
    multiple s.
    nodular s.
    progressive systemic s.
    systemic s.

SCO
    subcommissural organ

scoleciasis

scolex

Scopulariopsis

scopulariopsosis

scordinema

scratch
    s. skin test
    s. test

screening
    antibody s.
    family s.

scrofula

scrofuloderma

scrotum

scrub typhus

Scytalidium

SD
    sero-defined, serologically
        defined
            SD antigens

SDS
    sodium dodecyl sulfate
        SDS-PAGE (polyacryl-
            amide gel electropho-
            resis)

Seabright bantam syndrome

seasonal
    s. allergic rhinitis
    s. hay fever
    s. rhinitis

sebaceous glands

sebum

Seckel syndrome

second
    s. antigen
    s. messenger
    s. signal

secondary
    s. aldosteronism
    s. amenorrhea
    s. antibody affinity
    s. antibody interactions
    s. antibody response
    cell-mediated s. immune re-
        sponse
    s. coccidioidomycosis
    s. complications
    s. disease
    s. follicles
    s. hemochromatosis
    humoral s. immune re-
        sponse
    s. hyperaldosteronism
    s. hyperparathyroidism
    s. hypogonadism
    s. hypothyroidism
    s. immune response
    s. immunization
    s. immunodeficiency
    s. immunoglobulin defi-
        ciency
    s. impotence
    s. infection
    s. injection
    s. interaction
    s. lymphoid tissue
    s. myxedema
    s. nodule
    s. obesity
    s. osteoporosis
    s. response
    s. sex characters
    s. syphilis
    s. tuberculosis

second-set
    s.-s. graft rejection
    s.-s. phenomenon
    s.-s. reaction

second-set *(continued)*
  s.-s. rejection

secrete

secretin

secretion
  adrenaline s.
  adrenocorticotropic hor-
    mone s.
  androgen s.
  autocrine s.
  ectopic gastrin-releasing
    peptide s.
  estradiol s.
  external s.
  gastric acid s.
  gastrin s.
  hormone s.
  interleukin s.
  internal s.
  paracrine s.
  renin s.

secretoinhibitory

secretomotor
  s. control
  s. fibers

secretory
  s. cells
  s. component (SC)
  external s. system
  s. glands
  s. granules
  s. immunoglobulin (sIg)
  s. immunoglobulin A
  internal s. system
  s. isotype deficiencies
  s. piece
  s. system
  s. vesicles

section
  histologic s.
  stalk s.

sectioning
  thin s.

segment
  D (diversity) s's
  D (diversity) gene s's

segment *(continued)*
  framework s's
  gene s's
  J (joining) gene s's
  long terminal repeat s's
  rearranged gene s's
  V (variable) gene s's

segmental proportions

segregation
  mendelian s.

selected

selectin

selection
  clonal s.
  s. model
  negative s.
  positive s.
  s. process

selective
  s. IgA deficiency
  s. theory
  s. theory of antibody pro-
    duction

self

self-antigen
  sequestered s.-a's
  soluble s.-a's

self-infection

self-limiting

self-reactive
  s.-r. B cells

self-tolerance
  tolerance vs. s.-t.

sellar mass
  nonpituitary s. m.

sella turcica
  tomography of the s. t.

semen

semi-Lente insulin

seminal
  s. fluid

seminal *(continued)*
 s. fluid examination
 s. vesicle

seminiferous
 s. tubules
 s. tubule dysgenesis

seminoma

semiquantitative immunoassay

Semliki Forest virus

Semunya virus

Sendai virus

senescence

senile
 s. osteoporosis
 s. vaginitis

Sennetsu fever

sensibilization

sensitive

sensitivity
 anaphylactic-type s.
 contact s.
 ether s.
 gluten s.
 histamine s.
 nickel s.
 zirconium s.

sensitization
 antigen s.
 cytotoxic agent s.
 Rh s.

sensitized
 s. animal
 s. cell
 s. lymphocyte
 s. T lymphocyte

sensitizer

sensitizing
 s. antibody
 s. dose
 s. factor

sensory neuropathy

sentinel gland

Seoul virus

separation methods

Sepik virus

sepsis
 s. lenta

septan

septic
 s. arthritis
 s. necrosis
 s. shock

septicemia
 morphine injector's s.
 neonatal s.
 plague s.

septicemic plague

septo-optic dysplasia

sequela *pl.* sequelae
 neurologic sequelae
 postpolio s.
 postpoliomyelitis s.

sequence
 amino acid s.
 DNA s.
 intervening s's
 leader s.
 long terminal repeat s's
 s. motif
 recognition s.
 recombination signal s's
 RRE s.
 signal s.

sequential determinant

sequestered
 s. antigens
 s. antigen theory
 s. self-antigens

sera *(plural of* serum)

Sergent's white adrenal line

series
    lymphocyte s.
    lymphocytic s.
    monocyte s.
    monocytic s.
    plasmacyte s.
    plasmacytic s.

serine
    s. esterase
    s. protease

seroconversion
    HIV s.

seroconvert

sero-defined (SD)
    s. antigens

serodiagnosis

serodiagnostic

seroepidemiologic

seroflocculation

serogroup

serologic
    s. assay
    s. reaction
    s. test

serological

serologically defined (SD)
    s. d. antigens

serologist

serology
    diagnostic s.
    Mycoplasma s.

serolysin

seronegative

seronegativity

seropositive

seropositivity

seroprognosis

seroreaction

serorelapse

seroresistance

seroresistant

seroreversal

seroreversion

serositis

serotherapy

serotonin

serotoninergic
    s. pathways

serotype

serovaccination

serpiginous chancroid

Serratia
    S. liquefaciens
    S. marcescens
    S. odorifera

Sertoli
    S. cell
    S.-cell–only syndrome
    S. cell tumor
    S.-Leydig cell tumor

serum *pl.* serums, sera
    active s.
    s. amyloid protein
    s. antibodies
    anticomplementary s.
    antilymphocyte s. (ALS)
    antipneumococcus s.
    antirabies s.
    antitetanic s. (ATS)
    antitoxic s.
    bacteriolytic s.
    s. calcium
    s. complement
    convalescence s.
    convalescent s.
    convalescents' s.
    convalescent human s.

serum *(continued)*
  despeciated s.
  s. disease
  s. electrolyte
  s. electrophoresis
  foreign s.
  s. globulins
  s. growth hormone
  s. hepatitis
  s. hepatitis antigen
  heterologous s.
  homologous s.
  human s. factor
  hyperimmune s.
  immune s.
  inactivated s.
  leukocyte typing s.
  s. lipids
  lymphatolytic s.
  monovalent s.
  s. neutralization test
  normal s.
  s. osmolality
  s. paralysis
  s. peptide
  polyvalent s.
  pooled s.
  pregnancy s.
  s. protein
  s. reaction
  Sclavo's s.
  s. shock
  s. sickness
  s. sickness–like reaction
  s. sickness–like syndrome
  s. sickness syndrome
  specific s.
  s. therapy

seven-day fever

seven-up gene

severe
  s. combined immunodefi-
    ciency (SCID)
  s. combined immunodefi-
    ciency disease (SCID)
  s. combined immunodefi-
    cient mouse

severe *(continued)*
  s. diabetes
  X-linked s. combined immu-
    nodeficiency

sex
  s. chromosome
  s. cord neoplasm
  s. determination
  s. differentiation
  endocrinologic s.
  genital s.
  gonadal s.
  s. mesenchyma
  morphological s.
  phenotypic s.
  s. reassignment
  s. reversal
  s. steroid
  s. steroid–binding globulin
  somatic s.
  s. therapy

sex hormone
  s. h.–binding globulin
    (SHBG)
  female s. h.
  male s. h.

sex-linked
  s.-l. lymphopenic immuno-
    logic deficiency

sextan

sexual
  s. abuse
  s. behavior
  s. characteristics
  s. development
  s. differentiation
  s. dimorphism
  s. dwarf
  s. dysfunction
  s. function
  s. infantilism
  s. precocity
  s. reproduction

sexually transmitted disease

Sézary syndrome

SFO
    subfornical organ
S gene
SH
    serum hepatitis
        SH antigen
shared antigen
SHBG
    sex hormone–binding glob-
    ulin
SH3 domain
sheath
    myelin s.
    periarteriolar lymphatic s.
Sheehan's syndrome
sheep
    s. blood cell receptor
    s. cell agglutination
    s. cell agglutination test
    (SCAT)
    s. red blood cell receptor
sheet
    beta s's
shift
    antigen s.
    antigenic s.
Shigella
    S. ambigua
    *S. arabinotarda (types A and
    B)*
    S. boydii
    S. ceylonensis
    S. dysenteriae
    S. etousae
    S. flexneri
    S. newcastle
    S. paradysenteriae
    S. parashigae
    S. schmitzii
    S. shigae
    S. sonnei
shigellosis

shimamushi disease
shin bone fever
shingles
ship fever
shock
    anaphylactic s.
    anaphylactoid s.
    s. antigen
    endotoxic s.
    hemodynamic s.
    histamine s.
    hypoglycemic s.
    insulin s.
    s. organ
    septic s.
    serum s.
    s. tissue
Shohl solution
shop typhus
short
    s.-acting antiestrogen
    s. adrenocorticotropic hor-
        mone test
    s. consensus repeat (SCR)
    s.-incubation hepatitis
    s. stature
SHP phosphate
Shwartzman reaction
Shy-Drager syndrome
SIADH
    syndrome of inappropriate
        antidiuretic hormone
sialic acid
sialoprotein
Sialyl-Lewis X
    sulfated S.-L. X
Siberian tick typhus
sick euthyroid syndrome

sickle cell (SC)
    s. c. anemia
    s. c. disease

sickness
    serum s.
    serum s. syndrome
    sleeping s.

side-chain
    s.-c. cleavage defect
    s.-c. hypothesis
    s.-c. theory

siderating plague

siderophage

siderophore

SIF
    small, intensely fluorescent
        SIF cells

SIG
    specific immune serum
        globulin

sIg
    secretory immunoglobulin
    surface immunoglobulin

sign
    Abadie's s.
    Arroyo's s.
    Becker's s.
    Biederman's s.
    Boston's s.
    clavicular s.
    Cowen's s.
    Dalrymple's s.
    Darier s.
    Dixon Mann's s.
    Enroth's s.
    Filipovitch's s.
    Filipowicz's s.
    Graefe's s.
    Griffith's s.
    Higouménaki's s.
    Jendrassik's s.
    Knies' s.
    Kocher's s.

sign *(continued)*
    Koplik's s.
    Liddle s.
    Mann's s.
    Marfan's s.
    Marie's s.
    Mean's s.
    Mirchamp's s.
    Möbius' (Moebius') s.
    palmoplantar s.
    Pastia's s.
    Pemberton's s.
    Plummer's s.
    pseudo–Graefe's s.
    Riesman's s.
    rope s.
    Snellen's s.
    spine s.
    Stellwag's s.
    Suker's s.
    Thomson's s.
    Tresilian's s.
    von Graefe's s.
    Widowitz's s.
    Wilder's s.

signal
    costimulatory s's
    s. events
    s. hypothesis
    s. joint
    s. peptidase
    s. peptide
    receptor s's
    s. recognition
    s. recognition particle com-
        plex
    second s.
    s. sequence
    s. transducer
    s. transducers and activa-
        tors of transcription
        (STAT)
    s. transduction

signaling
    cell s.

silencer

silent
  s. carrier
  s. thyroiditis

Silver
  S. dwarf
  S's syndrome
  S.-Russell dwarfism
  S.-Russell syndrome

Silvestrini-Corda syndrome

Simbu
  S. group virus
  S. virus

simian
  s. immunodeficiency virus
    (SIV)
  s. virus 40 (SV40)

Simmonds
  S's disease
  S's syndrome

simple goiter

Simplexvirus

Sindbis
  S. fever
  S. virus

single
  s. chain Fv (fragment vari-
    able)
  s. diffusion
  s.-positive thymocyte
  s. radial diffusion
  s. radial immunodiffusion
    (SRID)

singlet oxygen

Sin Nombre virus

sinus
  carotid s.
  urogenital s.

sinusitis

Sipple's syndrome

site
  antibody s.
  antiestrogen binding s.
  antigen-binding s.
  antigen-combining s.
  antigen determinant s's
  combining s.
  immunologically privileged
    s's
  pseudosubstrate s.
  restriction s's
  triphenylethylene anties-
    trogen binding s. (TABS)

SIV
  simian immunodeficiency
    virus

size
  cell surface s.

Sjögren
  S's disease
  S's syndrome

skeletal
  s. age
  s. dysplasia
  s. growth
  s. growth factor
  s. mass
  s. modeling
  s. muscle
  s. remodeling
  s. system

skeleton

skin
  s. graft
  s. reaction
  s. reactive factor (SRF)
  s. testing
  s. window
  s. window test

skinfold measurement

skin graft
  s. g. experiment
  s. g. rejection

skin test
  Brucellergin s. t.
  coccidioidin s. t.
  delayed hypersensitivity
    s. t.
  Frei s. t.
  histoplasmin s. t.
  intradermal s. t.
  lymphogranuloma vene-
    reum s. t.
  patch s. t.
  pork trichina s. t.
  purified protein derivative
    (PPD) s. t.
  s. t. response
  Schick s. t.
  scratch s. t.
  toxoplasmin s. t.
  Trichinella spiralis s. t.
  tuberculin s. t.
  Vollmer's patch s. t.

Sklowsky's symptom

skull
  s. x-ray

SLE
  systemic lupus erythemato-
    sus

sleep

sleeping sickness

slime fever

slow
  s.-reacting substance of
    anaphylaxis (SRS-A)
  s. virus

SMA-12

small
  s. cleaved cell
  s. granule cells
  s. lymphocyte
  s. noncleaved cell
  s. pre-B cell
  s. uncleaved cell

smallpox
  s. complications

smallpox *(continued)*
  congenital s.
  flat s.
  fulminant s.
  hemorrhagic s.
  s. immunity
  s. incubation period
  s. inoculation
  malignant s.
  modified s.
  ordinary s.
  s. revaccination
  s. transmission
  s. vaccination
  s. vaccine
  s. virus

Sm antigen

smcy gene

smear
  buccal s.

Smith antibody

smoking

smooth muscle
  vascular s. m.

snake venom

Snellen's sign

sodium
  s. absorption
  s. alkali
  s. cellulose
  s. depletion
  s. deoxycholate
  s. diuresis
  s. dodecyl sulfate (SDS)
  s. escape
  s. iopanoate
  s. ipodate
  s. reabsorption

sodoku

soft
  s. chancre
  s. sore
  s. ulcer

sol
  s. particle
  s. particle immunassay
    (SPIA)

solid
  s. edema
  s. phase radioimmunoas-
    say

solitary myeloma

soluble
  s. antigen
  s. immune response sup-
    pressor
  s. mediator
  s. protein mediator
  s. self-antigens

solute
  s. permeability

solution
  compound iodine s.
  Lugol's s.
  Shohl s.
  strong iodine s.

somatic
  s. agglutinin
  s. antigens
  s. cell fusion
  s. diversification theory
  s. hypermutation
  s. mutation theory of anti-
    body production
  s. recombination
  s. sex

somatocrinin

somatoliberin

somatomammotropin
  chorionic s.
  human chorionic s. (hCS)

somatomedin
  s. A
  s. C
  s. hypothesis

somatomegaly

somatosexual

somatostatin
  s. cells

somatostatinoma

somatotrope
  s. adenoma
  s. cell
  s. hyperplasia

somatotroph
  s. adenoma
  s. cell

somatotrophic
  s. hormone

somatotrophin

somatotropic
  s. cell
  s. hormone

somatotropin
  s. release–inhibiting factor
    (SRIF)
  s. release–inhibiting hor-
    mone
  s.-releasing hormone

somatotropinoma

somatropin

somnolence

Somogyi
  S. effect
  S. phenomenon

SON
  supraoptic nucleus

Songo fever

sore
  cold s.
  hard s.
  mixed s.
  soft s.
  venereal s.

sor gene

Sorghum

sorter
  fluorescence-activated
    cell s. (FACS)

sorting
  fluorescence-activated cell
    s. (FACS)

Sotos' syndrome

South African tickbite fever

South American
  S. A. blastomycosis
  S. A. trypanosomiasis

Southern
  S. blot
  S. blot hybridization
  S. blot immunoassay
  S. blotting
  S. transfer

sowdah

soybean
  s. products

SP-40,40

SpA
  staphylococcal protein A

space
  lymphatic s's

spade hand

Spanish influenza

spare receptors

sparganosis

spasm
  canine s.
  cynic s.

species
  concordant s.
  discordant s.
  s. immunity
  s.-specific antigens

specific
  s. bactericide

specific (continued)
  s. immune globulin
  s. immune serum globulin
    (SIG)
  s. immunity
  s. polysaccharides
  s. serum
  s. staining
  s. urethritis

specificity
  antibody s.
  antigenic s.
  hormonal s.
  host s.
  private s.
  public s.
  receptor s.
  s. spillover

spectrophotometry
  dual-beam x-ray s.

Spengler's fragments

sperm
  s.-immobilizing antibody

spermatogenesis

spermatolysin

spermatotoxin

spermatozoon pl. spermatozoa

spermatoxin

spermicidal
  s. agent

spermolysin

spermotoxin

spherulin

sphingolipid

sphingolipidosis

SPIA
  sol particle immunoassay

spillover
  specificity s.

spinal
  s. cord
  s. cord damage
  s. cord injury
  s. paralytic poliomyelitis

spine sign

spirillemia

spirillosis

Spirillum
  S. minus

spirillum *pl.* spirilla
  s. fever

Spirochaeta

spirochete

spirochetal jaundice

spirochetemia

spirochetogenous

spirochetosis
  s. arthritica

spirocheturia

spironolactone

spleen
  s. index
  s. removal

splenectomy

splenic
  s. fever
  s. index

splenocyte

splenolysin

splenomegaly
  infectious s.
  infective s.

splenometric index

spliceome

splicing
  RNA s.

split
  s. tolerance
  s.-virus vaccine

Spondweni virus

spondylitis
  ankylosing s.

spongiocyte

spontaneous
  s. allergy
  s. autoimmune disease
  s. cretinism
  s. phagocytosis

sporadic
  s. cretinism
  s. goitrous cretinism
  s. nongoitrous cretinism

spore

Sporobolomyces

Sporothrix
  S. schenckii

sporotrichin

sporotrichosis

sporotrichotic

sporozoa (*plural of* sporozoon)

sporozoan

sporozoite

sporozoon *pl.* sporozoa

sporozoosis

spot
  Christopher's s's
  Forschheimer s's
  Koplik's s's
  Maurer's s's
  rose s's
  Stephen's s's
  typhoid s's

spotted fever

spreading
  epitope s.

spreading *(continued)*
    s. factor

S protein

Spumavirus

spumavirus

spurious hermaphroditism

spurt
    adolescent growth s.
    pubertal growth s.

squamous epithelium

SR
    stimulation ratio

src oncogene

SRE
    steroid response element

SRF
    skin reactive factor

SRID
    single radial immunodiffu-
      sion

SRIF
    somatotropin release–
      inhibiting factor

SRS-A
    slow-reacting substance of
      anaphylaxis

SS-A antigen

SS-B antigen

SSP
    subacute sclerosing panen-
      cephalitis

stabile
    heat s.

stability
    peptide s.

stage
    s. I thymocyte
    s. II thymocyte
    s. III thymocyte

stage *(continued)*
    amphibolic s.
    incubative s.
    latency s.
    preeruptive s.
    prodromal s.
    Ranke's s's
    stepladder s.
    Tanner s's

stain
    Lugol's iodine s.
    Wright's s.

staining
    immunohistochemical s.
    negative s.
    nonspecific s.
    phosphotungstic acid nega-
      tive s.
    specific s.

stalk
    hypophysial s.
    infundibular s.
    neural s.
    pituitary s.
    s. section

stanolone

staphylococcal
    s. bacteriophage lysate
    s. enterotoxin
    s. parotitis
    s. protein A (SpA)
    s. toxin
    s. toxoid

staphylococcemia

staphylococci *(plural of* staphy-
    lococcus)

staphylococcosis

Staphylococcus
    S. albus
    S. aureus
    S. aureus enterotoxin
    S. aureus esterase
    S. epidermidis
    S. haemolyticus
    S. hominis

Staphylococcus (continued)
    S. hyicus
    S. pyogenes
    S. saprophyticus
    S. simulans

staphylococcus *pl.* staphylococci
    avirulent s.
    pathogenic s.
    virulent s.

staphylolysin
    α s.
    alpha s.
    β s.
    beta s.
    δ s.
    delta s.
    ε s.
    epsilon s.
    γ s.
    gamma s.

starch

starvation
    accelerated s.

stasis

STAT
    signal transducers and acti-
        vators of transcription
        STAT-6

state
    carrier s.

station test

statistical mechanical hypothe-
    sis

stature
    adult s. prediction
    constitutional short s.
    hereditary short s.
    short s.
    tall s.

status
    immune s.

Staub
    S.-Traugott effect

Staub *(continued)*
    S.-Traugott phenomenon

steady-state
    s.-s. viral infection

Steel factor

Stein-Leventhal syndrome

Stellwag's sign

stem
    s. bromelain
    infundibular s.

stem cell
    s. c. deficiency
    s. c. factor (SCF)
    hematopoietic s. c.
    hemopoietic s. c.
    lymphoid s. c.
    multiple s. c. (MSC)
    multipotential s. c.
    peripheral blood s. c's
    pluripotent s. c.
    primitive s. c.

Stenotrophomonas

Stephen's spots

stepladder stage

steric hindrance

sterile
    s. immunity

sterilization
    Quinacrine s.

steroid
    adrenal cortical s.
    adrenocortical s.
    s. affinity chromatography
    anabolic s.
    s. diabetes
    gonadal s.
    s. hormones
    s. hormone antagonism
    s. hormone receptor
    ovarian s.
    s. receptor
    s. response element (SRE)
    sex s.

steroid *(continued)*
  s.-site activation

steroidogenesis

steroidogenic
  s. diabetes

Sticker's disease

stilbestrol

Still-Chauffard syndrome

stimulation
  autocrine s.
  s. index
  s. ratio (SR)
  T cell s.
  s. test

stimulator
  human thyroid adenylate
    cyclase s's (HTACS)
  long-acting thyroid s.
    (LATS)

stimulatory
  s. hypersensitivity

stimulon

stimulus *pl.* stimuli
  immunogenic stimuli
  osmotic stimuli

sting
  insect s.

stippling
  malarial s.
  Maurer's s.
  Schüffner's s.

stochastic model

stomach

stomatomycosis

stone
  kidney s.
  renal s.

stool
  caddy s.

stool *(continued)*
  pea soup s.
  rice-water s's

storage
  insulin s.

storm
  thyroid s.
  thyrotoxic s.

strain
  congenic resistant s's
  Edmonston s. (*of measles*)
  El Tor s. (*of Vibrio chol-
    erae*)
  inbred mouse s.
  Moraten s. (*of measles*)
  recombinant s's
  recombinant inbred s's
  Schwartz s. (*of measles*)

streak gonads

street virus

streptavidin

strepticemia

Streptobacillus
  S. moniliformis

streptocerciasis

streptococcal
  s. antibody
  s. antigen cross reactivity
  s. enterotoxin
  s. infection
  s. pharyngitis
  s. skin infection
  s. upper respiratory infec-
    tion

streptococcemia

streptococci (*plural of* streptococcus)

streptococcosis

Streptococcus
  S. acidominimus

Streptococcus (continued)
  S. agalactiae
  S. anaerobius
  S. anginosus
  S. avium
  S. bovis
  S. cremoris
  S. epidemicus
  S. equi
  S. equinus
  S. equisimilis
  S. erysipelatis
  S. faecalis
  S. faecium
  S. foetidus
  S. hemolyticus
  S. lacticus
  S. lactis
  S. lanceolatus
  S. mastitidis
  S. micros
  S. mitis
  S. mutans
  S. pneumoniae
  S. pyogenes
  S. salivarius
  S. sanguis
  S. scarlatinae
  S. suis
  S. thermophilus
  S. uberis
  S. viridans
  S. zooepidemicus
streptococcus *pl.* streptococci
  group A streptococci
  s. MG agglutinin
streptokinase
  s.-streptodornase
streptolysin
  s. O
  s. S
Streptomyces
  S. paraguayensis
  S. somaliensis
streptomycin
  s.-resistant gonococci

streptomycosis

streptosepticemia

streptozyme test

stress
  s. hyperglycemia
  s. hypertension
  s. reaction

striated muscle

stroke

stroma *pl.* stromata
  s. glandulae thyroideae
  ovarian s.
  thymic s.
  s. of thyroid gland

stromal
  s. hyperplasia
  s. tumor
  testicular s. tumor

strong iodine solution

Strongyloides stercoralis

strongyloidiasis
  intestinal s.
  pulmonary s.

structure
  antigenic s.
  arsonate group s.
  bone s.
  carboxylate group s.
  four-peptide s.
  hairpin s's
  HIV s.
  isotype s.
  polypeptide s's
  thyroid s.

struma
  s. aberrata
  cast iron s.
  s. colloides
  s. endothoracica
  s. fibrosa
  s. follicularis

struma *(continued)*
 s. gelatinosa
 Hashimoto's s.
 ligneous s.
 s. lymphomatosa
 s. nodosa
 s. parenchymatosa
 Riedel s.

strumectomy
 median s.

strumitis

Strümpell's disease

study
 immunologic s's
 population s.

subacute
 s. granulomatous thyroiditis
 s. inguinal poradenitis
 s. lymphocytic thyroiditis
 s. sclerosing panencephalitis (SSP)
 s. spongiform encephalopathy
 s. thyroiditis

subclass
 immunoglobulin s's

subclinical
 s. diabetes
 s. hypothyroidism
 s. infection

subcommissural organ (SCO)

subcutaneous
 s. fungus
 s. phycomycosis
 s. zygomycosis

subfornical organ (SFO)

sublymphemia

subnormal intelligence

subperiosteal resorption of the
 middle phalanx

subpopulation
 T cell s.

subset
 helper/inducer s.
 T cell s.

substance
 blood group s's
 depressor s.
 ground s.
 H s.
 s. K
 müllerian inhibiting s.
 s. P
 precursor s.
 pressor s.
 slow-reacting s. of anaphylaxis (SRS-A)
 vasoactive s's

substernal
 s. goiter
 s. thyroid

substitution therapy

substrate
 s. cycling
 insulin receptor s.-1
 renin s.

subtilisin

subtractive hybridization

subtype
 thymocyte s's

subunit
 alpha s.
 beta s.
 s. vaccine

subventricular nucleus

subvirion vaccine

successful pathogen

suckling reflex

sucrose
 s. density gradient ultracentrifugation
 s. polyester

sudanophobic
    s. unit
    s. zone

suffocative goiter

sugar
    blood s. (glucose)
    chlorinated s.
    diabetic s.
    fasting blood s. (FBS)
    s. test
    threshold s.

Suker's sign

sulfanilamide

sulfatase
    placental s.

sulfate
    sodium dodecyl s. (SDS)

sulfated Sialyl-Lewis X

sulfation factors

sulfonamide

sulfonylurea

sulfotransferase

sulfur granules

Sulzberger-Chase phenomenon

sunlight

superantigen
    bacterial s.
    s.-binding T cells
    endogenous viral s.
    Epstein-Barr virus s.

superfamily
    immunoglobulin s.
    transmembrane receptor s.

supergroup

superinfection

superior
    s. border of adrenal gland
    s. border of body of pan-
        creas

superior (continued)
    s. border of pancreas
    s. border of suprarenal
        gland
    s. margin of adrenal
        gland
    s. margin of suprarenal
        gland

supernatant

superoxide
    s. anion
    s. dismutase

supersensitization

supplementation
    potassium s.

supporting medium
    agar gel
    starch
    Whatman paper

suppression
    pituitary-adrenal s.
    s. test

suppressor
    s. cells
    s. gene
    s. lymphocyte
    soluble immune re-
        sponse s.
    s. T cells

suprachiasmatic nucleus (SC)

suprahyoid thyroid

supraoptic
    s. crest
    s. nucleus (SON)

suprarenal
    accessory s. glands
    s. body
    s. capsule
    s. cortex
    s. gland
    s. medulla
    s. rests

suprarenalectomy

suprarenalism

suprarenalopathy

suprarenogenic

suprarenopathy

suprarenotropic

suprasellar cyst

surface
  activator s.'s
  anterior s. of adrenal gland
  anterior s. of pancreas
  anterior s. of suprarenal
    gland
  anteroinferior s. of body of
    pancreas
  anterosuperior s. of body
    of pancreas
  s. antigen
  s. epithelium
  s. immunoglobulin (sIg)
  s. macrophage
  s. marker
  s. molecules
  s. monocyte
  mucosal s.'s
  s. phagocytosis
  posterior s. of adrenal
    gland
  posterior s. of body of pan-
    creas
  posterior s. of suprarenal
    gland
  renal s. of adrenal gland
  renal s. of suprarenal gland

surfactant
  s. protein A
  s. protein D

surgery
  transsphenoidal s.

surgical
  s. abortion
  s. tuberculosis

surrogate
  s. light chains
  s. testing

surveillance
  immune s.
  immunologic s.
  immunological s.

susceptibility
  Mycobacterium s.

sushi domain

suspension
  virus s.

Suttonella
  S. indologenes

SV40
  simian virus 40

S value

swamp fever

sweat
  s. glands
  night s.

swelling
  Calabar s.'s
  cloudy s.
  Kamerun s.'s
  tropical s.'s

swine influenza virus

Swiss-type agammaglobulinemia

switch
  class s.
  isotype s.
  s. recombination
  s. regions

switching
  class s.
  isotype s.

Swyer syndrome

Syk kinase

sylvatic plague

Sylvest's disease

symbiosis
    bacteria s. with viruses

Symmers' fibrosis

symmetrical peripheral poly-
    neuropathy

sympathetic
    s. blockers
    s. nervous system
    s. nerve ending storage
        pools
    s. ophthalmia
    s. stress reaction

sympathoadrenal
    s. system

sympathoblast

sympathogonium *pl.* sympatho-
gonia

sympathomimetic
    s. amines

symptom
    Castellani-Low s.
    Colliver's s.
    deficiency s.
    gastrointestinal s.
    Sklowsky's s.

symptomatic
    s. dwarfism

symptothermal
    s. method of natural family
        planning

synalbumin

synapse

synaptic
    s. cleft
    s. vesicles

Syncephalastrum

syncytiolysin

syncytiotoxin

syncytium

syndrome
    Achard-Thiers s.
    acquired immune deficien-
        cy s. (AIDS)
    acquired immunodeficien-
        cy s. (AIDS)
    acro-osteolysis s.
    addisonian s.
    adiposogenital s.
    adrenogenital s.
    Albers-Schönberg s.
    Aldrich's s.
    Alström s.
    androgen insensitivity s.
    apparent hyperprolactine-
        mia s.
    Asherman s.
    ataxia-telangiectasia s.
    autoimmune polyendo-
        crine-candidiasis s.
    autoimmune polyglandu-
        lar s.
    Babinski-Fröhlich s.
    Bannwarth's s.
    bare lymphocyte s.
    Bartter's s.
    Beckwith s.
    Beckwith-Wiedemann s.
    Bernard-Sergent s.
    Bloom s.
    Bonnevie-Ullrich s.
    brittle bone s.
    bronchial carcinoid s's
    Buckley's s.
    candidiasis endocrinopa-
        thy s.
    carcinoid s.
    Carpenter s.
    Chauffard's s.
    Chauffard-Still s.
    Chédiak-Higashi s.
    Chiari-Frommel syndome
    chronic diarrheal s.
    chronic fatigue s.
    Churg-Strauss s.

syndrome *(continued)*
 Cockayne s.
 Cohen s.
 cold agglutinin s.
 congenital rubella s.
 Conn's s.
 cortisol hyperreactive s.
 CREST s.
 Cushing's s.
 Cushing's s. medicamento-
  sus
 de Lange s.
 del Castillo's s.
 de Morsier's s.
 dengue shock s.
 maternal deprivation s.
 diabetes insipidus–like s.
 diabetic foot s.
 diarrheogenic s.
 DIDMOAD s.
 diencephalic s.
 DiGeorge s.
 Down s.
 Drash s.
 Dressler's s.
 Duncan's s.
 ectopic ACTH s.
 ectopic corticotropin-releasing hormone s.
 Ellis-van Creveld s.
 embryonic testicular re-
  gression s.
 empty sella s.
 epiphyseal s.
 euthyroid sick s.
 excited skin s.
 familial medullary thyroid
  carcinoma–pheochromo-
  cytoma s.
 Fanconi s.
 feminizing testes s.
 fertile eunuch s.
 Fitz-Hugh–Curtis s.
 Forbes-Albright s.
 fragile X s.
 Fraser s.
 Fröhlich's s.
 functional prepubertal cas-
  trate s.

syndrome *(continued)*
 galactorrhea-amenorrhea s.
 gastric carcinoid s's
 gay bowel s.
 genital ulcer s.
 Gitelman's s.
 glucagonoma s.
 Good's s.
 Goodpasture's s.
 Gordon's s.
 Guillain-Barré s.
 Hajdu-Cheney s.
 hantavirus pulmonary s.
 Harris' s.
 hemophagocytic s.
 Hoffman s.
 hungry bone s.
 Hunter s.
 Hurler s.
 Hutchinson-Gilford s.
 17-hydroxylase deficien-
  cy s.
 hyperdynamic β-adrenerg-
  ic s.
 hypereosinophilic s's
 hyper-IgM s.
 hyperimmunoglobulinemia
  E s.
 hyperimmunoglobulin E s.
  (HIE)
 hyperimmunoglobulin M
  (hyper-IgM) s.
 hyperviscosity s.
 hypotonic s's
 iatrogenic Cushing's s.
 idiopathic postprandial s.
 immobile cilia s.
 immunoendocrinopathy s.
 s. of inappropriate antidiuretic hormone (SIADH)
 s. of inappropriate somatotropin secretion
 inferior s. of red nucleus
 inhibitory s.
 Job's s.
 Kallmann's s.
 Kearns-Sayre s.
 Klinefelter's s.
 Kocher-Debré-Sémélaigne s.

syndrome *(continued)*
    Laron s.
    Launois' s.
    Laurence-Moon-Bardet-
      Biedl s.
    lazy leukocyte s.
    Lesch-Nyhan s.
    Lorain-Lévi s.
    Louis-Bar's s.
    low T_3 (triiodothyronine) s.
    lupus erythematosus–
      like s.
    lymphadenopathy s.
    lymphoproliferative s.
    McCune-Albright s.
    malabsorption s.
    Marfan's s.
    Maroteaux-Lamy s.
    maternal deprivation s.
    Mauriac s.
    menopausal s.
    milk-alkali s.
    Morquio s.
    Morris s.
    mucosal neuroma s.
    multiple endocrine defi-
      ciency s.
    multiple glandular deficien-
      cy s.
    myasthenic s.
    Nelson's s.
    nephritic s.
    nephrotic s.
    neutrophil dysfunction s.
    Nezelof s.
    Noonan's s.
    obstructive sleep apnea s.
    overlap s.
    pancreatic cholera s.
    paraneoplastic s.
    Parinaud s.
    Pellizzi's s.
    Pendred's s.
    persistent estrus s.
    persistent müllerian duct s.
    pertussis s.
    pertussis-like s.
    Peutz-Jeghers s.
    pharyngeal pouch s.

syndrome *(continued)*
    phosphate deficiency s.
    Picchini's s.
    pickwickian s.
    pineal s.
    pituitary isolation s.
    POEMS s.
    polycystic ovary s. (PCOS)
    polyglandular autoimmune
      s's
    postcardiotomy s.
    post–myocardial infarc-
      tion s.
    postpartum thyroiditis s.
    postperfusion s.
    postpoliomyelitis s.
    posttransfusion s.
    Prader-Willi s.
    premenstrual s. (PMS)
    premenstrual tension s.
    pseudo–Cushing's s.
    pseudo–Turner s.
    psychosocial deprivation s.
    Purtilo's s.
    Rabson-Mendenhall s.
    Reifenstein's s.
    Reiter's s.
    respiratory distress s.
    Reye's s.
    Riley-Day s.
    Rosewater's s.
    rubella s.
    rudimentary testis s.
    Russell s.
    Russell-Silver s.
    Sanfilippo s.
    Scheie s.
    Schmidt's s.
    Seabright bantam s.
    Seckel s.
    Sertoli-cell–only s.
    serum sickness s.
    serum sickness–like s.
    Sézary s.
    Sheehan's s.
    Shy-Drager s.
    sick euthyroid s.
    Silver's s.

syndrome *(continued)*
    Silver-Russell s.
    Silvestrini-Corda s.
    Simmonds' s.
    Sipple's s.
    Sjögren's s.
    Sotos' s.
    Stein-Leventhal s.
    Still-Chauffard s.
    Swyer s.
    testicular feminization s.
    toxic shock s.
    Turner s.
    Ullrich s.
    vanishing testes s.
    Verner-Morrison s.
    wasting s.
    Waterhouse-Friderichsen s.
    watery diarrhea s.
    WDHA s.
    WDHH s.
    Weil's s.
    Wermer's s.
    Wernicke-Korsakoff s.
    Wiskott-Aldrich s.
    Wolfram s.
    X-linked hyper IgM s.
    X-linked lymphoprolifera-
      tive s.
    XX male s.
    XXY s.
    Zahorsky's s.
    Zollinger-Ellison s.

synergism

synergistic

syngeneic
    s. graft
    s. mouse
    s. transplantation

syngenesioplastic
    s. transplantation

syngenesiotransplantation

syngraft

synovitis

synthase
    fatty acid s.

synthesis
    acetylcholine s.
    adrenaline s.
    aldosterone s.
    antibody s.
    catecholamine s.
    fatty acid s.
    hemoglobin s.
    hormone s.
    humoral s.
    insulin s.
    protein s.

synthetase
    prostaglandin s.

synthetic
    s. antigen
    s. steroid
    s. vaccine

syphilis
    congenital s.
    early s.
    early latent s.
    endemic s.
    gummatous s.
    late s.
    late benign s.
    late latent s.
    latent s.
    nonvenereal s.
    primary s.
    rabbit s.
    secondary s.
    tertiary s.

syphilitic
    s. bubo
    s. necrosis
    s. reagin

syphiloma

system
    ABO blood group s.
    adrenergic nervous s.
    alimentary s.
    aminergic nervous s.

system *(continued)*
    APUD s.
    biological amplification s's
    biological insulin delivery s.
    cardiovascular s.
    CD s.
    central nervous s. (CNS)
    chromaffin s.
    closed-loop glycemic insulin delivery s.
    complement s.
    cutaneous immune s.
    dopaminergic s.
    endocrine s.
    endothelial s.
    enteric nervous s.
    external secretory s.
    gastrointestinal s.
    glucose transport s.
    H-2 antigen s.
    hematopoietic s.
    HLA s.
    host immune s's
    humoral amplification s's
    hypophyseal portal s.
    hypophyseoportal s.
    hypophysioportal s.
    hypothalamic hypophysial portal s.
    hypothalamic-pituitary s.
    hypothalamic-pituitary portal s.
    hypothalamo-hypophysial portal s.
    immune s.
    implanted biological insulin delivery s.
    internal secretory s.
    kinin s.
    lymphatic s.
    lymphoid s.
    lymphoreticular s.
    macrophage s.

system *(continued)*
    mononuclear phagocyte s. (MPS)
    mucosal immune s.
    musculoskeletal s.
    nervous s.
    neuroendocrine s.
    parasympathetic nervous s.
    P1 bacteriophage recombination s.
    peptidergic nervous s.
    pituitary portal s.
    prolactin receptor s.
    properdin s.
    receptor-effector s.
    renin-angiotensin s.
    renin-angiotensin-aldosterone s.
    reproductive s.
    respiratory s.
    reticuloendothelial s. (RES)
    salivary gland s.
    secretory s.
    skeletal s.
    sympathetic nervous s.
    sympathoadrenal s.
    T cell s.
    three host cascade s's
    thymus-independent lymphoid s.
    urogenital s.

systemic
    s. anaphylaxis
    s. autoimmune disease
    s. autoimmunity
    s. blastomycosis
    s. calciphylaxis
    s. circulation
    s. fungus
    s. infection
    s. lupus erythematosus (SLE)
    s. sclerosis

T
  T agglutinin
  T cell
  tetanus toxoid
  T lymphocyte

T_3
  triiodothyronine
    low T_3 syndrome
    T_3 neogenesis
    reverse T_3 (rT3)
    T_3 toxicosis

T_4
  thyroxine
    T_4-binding inter-α globulin
    T_4-binding prealbumin (TBPA)
    T_4 level
    T_4 toxicosis

T15

T-200 (CD45)

TA
  toxin-antitoxin

TAA
  tumor-associated antigen

tabardillo

tabes dorsalis

table
  Gaffky t.
  weight/height t's

TABS
  triphenylethylene antiestrogen binding site

Tac antigen

Tacaribe
  T. complex
  T. virus

tache
  t. noire

tachycardia
  t. in thyrotoxicosis

tachykinin
  t. family

tachyphylaxis

tachyzoite

tacrolimus (FK506)

taeniasis

TAF
  tumor angiogenesis factor

T agglutinin

Tahyna virus

tail
  t. of pancreas

tailpiece
  t's of immunoglobulins

Takayasu's disease

tall stature

TAM
  tumor-associated macrophage

Tamiami virus

tanapox virus

Tanner stages

T antigen

θ antigen

TAP
  transporter in antigen processing
    TAP1
    TAP2

TAPA-1 (CD81)

tapasin

tarbadillo

target
  t. cell
  t. gland
  t. organ
  t. tissue

targeting
    gene t.

tart cell

tat gene (*of HIV virus*)

tat protein

TATA box

Tatlockia micdadei

Tatumella

taurocholic

Tay-Sachs disease

TBE
    tick-borne encephalitis

TBG
    thyroxine-binding globulin

TBII
    thyroid-binding inhibitory
        immunoglobulins
    thyrotropin-binding inhibi-
        tory immunoglobulins

T₄-binding prealbumin (TBPA)

TBPA
    T₄-binding prealbumin

Tc cells
    Tc1 cells
    Tc2 cells

T cell
    T c. activation
    T c. antigen receptor (TCR)
    armed effector T c's
    autoreactive T c's
    T c. clones
    cloned T c. line
    cytotoxic T c.
    T c. defects
    dendritic epidermal T c.
        (dETC)
    T c.–dependent antigen
    T c. diversity
    effector T c's
    effector T c. function

T cell (*continued*)
    T c. function
    T c. growth factor
    helper T c's
    T c. hybrids
    T c.–independent antigen
    T c. lines
    T c. lymphoma
    mature T c's
    T c.–mediated hypersensi-
        tivity
    T c.–mediated hypersensi-
        tivity reaction
    T c.–mediated immunity
    T c. memory
    memory T c's
    T c. receptor (TCR) (T cell
        antigen receptor)
    T c. receptor complex
    T c. replacing factor
    T c. stimulation
    T c. subpopulation
    T c. subset
    superantigen-binding T c's
    suppressor T c's
    T c. system
    tumor-infiltrating T c.
    unipotent precursor T c.
    variable T c. receptor

T_DTH cell

TCGF
    T cell growth factor

TCID₅₀
    median tissue culture infec-
        tive dose

TCMI
    T cell–mediated immunity

TCR
    T cell antigen receptor

Td
    tetanus and diphtheria tox-
        oids

TDA
    TSH-displacing antibody

TD cell (*same as* sensitized lymphocyte)

T-dependent
  T-d. antigen
  T-d. area

Tdt
  terminal deoxynucleotidyl transferase

TDX immunoassay

TeBG
  testosterone-binding globulin

technique
  antiglobulin coprecipitation t.
  aseptic t.
  clamp t.
  direct immunofluorescence t.
  dot blot t.
  double isotope derivative t.
  enzyme-multiplied immunoassay t.
  Farr t.
  fluorescent antibody t.
  gene knockout t's
  hemagglutination inhibition t.
  horseradish peroxidase t.
  immunocytoadherence t.
  immunofluorescent t's
  immunogold t.
  immunoperoxidase t.
  immunoprecipitation t's
  inhibition t.
  Jerne plaque t.
  kinetic t.
  Kleinschmidt t.
  Laurell t.
  leukocyte adherence inhibition t.
  Oakley-Fulthorpe t.
  Ouchterlony t.
  Oudin t.
  PAP t. (peroxidase-antiperoxidase technique)

technique (*continued*)
  passive hemagglutination t.
  peroxidase-antiperoxidase t. (PAP technique)
  plaque t.
  polymerase chain reaction t.
  Rebuck skin window t.
  Western blot t.

tegument

teichoic acid
  mucopolysaccharide-t. a.
  mucopolysaccharide-t. a. layer (*of Staphylococcus aureus cell wall*)

telangiectasia
  ataxia-t.
  t. macularis eruptiva perstans

telobranchial bodies

temperate
  t. bacteriophage
  t. virus

temperature
  body t.

template theory

tempolabile

temporal
  t. alopecia

tempostabile

teniasis

teratogenesis

teratoma
  testicular t.

terminal
  t. complement components
  t. deoxynucleotidyl transferase (Tdt)

terminology
  transplantation t.

tertiary
  t. cortex

tertiary *(continued)*
   t. hyperparathyroidism
   t. hypothyroidism
   t. immunization
   t. response
   t. syphilis

Teschen
   T. disease
   T. virus

test
   acid-lability t.
   ACTH infusion t.
   adrenocorticotropic hormone infusion t.
   adrenolytic t's
   agar gel diffusion t.
   agglutination t.
   AHG t.
   AL t.
   Allen-Doisy t.
   anti-deoxyribonuclease B t.
   antiglobulin t.
   antiglobulin consumption t.
   antihuman globulin t.
   anti-hyaluronidase t.
   antistreptolysin O neutralization t.
   arm-raising t.
   assay validity t. (AVT)
   autoantibody t's
   bacteriolysin t.
   basophil degranulation t.
   bentonite flocculation t.
   bronchial challenge t.
   Brucellergin skin t.
   challenge t.
   chemiluminescence t.
   coccidioidin t.
   coccidioidin skin t.
   combined anterior pituitary t.
   competitive radioimmunosorbent t.
   complement fixation t.
   complement fixation inhibition t.
   conglutinating complement absorption t.

test *(continued)*
   contact t's
   Coombs' t.
   Corner-Allen t.
   cortisone-oral glucose tolerance t.
   corzyme EIA t.
   Davidsohn differential t.
   D-dimer t.
   dehydroepiandrosterone loading t.
   delayed hypersensitivity skin t.
   dexamethasone suppression t.
   dextrose t.
   DHEA loading t.
   diabetes t.
   direct antiglobulin t. (DAT)
   direct antihuman globulin t.
   direct Coombs' t.
   direct t. of immunofluorescence
   Donath-Landsteiner t.
   double diffusion t.
   double glucagon t.
   Du rosette t.
   dye t.
   dynamic t.
   edrophonium t.
   Elek's diffusion t.
   Elek's double diffusion t.
   ELISA t.
   endpoint diffusion t.
   FAB t.
   Fahey t.
   Farr t.
   fermentation t.
   Finn chamber t.
   flocculation t.
   fluorescent antibody t.
   fluorescent treponemal antibody absorption t. (FTA-ABS)
   food challenge t.
   Foshay's t.
   Francis' t.
   Frei t.

test *(continued)*
Frei skin t.
gel diffusion t.
glucagon stimulation t.
glucose t.
glucose tolerance t. (GTT)
GnRH (gonadotropin-releasing hormone) t.
HAI t. (hemagglutination inhibition test)
hapten inhibition t.
hemadsorption t.
hemagglutination t.
hemagglutination inhibition t.
HI t. (hemagglutination inhibition test)
Hickey-Hare t.
high-dose dexamethasone suppression t.
histamine t.
histamine flare t.
histoplasmin skin t.
IFA t.
immobilization t.
indirect antihuman globulin t.
indirect Coombs' t.
indirect fluorescent antibody (IFA) t.
indirect t. of immunofluorescence
inhalational challenge t.
insulin tolerance t.
intracutaneous t.
intradermal t.
intradermal skin t.
intravenous glucose tolerance t.
Jerne plaque t.
kinetic diffusion t.
Kleihauer-Betke t.
Kober t.
Kveim t.
latex agglutination t.
latex fixation t.
leishmanin t.
lepromin t.
leucine t.

test *(continued)*
low-dose dexamethasone suppression t.
lupus band t.
lymphocyte proliferation t.
lymphogranuloma venereum skin t.
Machado t.
Machado-Guerreiro t.
mallein t.
Mancini t.
Mantoux t.
metabolic inhibition t.
metyrapone t.
microprecipitation t.
MIF t.
migration inhibitory factor t.
Mitsuda t.
mixed lymphocyte culture t.
Molisch's t.
Moloney t.
Monospot t.
Montenegro t.
multiple-puncture t.
mumps skin t.
Mycoplasma hemagglutination inhibition t.
NBT t.
neutralization t.
Nickerson-Kveim t.
nitroblue tetrazolium t.
Oakley-Fulthorpe t.
opsonocytophagic t.
oral glucose tolerance t. (OGTT)
oral leucine t.
Ouchterlony t.
Oudin t.
paper radioimmunosorbent t. (PRIST)
passive cutaneous anaphylaxis t.
passive protection t.
passive transfer t.
patch t.
patch skin t.
Paul-Bunnell t.

test *(continued)*
PCA t.
perchlorate discharge t.
phentolamine t.
Pirquet t.
P-K (Prausnitz-Küstner) t.
plaque reduction t.
platelet immunofluores-
  cence t.
pork trichina skin t.
Prausnitz-Küstner (P-K) t.
precipitation t.
precipitin t.
prick t.
protection t.
protein-bound iodine t.
provocation t.
provocative t.
purified protein derivative
  (PPD) skin t.
radial immunodiffusion t.
  (RID test)
radioactive antiglobulin t.
radioactive iodine uptake t.
radioallergosorbent t.
radioimmunosorbent t.
radioiodine uptake t.
Ramon flocculation t.
rapid plasma reagin (RPR)
  card t.
rapid slide t.
reagin screen t.
Rebuck t.
rheumatoid arthritis t.
RID t.
Rose-Waaler t.
RPR (rapid plasma reagin)
  card t.
Rubner's t.
Sabin-Feldman dye t.
saccharimeter t.
saline suppression t.
sandwich t.
scarification t.
Schick t.
Schick skin t.
scratch t.
scratch skin t.
serologic t.

test *(continued)*
serum neutralization t.
sheep cell agglutination t.
short adrenocorticotropic
  hormone t.
skin t.
skin t. response
skin window t.
station t.
stimulation t.
streptozyme t.
sugar t.
suppression t.
thin layer rapid use epicutaneous (TRUE) t.
thyroid function t. (TFT)
thyroid-releasing hormone
  stimulation t.
thyroid-stimulating hor-
  mone t.
thyroid-stimulating hor-
  mone stimulation t.
thyroid stimulation t.
thyroid suppression t.
thyrotropin-releasing hormone stimulation t.
tolbutamide t.
toxoplasmin skin t.
treponemal agglutination t.
TRH t.
TRH stimulation t.
Trichinella spiralis skin t.
trichophytin t.
triiodothyronine resin uptake t.
TRUE (thin layer rapid use
  epicutaneous) t.
TSH stimulation t.
tuberculin skin t.
tyramine t.
unheated serum reagin
  (USR) t.
vasopressin t.
VDRL slide t.
Vollmer's patch t.
Vollmer's patch skin t.
von Pirquet t.
Waaler-Rose t.
Wassermann t.

test *(continued)*
    water deprivation t.
    Weil-Felix t.
    Western blot t.
    Widal t.
    yeast cell t.

testicle

testicular
    t. agenesis
    t. feminization
    t. feminization syndrome
    t. function
    t. hormone
    incomplete t. feminization
    t. stromal tumor
    t. teratoma
    t. tumors

testing
    cytotoxicity t.
    paternity t.
    skin t.
    surrogate t.

testis *pl.* testes
    cryptorchid t.
    t. hormone
    rudimentary t.

testoid

testosterone
    t.-binding globulin (TeBG)
    t. cypionate
    t. enanthate
    t.-estradiol–binding globu-
        lin
    t.-estrogen–binding globu-
        lin
    ethinyl t.
    t. pellets
    t. undeconate

testotoxicosis
    familial t.

tetanic

tetaniform

tetanigenous

tetanus
    t. antitoxin

tetanus *(continued)*
    cephalic t.
    cerebral t.
    cryptogenic t.
    t. and diphtheria toxoids
    t. immune globulin
    t. toxin
    t. toxoid
    t. toxoid vaccine

tetany

tetrahydrobiopterin

tetraiodothyronine (T_4)
    L-3,5,3′,5′-t.

tetrazolium

Texas tick fever

TF
    transfer factor

TFT
    thyroid function test

Tγ cells

TGF
    transforming growth factor
        TGF a
        TGF β

TH
    tyrosine hydroxylase

Thai hemorrhagic fever

TH cell (helper T lymphocyte)
    TH1 cell (inflammatory CD4
        T cell)
    TH2 cell (helper CD4 T
        cell)
    TH3 cell

theca
    t. cell
    t. cell tumor
    t.-lutein cell of corpus lu-
        teum

thecosis

Theiler
    T's virus

theileriasis

theileriosis

thelarche
  premature t.

thelaziasis

theliolymphocyte

theophylline

theory
  Cannon's t.
  Cannon-Bard t.
  cellular immunity t.
  cellular t. of immunity
  clonal deletion t.
  clonal selection t.
  Darlington plasmagene t.
  Ehrlich's t.
  Ehrlich's side-chain t.
  emergency t.
  Fisher-Race t.
  forbidden clone t.
  germ t.
  germline t.
  humoral t. of immunity
  immunologic deficiency t.
  inactive X t.
  instructive t. of antibody
    synthesis
  Metchnikoff's (Mechni-
    kov's) cellular immunity t.
  natural selection t.
  network t.
  Pasteur's t.
  recombinational germline t.
  selective t.
  sequestered antigen t.
  side-chain t.
  somatic diversification t.
  somatic mutation t. of anti-
    body production
  template t.
  Weiner t.

therapy
  adjunctive t.
  androgen replacement t.
  autolymphocyte t.
  autoserum t.
  behavioral t.
  biological t.

therapy *(continued)*
  desensitization t.
  diet t.
  drug t.
  endocrine t.
  endocrine breast cancer t.
  estrogen t.
  gene t.
  heterovaccine t.
  hormonal t.
  hormone t.
  immunization t.
  immunosuppressive t.
  insulin t.
  nonhormonal t.
  radiation t.
  replacement t.
  serum t.
  sex t.
  substitution t.
  thyroid replacement t.
  thyroxine replacement t.
  vaccine t.

Thermoactinomyces
  T. vulgaris

thermogenesis

thermogenin

thermography

thermoregulation

thermostabile

thermostability

theta antigen

thiazide diabetes

thick
  t. ascending loop of Henle

thickening
  capillary t.

thin
  t. layer rapid use epicuta-
    neous (TRUE) test
  t. sectioning

thiocyanate

thionamide

thirst
    t. satiation
    volume-mediated t.

Thogoto
    T. virus
    T.-like viruses

Thomsen-Friedenreich antigen

Thomson's sign

thoracic duct

threading concept

three
    t.-day fever
    t.-day measles
    t. host cascade systems

threshold
    osmotic t.
    t. sugar

thrombin

thromboagglutinin

thrombocyte

thrombocytopenia
    antibody-mediated t.
    autoimmune t.
    immune t.

thrombocytopenic purpura
    drug-induced t. p.
    idiopathic t. p.

thromboembolic disease

thromboembolism

thrombophlebitis

thrombosis
    infective t.
    venous t.

thrombospondin

thromboxane
    t. synthetase

thrombus *pl.* thrombi
    infective t.

thrush

Thy 1
    T. 1 antigen
    T. 1 molecule

thymectomy
    neonatal t.

thymic
    t. alymphoplasia
    t. anlage
    t. aplasia
    t. cortex
    t. cortical epithelial cells
    t. factor
    t. humoral factor
    t. hypoplasia
    t. lobule
    t. macrophage
    t.-parathyroid aplasia
    t. stroma
    t. tumor

thymidine
    t. incorporation
    t. kinase
    tritiated t.

thymidylate

thymin

thymocyte
    common t.
    t. death
    double-negative t.
    double-positive t.
    early t.
    intermediate t.
    mature t.
    t. organization
    single-positive t.
    t.-specific surface marker
    stage I t.
    stage II t.
    stage III t.
    t. subtypes

thymoma

thymopoietin

thymosin

thymus
  parathyroid adenoma of t.

thymus-dependent (TD)
  t.-d. antigen
  t.-d. area
  t.-d. lymphocyte
  t.-d. protein antigen
  t.-d. region
  t.-d. zone

thymus-independent (TI)
  t.-i. antigen
  t.-i. area
  t.-i. lymphocyte
  t.-i. lymphoid system
  t.-i. region
  t.-i. zone

thyroactive

thyroadenitis

thyroaplasia

thyrocalcitonin

thyrocardiac

thyrocele

thyrocolloid

thyrogenic

thyrogenous

thyroglobulin

thyroid
  aberrant t's
  accessory t's
  t. adenoma
  t. autoantibodies
  benign t. tumor
  t.-binding inhibitory immu-
    noglobulins
  t. cancer
  t. carcinoma
  t. cartilage
  t. disease
  ectopic t's
  t. follicular cells

thyroid *(continued)*
  t. function test
  t. gland
  t. hormones
  t. hormone economy
  intrathoracic t.
  lingual t.
  t. lymphoma
  pituitary-t. axis
  t. radiodine turnover
  t. radioiodine uptake
  t. reserve
  retrosternal t.
  t. scan
  t.-stimulating immunoglob-
    ulins
  t. stimulation test
  t. storm
  t. structure
  substernal t.
  t. suppression test
  suprahyoid t.

thyroidal hypothyroidism

thyroidectomize

thyroidectomy
  t. cells
  medical t.

thyroiditis
  acute pyogenic t.
  acute suppurative t.
  atrophic t.
  atrophic autoimmune t.
  autoimmune t.
  chronic t.
  chronic fibrous t.
  chronic lymphadenoid t.
  chronic lymphocytic t.
  chronic sclerosing t.
  de Quervain's t.
  giant cell t.
  giant follicular t.
  goitrous t.
  granulomatous t.
  Hashimoto's t.
  invasive t.
  invasive fibrous t.

thyroiditis *(continued)*
　ligneous t.
　lymphocytic t.
　lymphoid t.
　nongoitrous autoimmune t.
　painless t.
　postpartum t.
　pseudotuberculous t.
　radiation t.
　Riedel t.
　sclerosing t.
　silent t.
　subacute t.
　subacute granulomatous t.
　subacute lymphocytic t.
　woody t.

thyroidization

thyroidotherapy

thyroidotomy

thyroidotoxin

thyroid-releasing hormone (TRH)
　t.-r. h. stimulation test

thyroid-stimulating hormone
　t.-s. h. level
　t.-s. h.–secreting adenoma
　t.-s. h. stimulation test
　t.-s. h. test

thyrointoxication

thyroliberin

thyrolytic

thyromegaly

thyromimetic

thyronine
　t.-binding globulin

thyroparathyroidectomy

thyroparathyroprivic

thyropathy

thyroprival

thyroprivia

thyroprivic
　t. hypothyroidism

thyroprivous

thyroptosis

thyroregulatory mechanism

thyrotherapy

thyrotomy

thyrotoxic
　t. crisis
　t. exophthalmos
　t. myopathy
　t. periodic paralysis
　t. storm

thyrotoxicosis
　adolescent t.
　bowel function in t.
　dyspnea in t.
　t. factitia
　hamburger t.
　tachycardia in t.

thyrotrope
　t. adenoma
　t. cell
　t. tumor

thyrotroph

thyrotrophic

thyrotrophin

thyrotropic
　t. cell
　t. exophthalmos
　t. hormone

thyrotropin
　t.-binding inhibitory immu-
　　noglobulins (TBII)
　chorionic t.
　human chorionic t. (hCT)
　t. level
　t.-releasing hormone
　　(TRH)
　t.-releasing hormone stimu-
　　lation test

thyrotropinoma

thyroxin

thyroxine (T₄)
t.-binding globulin (TBG)
free t.
t. level
t. replacement therapy
total t.
total serum t.

thyroxinic

TI-1 antigen

tick
t. fever
Ixodes t.
t. paralysis
t. typhus

tick-borne
t.-b. encephalitis (TBE)
t.-b. encephalitis viruses
t.-b. typhus
t.-b. viruses

tickover

tight junction

TIL
tumor-infiltrating lymphocyte

time
Achilles reflex t.
Achilles tendon reflex t.
activated partial thromboplastin t. (APTT)
generation t.
partial thromboplastin t. (PTT)
prothrombin t. (PT)

timothy

T-independent
T-i. antigen
T-i. area

tinea
t. axillaris

tinea *(continued)*
t. barbae
t. capitis
t. ciliorum
t. circinata
t. circinata tropical
t. corporis
t. cruris
t. faciei
t. favosa
t. glabrosa
t. imbricata
t. manus
t. manuum
t. nigra
t. pedis
t. profunda
t. sycosis
t. tonsurans
t. unguium

tingible body macrophages

TIP
translation inhibitory protein

tissue
adipose t.
adrenogenic t.
allografted t.
t. antigen
bronchial-associated lymphoid t. (BALT)
brown adipose t. (BAT)
bursa-equivalent t.
bursal equivalent t.
cardiac t.
central lymphoid t's
chromaffin t.
connective t.
t. culture
t. damage
t. dendritic cells
ectopic adrenal t.
ectopic lymphoid t.
t. engineering
glandular t.
t. grafts

tissue *(continued)*
 gut-associated lymphoid t. (GALT)
 t. immunity
 lymphoid t.
 lymphoreticular t.
 t. matching
 mucosa-associated lymphoid t. (MALT)
 mucosal t's
 mucosal-associated lymphoid t. (MALT)
 t. necrosis
 parathyroid t.
 peripheral lymphoid t.
 t. phagocyte
 primary lymphoid t's
 t. regeneration
 secondary lymphoid t.
 shock t.
 target t.
 tuberculosis granulation t.
 t. typing
 white adipose t.
 Xenopus lymphomyeloid t's

tissue-specific
 t.-s. antigen
 t.-s. autoimmune disease

titer
 agglutination t.
 antibody t.
 antistreptolysin O t.
 bacteriophage t.
 t. changes
 whole complement t.

titration
 chessboard t.
 Dean and Webb t.
 virus t.

TLA gene

T$_4$ level

TLI
 total lymphoid irradiation

T lymphocyte
 alloreactive T l's

T lymphocyte *(continued)*
 T l. hybridoma
 T l. tolerance

Tμ cells

TMV
 tobacco mosaic virus

TNF
 tumor necrosis factor

tobacco mosaic virus (TMV)

Tobia fever

Togaviridae

togavirus

tokelau

Tokelau ringworm

tolbutamide test

tolerance
 acquired t.
 adoptive t.
 B cell t.
 cellular t.
 central t.
 drug-induced t.
 endotoxin t.
 fetal t.
 glucose t.
 high-dose t.
 high-zone t.
 immunologic t.
 impaired glucose t.
 low-dose t.
 low-zone t.
 lymphocyte t.
 natural t.
 neonatally-induced t.
 oral t.
 peripheral t.
 self-t.
 split t.
 T lymphocyte t.
 t. vs. self-t.
 transplantation t.

tolerant

toleration

tolerogen

tolerogenesis

tolerogenic
  t. antigen
  t. protein antigen

tomboyism

tomography
  computed t. (CT)
  t. of the sella turcica

tonsil
  palatine t.
  pharyngeal t.

tonsillitis
  diphtherial t.

tonsillotyphoid

topical calciphylaxis

topoisomerase

TOPV
  poliovirus vaccine live oral
    trivalent

Torovirus

torovirus

Torres-Teixeira bodies

Torulopsis
  T. glabrata

torulopsosis

torulosis

Toscana virus

total
  t. body potassium
  t. body water
  t. complement assay
  t. hemolytic complement
    (CH50)
  t. lymphoid irradiation
    (TLI)
  t. serum thyroxine
  t. serum triiodothyronine

total *(continued)*
  t. thyroxine
  t. triiodothyronine

Toulon typhus

toxemia
  hydatid t.
  intraperitoneal t.

toxic
  t. adenoma
  t. atrophy
  diffuse t. goiter
  t. goiter
  t. multinodular goiter
  t. shock syndrome
  t. shock syndrome toxin-1
    (TSST-1)

toxicosis
  liothyronine t.
  T_3 (triiodothyronine) t.
  T_4 (thyroxine) t.

toxin
  bacterial t.
  t.-based vaccine
  cholera t.
  clostridial t.
  diphtheria t.
  heat-labile t.
  inactivated t.
  t. neutralization
  pertussis t.
  staphylococcal t.
  tetanus t.
  toxic shock syndrome t.-1
    (TSST-1)
  whooping cough t.

toxin-antitoxin (TA)
  t.-a. reaction

Toxocara canis

toxocariasis
  human t.

toxoid
  t.-antitoxin floccule
  diphtheria t.
  diphtheria and tetanus t's

toxoid *(continued)*
    t. immunization
    Panton-Valentine leukoci-
      din t.
    staphylococcal t.
    tetanus t.
    tetanus and diphtheria t's

toxoid-antitoxoid

Toxoplasma gondii

toxoplasmic meningoencephalitis

toxoplasmin skin test

toxoplasmosis

Tp4 antigen

TPHA (*Treponema pallidum*
  hemagglutination assay)

TPI test (*Treponema pallidum*
  immobilization test)

TRAb
    TSH receptor antibodies

trabecular adenoma

tracheobronchial tuberculosis

trachoma

tract
    biliary t.
    gastrointestinal t.
    genital t.
    müllerian t.
    reproductive t.
    respiratory t.
    urinary t.

trait
    recessive t.

trans-acting factor

transactivating response element

transactivator
    class II t.
    class II MHC t. (CIITA)

transaminase

transcobalamin
    t. I
    t. II
    t. III

transcortin

transcriptase
    reverse t.

transcription
    t.-activating factor
    t. activation
    t. activator
    t. factor
    Ig gene t.
    t. rate
    signal transducers and acti-
      vators of t. (STAT)

transcriptional
    t. activation
    t. activation region
    t. activity
    t. control
    t. regulation

transcytosis

transducer
    neuroendocrine t.
    signal t.
    signal t's and activators of
      transcription (STAT)

transduction
    rhodopsin signal t.
    signal t.

transfectoma

transfer
    adoptive t.
    cellular t.
    Northern t.
    Northern RNA t.
    passive t.
    passive t. of cellular resis-
      tance
    pronuclear stage tubal t.
      (PROST)
    resistance t.
    Southern t.

transfer *(continued)*
zygote intrafallopian t. (ZIFT)

transference of immunity

transfer factor
antigen-liberated t. f.
Lawrence-type dialyzable t. f.

transferrin
t. receptor

transformation
blast t.
genetic t.
lymphocyte t.
tumor t.
virus-mediated t.
von Krogh t.

transformed cell

transforming growth factor (TGF)

transfusion
allogeneic t.
blood t.
exchange t.
t. hepatitis
intraperitoneal fetal t.
t. reaction

transgene

transgenesis

transgenic
t. animal
t. mouse
t. pig

transient autoimmunity

transient hypogammaglobulin-emia of infancy

transillumination

translation
t. inhibitory protein

translocation
chromosomal t.

translocation *(continued)*
X autosome t.
X–X t.

transmembrane
t. receptor
t. receptor superfamily

transmissible
t. neurodegenerative disease
t. spongiform encephalopathy

transmission
HIV t.
horizontal t.
smallpox t.
vertical t.

transmitted light microscope

transovarial

transovarian

transplacental
t. hemorrhage

transplant
t. antigen

transplantation
allogeneic t.
antigen t.
t. antigens
autologous t.
bone marrow t.
cadaveric donor t.
cornea t.
heart t.
heterotopic t.
homotopic t.
kidney t.
liver t.
living nonrelated donor t.
living related donor t.
living unrelated donor t.
lung t.
organ t.
orthotopic t.
pancreas t.
syngeneic t.
syngenesioplastic t.

transplantation *(continued)*
 t. terminology
 t. tolerance
 xenogeneic t.

transplanted organ

transport
 electrogenic t.
 electroneutral t.
 iodide t.
 ion t.
 peptide t.
 t. proteins

transporter (in antigen processing)

transposon

transsexualism

transsphenoidal surgery

transthyretin
 amyloid t.

transudate

transurethral prostatectomy

transverse hermaphroditism

trauma

traumatic
 t. herpes
 t. myiasis

treatment
 allergy t.
 anorexia t.
 atherosclerosis t.
 Brown-Séquard's t.
 Kenny t.
 obesity t.
 rejection t.

trematode

trematodiasis

tremor
 parkinsonian t.

trench fever

Treponema
 T. carateum

Treponema (continued)
 T. cuniculi
 T. genitalis
 T. herrejoni
 T. pallidum
 T. pallidum hemagglutination assay (TPHA)
 T. pallidum immobilization test (TPI test)
 T. pallidum subsp. *pertenue*
 T. pertenue

treponemal
 t. agglutination test
 t. antigens
 t. immobilizing antibody

treponematosis

treponeme

treponemiasis

Tresilian's sign

TRH
 thyrotropin-releasing hormone
  TRH stimulation test
  TRH test
 TSH-releasing hormone
  TRH stimulation test

triad
 adrenomedullary t.
 Grancher's t.
 hutchinsonian t.
 Whipple's t.

triangulation number

Trichinella spiralis
 T. spiralis skin test

trichinelliasis

trichinellosis

trichiniasis

trichiniferous

trichinization

trichinosis

trichinous
 t. myositis

trichinous *(continued)*
    t. polymyositis

trichocephaliasis

trichocephalosis

Trichomonas vaginalis

trichomoniasis
    t. vaginalis

trichomycosis

trichophytic

trichophytid

trichophytin test

Trichophyton
    T. concentricum
    T. mentagrophytes
    T. rubrum
    T. schoenleinii
    T. simii
    T. tonsurans
    T. verrucosum
    T. violaceum

trichophytosis

Trichosporon

trichosporonosis

trichosporosis

trichostrongyliasis

trichostrongylosis

trichotoxin

Trichuris trichiura

trichuriasis

Triglochin

triglyceride
    t. metabolism

trihydroxyestrin

triiodothyronine (T_3)
    free t.
    t. resin uptake
    t. resin uptake test
    reverse t. (rT3)

triiodothyronine *(continued)*
    total t.
    total serum t.

trimer

Tripedia

triphenylethylene
    t. antiestrogen
    t. antiestrogen binding site
    (TABS)

triple response (*of Lewis*)

trisomy
    t.-21

Trizivir

trombiculiasis

trombiculid
    t. mite

trombiculidiasis

trombidiiasis

trombidiosis

Tropheryma
    T. whippelii

trophoblast cells

trophoblastic
    t. cells
    t. disease
    t. tumors

trophoprivic hypothyroidism

tropical
    t. bubo
    t. spastic paraparesis
    t. spastic paraplegia
    t. swellings
    t. typhus

TRUE
    thin layer rapid use epicu-
       taneous
          TRUE test

true
    t. chancre
    t. dwarf

true *(continued)*
    t. hermaphrodite
    t. hermaphroditism
    t. intersex

Trypanosoma
    T. brucei
    T. cruzi
    T. rhodesiense

trypanosomiasis
    African t.
    American t.
    East African t.
    Gambian t.
    Rhodesian t.
    South American t.
    West African t.

trypomastigote

trypsin

tryptase

tryptophan
    t. hydroxylase

TSA
    tumor-specific antigen

TS cell

TSH
    thyroid-stimulating hormone
        TSH-binding inhibitory
            immunoglobulins
        TSH-displacing anti-
            body (TDA)
        TSH-secreting ade-
            noma
        TSH stimulation test

TSI
    thyroid-stimulating immu-
       noglobulins

TSTA
    tumor-specific transplanta-
       tion antigen

tsutsugamushi
    t. disease (chigger-borne
       typhus)

tsutsugamushi *(continued)*
    t. fever

T_3 toxicosis

T_4 toxicosis

tube
    fallopian t.

tuber
    t. cinereum
    omental t. of body of pan-
       creas
    t. omentale corporis pan-
       creatis

tubercle
    t. bacillus
    t. bacillus wax
    caseous t.
    fibrous t.
    gray t.
    miliary t.

tubercular

tuberculate

tuberculated

tuberculation

tuberculin
    t. skin test
    t. skin test reaction
    t. testing schedule
    t.-type hypersensitivity

tuberculization

tuberculoid
    t. leprosy
    t. lymphadenitis

tuberculoma

tuberculosis
    adult t.
    aerogenic t.
    atypical t.
    basal t.
    t. of bones and joints
    cestodic t.
    childhood t.

tuberculosis *(continued)*
   t. colliquativa
   t. colliquativa cutis
   t. cutis orificialis
   disseminated t.
   exudative t.
   genital t.
   genitourinary t.
   t. granulation tissue
   hematogenous t.
   hilus t.
   inhalation t.
   t. of intestines
   laryngeal t.
   t. of larynx
   t. of lungs
   miliary t.
   Mycobacterium t.
   open t.
   orificial t.
   postprimary t.
   primary t.
   primary inoculation t.
   productive t.
   pulmonary t.
   reactivation t.
   reinfection t.
   secondary t.
   t. of serous membranes
   surgical t.
   tracheobronchial t.
   t. ulcerosa
   t. vaccine

tuberculotic

tuberculous
   t. chancre
   t. gumma
   t. infiltration
   t. laryngitis
   t. lymphadenitis
   t. lymphadenopathy

tuberohypophyseal neuron

tuberoinfundibular pathway

tubular
   t. basement membrane
   t. cell injury

tubular *(continued)*
   t. reabsorption of phos-
     phate (TRP)

tubule
   annular t.
   collecting t.
   distal t.
   distal renal t.

tuftsin

tularemia
   gastrointestinal t.
   glandular t.
   oropharyngeal t.
   pulmonary t.
   pulmonic t.
   typhoidal t.
   ulceroglandular t.

tumescence
   nocturnal penile t. (NPT)

tumor
   adrenal t.
   adrenal rest t.
   adrenocortical t.
   aldosterone-producing t.
   aldosterone-secreting t.
   t. angiogenesis factor
   annular tubule t.
   t. antigen
   t. antigenicity
   t.-associated antigen (TAA)
   t.-associated macrophage
   B cell t.
   benign t.
   Brenner t.
   calcitonin-producing t.
   candidate t.
   carcinoid t.
   catecholamine-secreting t.
   t. cell
   central nervous system t.
   chorionic gonadotropin–
     secreting t.
   chromaffin cell t.
   t. complement receptor
   corticotrope t.
   corticotroph t.

tumor *(continued)*
    craniopharyngeal duct t.
    dermoid t.
    t. diagnosis
    diarrheogenic t.
    eosinophil t. with acromeg-
      aly
    t. escape
    feminizing t.
    functional t.
    functioning t.
    gastroenteropancreatic,
      non–insulin-secreting t.
    granulosa-theca cell t.
    growth hormone–produc-
      ing t.
    growth hormone–releasing
      hormone releasing t.
    gummy t.
    headache manifestation of
      pituitary t.
    hilar cell t.
    hormone-producing t.
    Hürthle cell t.
    t. immunity
    t. immunology
    t. immunotherapy
    t.-infiltrating lymphocytes
    interstitial cell t.
    intracranial t.
    islet cell t.
    Leydig cell t.
    malignant t.
    t. markers
    multiple hormone–secret-
      ing t.
    t. necrosis factor
    t. necrosis factor-α
    t. necrosis factor-β
    non–beta cell t.
    nonfunctional t.
    opportunistic t.
    t. origin
    t. osteomalacia
    ovarian t.
    oxyphil cell t.
    pancreatic t.

tumor *(continued)*
    pancreatitic polypeptide–
      producing t.
    passive t.
    pineal t.
    pituitary t.
    plasma cell t.
    prolactin-secreting t.
    prostate t.
    pure theca cell t.
    Rathke's t.
    Rathke's pouch t.
    t. rejection antigen
    renin-secreting t.
    Sertoli cell t.
    Sertoli-Leydig cell t.
    t.-specific antigen (TSA)
    t.-specific transplantation
      antigen (TSTA)
    t.-suppressor genes
    testicular t.
    testicular stromal t.
    theca cell t.
    theca lutein of corpus lu-
      teum cell t.
    thymic t.
    thyrotrope t.
    thyrotroph t.
    t. transformation
    trophoblastic t's
    unclassifiable sex mesen-
      chymal t.
    virilizing t.
    t. virus

tumorigenesis

TUNEL
    TdT-dependent dUPT-bio-
      tin nick end labeling
        TUNEL assay

tunica
    ovarian t.

tunicate

turbidimetry

Turlock virus

Turner syndrome

turnover
  phosphatidylinositol t.
  thyroid radiodine t.

two-dimensional gel electrophoresis

Twort-d'Herelle phenomenon

type
  buffalo t.
  t. 1 diabetes mellitus
  t. 2 diabetes mellitus
  t. I hypercalciuria
  t. I hypersensitivity
  t. I hypersensitivity reaction
  t. II hypersensitivity
  t. II hypersensitivity reaction
  t. III hypersensitivity
  t. III hypersensitivity reaction
  t. IV hypersensitivity
  t. IV hypersensitivity reaction
  monoclonal gammopathy t.
  pathogen t's
  vaccine t's

typhic corpuscles

typhoid
  t. fever
  t. nodule
  t. osteomyelitis
  provocation t.
  t. spots
  t. vaccine

typhoidal
  t. tularemia

typhous

typhus
  Australian tick t.
  cat flea t.
  chigger-borne t.

typhus (continued)
  classic t.
  endemic t.
  epidemic t.
  European t.
  exanthematic t. of São Paulo
  t. exanthématique
  exanthematous t.
  t. fever
  flea-borne t.
  flying squirrel t.
  flying squirrel–associated t.
  Gubler-Robin t.
  Indian tick t.
  Kenya tick t.
  latent t.
  louse-borne t.
  Manchurian t.
  Mexican t.
  mite-borne t.
  Moscow t.
  murine t.
  t. nodules
  North Asian tick t.
  North Queensland tick t.
  Queensland tick t.
  recrudescent t.
  São Paulo t.
  scrub t.
  shop t.
  Siberian tick t.
  tick t.
  tick-borne t.
  Toulon t.
  tropical t.
  urban t.
  t. vaccine

typing
  ABO t.
  blood t.
  HLA t.
  primed lymphocyte t. (PLT)
  tissue t.

tyramine
    t. test

tyrosinase

tyrosine
    Bruton's t. kinase (Btk)

tyrosine *(continued)*
    t. hydroxylase (TH)
    t. kinase

Tyzzer's disease

U
   U virus

ubiquitous

Uganda S virus

ulcer
   chancroid u.
   gummatous u.
   pudendal u.
   peptic u.
   soft u.
   venereal u.

ulceration

ulcerative
   u. colitis
   u. lesion

ulceroglandular tularemia

ulcerogranuloma

Ullrich syndrome

ultimobranchial
   u. bodies
   u. cells

ultracentrifugal analysis

ultracentrifugation
   density gradient u.
   sucrose density gradient u.

ultradian rhythm

ultrasensitivity

ultrasonography

ultrasound

ultraviolet (UV)
   u. light

umbilical
   u. diphtheria
   u. granuloma

uncinarial dermatitis

uncinariasis

uncinariatic

uncinate process of pancreas

unclassifiable
   u. sex mesenchymal tumor

unc mutation

uncomplemented

uncoupling protein

underactivity

undernutrition

undifferentiated carcinoma of
   thyroid gland

undulant fever

unfavorable
   u. microenvironment

unheated serum reagin (USR)
   test

unicellular organism

unilateral
   u. blindness
   u. hermaphroditism

unilocular hydatid disease

unipotent
   u. precursor T cell

unisexual

unit
   Allen-Doisy u.
   amboceptor u.
   antigen u.
   antitoxic u.
   CH50 u.
   complement u.
   Corner-Allen u.
   Felton's u.
   hemolytic u.
   hypothalamic-pituitary u.
   international insulin u.
   Lf u.
   mouse u.
   Noon pollen u.
   u. of oxytocin
   plaque-forming u.
   sudanophobic u.

unitarian hypothesis

universal
  u. blood and body fluid
    precautions
  u. donor
  u. infantilism
  u. recipient

unresponsiveness
  immunologic u.

unstable nucleus

upgrading reaction

Uppsala virus

upright plasma renin activity

uptake
  catecholamine u.
  pertechnetate u.
  radioactive iodine u.
  radioiodine u.
  thyroid radioiodine u.
  triiodothyronine resin u.

urban typhus

urea cycle

Ureaplasma
  U. urealyticum

uremia

uremic
  u. osteodystrophy
  u. pseudodiabetes mellitus

urethra

urethritis
  gonococcal u.
  gonorrheal u.
  specific u.
  u. venerea

uric acid
  u. a. lithiasis

urinary
  u. androgen
  u. calcium
  u. cortisol

urinary *(continued)*
  u. cyclic AMP (UcAMP)
  u. mineralocorticoid
  u. phosphate
  u. schistosomiasis
  u. tract

urine
  u. concentration
  u. osmolality
  u. pH
  u. volume

uroanthelone

uroenterone

urofollitropin

urogastrone

urogenital
  u. sinus
  u. system

urolithiasis
  idiopathic calcium u.

urography
  intravenous u.

uroxin

urticaria
  u. pigmentosa

urticarial vasculitis

USR
  unheated serum reagin
    USR test

uterine
  u. bleeding
  u. cancer
  u. prolapse

uterotonin

uterotropin

uterus

Uukuniemi virus

uveitis

U virus

V
variable
V domain
V gene segments
V region

vaccina

vaccinal

vaccinate

vaccination
active v.
v. considerations
DNA v.
HIV v.
measles v.
passive v.
smallpox v.

vaccinator

vaccine
acellular v.
acellular pertussis v.
anthrax v.
antifertility v.
anti-idiotype v.
antitumor v.
attenuated v.
attenuated live v.
autogenous v.
bacterial v.
BCG v.
bivalent attenuated v.
Calmette's v.
cancer v.
capsular polysaccharide v.
cholera v.
combined v.
commercially available v.
conjugate heptavalent
pneumococcal v.
current v.
dead v.
diphtheria-pertussis-tetanus v. (DPT)
diphtheria and tetanus toxoids and acellular pertussis v. (DTaP)

vaccine *(continued)*
diphtheria and tetanus toxoids and pertussis
v. (DTP)
Edmonston measles vi-
rus v.
Haemophilus b conjugate v.
(HbCV)
Haemophilus b polysac-
charide v. (HbPV)
hepatitis v.
hepatitis A v. inactivated
hepatitis B v.
hepatitis B v. (recombinant)
heterologous v.
heterotypic v.
human diploid cell v.
inactivated v.
influenza virus v.
Jeryl Lynn live attenuated
mumps v.
killed v.
live v.
live attenuated v.
Lyme disease v. (recombi-
nant OspA)
measles v.
measles, mumps, and ru-
bella virus v. live (MMR)
measles and mumps virus
v. live
measles and rubella virus
v. live
measles virus v. live
meningococcal polysac-
charide v.
mixed v.
mumps v.
mumps virus v. live
Mycoplasma v.
natural live v.
nonreplicative v.
pertussis v.
plague v.
pneumococcal v. polyva-
lent
polio v.
poliomyelitis v.

vaccine *(continued)*
    poliovirus v.
    poliovirus v. inactivated
      (IPV)
    poliovirus v. live oral
      (OPV)
    poliovirus v. live oral triva-
      lent (TOPV)
    polysaccharide v.
    polyvalent v.
    polyvalent attenuated v.
    purified chick embryo
      cell v. (PCEC)
    rabies v.
    rabies v. adsorbed (RVA)
    recombinant v.
    v. regimen
    replicative v.
    Rocky Mountain spotted
      fever v.
    rotavirus v. live oral
    rubella v.
    rubella and mumps virus v.
      live
    rubella virus v. live
    rubeola v.
    Sabin v.
    Sabin poliovirus v.
    Sabin-type v.
    Salk v.
    Salk-type v.
    Schwartz measles virus v.
    smallpox v.
    split-virus v.
    subunit v.
    subvirion v.
    synthetic v.
    tetanus toxoid v.
    v. therapy
    toxin-based v.
    tuberculosis v.
    v. types
    typhoid v.
    typhus v.
    varicella-zoster v.
    viral v.
    virus v.
    whole organism v.
    yellow fever v.

vaccinia
    fetal v.
    v. gangrenosa
    generalized v.
    v. immune globulin (VIG)
    progressive v.
    v. virus

vaccinial

vacciniform

vaccinogen

vaccinogenous

vaccinostyle

vaccinotherapy

vacuole

vagabonds' disease

vagina

vaginal
    v. bleeding
    v. candidiasis
    v. contraceptive
    v. diaphragm
    v. dryness
    v. epithelium
    v. flora
    v. mucosa
    v. outlet
    v. papillae
    relaxed v. outlet
    v. rings
    v. rugae

vaginitis
    Candida v.
    candidal v.
    senile v.

vagrants' disease

vagus nerve

valence

valency
    antigen v.
    antigenic v.

value
    S v.

van der Waals forces

van Dyke protein

vanillylmandelic acid (VMA)

vanishing testes syndrome

variability
    antibody v.
    v. plot

variable (V)
    v. antibody
    v. domain
    v. genes
    v. gene segments
    v. lymphocyte
    v. region
    v. surface glycoprotein
      (VSG)
    v. T cell receptor

variant
    isotypic v.

variation
    allotypic v.
    antigenic v.
    idiotypic v.
    isotypic v.
    normal v.
    precipitin test ring v's

varicella
    v. gangrenosa
    v. immunization
    v. virus
    v.-zoster immune globulin
      (VZIG)
    v.-zoster vaccine
    v.-zoster virus

Varicellovirus

varicelliform

varicelloid

varicocele

varicosity

variola
    v. haemorhagica
    v. major
    v. minor
    v. sine eruptione
    v. virus

variolar

variolate

variolation

variolic

varioliform

variolization

varioloid

variolous

vascular
    v. addressins
    v. cell adhesion molecule
      (VCAM)
    v. cell adhesion molecule 1
      (VCAM-1)
    v. goiter
    hypertrophic v. disease
    v. lesions
    v. permeability
    v. rejection
    v. response
    v. smooth muscle

vasculitis
    allergic v.
    Churg-Strauss v.
    hypersensitivity v.
    hypocomplementemic v.
    immunologic v.
    leukocytoclastic v.
    necrotizing v.
    urticarial v.

vas deferens

vasectomy

vasoactive
    v. amines
    v. intestinal peptide (VIP)

vasoactive *(continued)*
   v. intestinal polypeptide
      (VIP)
   v. substances

vasoamine

vasoconstriction

vasoconstrictor

vasodilatation

vasodilation

vasodilator
   v. hormones

vasomotor
   v. conditioning
   v. instability

vasopermeability factor

vasopressin
   aqueous v.
   arginine v.
   lysine v.
   v. response
   v. test

vasopressinase

vasotocin
   arginine v. (AVT)

vasotonin

vasovasostomy

VCAM
   vascular cell adhesion mol-
      ecule
      VCAM-1

V (variable) domain

VDRL
   Venereal Disease Research
      Laboratory
      VDRL antigen
      VDRL slide test

vection

vector
   biological v.
   mechanical v.

vector-borne
   v.-b. infection

vectorial

VEE
   Venezuelan equine enceph-
      alomyelitis
      VEE virus

veil cells

veiled cells

vein
   hypophyseoportal v's
   ovarian v.
   portal v's of hypophysis

vena *pl.* venae
   venae portales hypophy-
      siales

venereal
   v. disease
   V. Disease Research Labo-
      ratory (VDRL)
   v. route
   v. sore
   v. ulcer

venereologist

venereology

Venezuelan
   V. equine encephalomyeli-
      tis (VEE)
   V. equine encephalomyeli-
      tis virus (VEE virus)

venoconstriction

venom
   insect v.
   snake v.

venous
   v. thrombosis

ventriculoarterial shunt

venule
   high endothelial v. (HEV)
   postcapillary high endothe-
      lial v.

vermination

verminosis

verminotic

verminous abscess

Verner-Morrison syndrome

Vero cells

verotoxin

verruca *pl.* verrucae
  v. peruana
  v. peruviana

verruga
  v. peruana

vertebral osteophyte

vertical
  v. transmission

very late antigens (VLA) (1–6)

very late activation (VLA)
  v. l. a. antigen
  v. l. a. molecules

very-low-density lipoprotein (VLDL)

vesical
  v. schistosomiasis

vesicle
  coated v's
  multilaminar v.
  phagocytotic v.
  pituitary v.
  secretory v's
  seminal v.
  synaptic v's

vesicular
  v. pharyngitis
  v. stomatitis virus
  v. stomatitis–like viruses

Vesiculovirus

vessel
  afferent lymph v's
  blood v.

vessel *(continued)*
  efferent lymph v's
  lymph v's
  lymphatic v's

veto cells

Vi
  V. agglutination
  V. antigen

Vibrio
  V. alginolyticus
  V. cholerae
  V. cholerae biotype *albensis*
  V. cholerae biotype *cholerae*
  V. cholerae biotype *eltor*
  V. cholerae biotype *proteus*
  V. comma
  V. damsela
  V. danubicus
  V. eltor
  El Tor strain of *V. cholerae*
  V. fluvialis
  V. ghinda
  V. massauah
  V. metschnikovii
  V. mimicus
  V. parahaemolyticus
  V. phosphorescens
  V. vulnificus

vibriosis

vif gene (*of HIV*)

VIG
  vaccinia immune globulin

villikinin

VIP
  vasoactive intestinal peptide
  vasoactive intestinal polypeptide

VIPoma

viral
  v. antibody
  v. capsid antigen
  v. disease

viral *(continued)*
    v. envelope
    v. hemagglutination
    v. hemorrhagic fevers
    v. hepatitis
    v. neutralization
    v. oncogene
    v. orchitis
    v. particle
    v. proteins
    v. superantigen
    v. vaccine

viral infection
    congenital v. i.
    cytolytic v. i.
    generalized v. i.
    inapparent v. i.
    integrated v. i.
    localized v. i.
    steady-state v. i.

Virchow's gland

viremia

viricidal

viricide

virile

virilescence

virilism
    adrenal v.

virility

virilization

virilizing
    v. tumor

virion
    adenovirus v.
    hepatitis B v.

virogene

virogenetic

viroid

virologist

virology

viromicrosome

viropexis

viroplasm

virosis *pl.* viroses

virostatic

virucidal

virucide

virulence
    established v.
    v. factors
    v. measurement
    virus v.

virulent
    v. bubo
    v. staphylococcus

virulicidal

viruliferous

virus
    Absettarov v.
    acute laryngotracheobron-
      chitis v.
    adeno-associated v.
    African horse sickness v.
    Amapari v.
    Anopheles A v.
    Anopheles B v.
    antibody-binding v.
    arbovirus
    Argentine hemorrhagic fe-
      ver v.
    attenuated v.
    Australian X disease v.
    B v.
    B19 v.
    bacterial v.
    Bakau v.
    Bayou v.
    Belgrade v.
    beneficient v.
    Berne v.
    BK v.
    v. blockade

virus *(continued)*
    Bolivian hemorrhagic fe-
      ver v.
    Borna disease v.
    Bunyamwera v.
    Bussuquara v.
    Bwamba v.
    C v.
    CA v.
    California encephalitis v.
    cancer-inducing v.
    Capim v.
    Catu v.
    Central European encephal-
      itis v.
    Chagres v.
    Changuinola v.
    chikungunya v.
    Coe v.
    Colorado tick fever v.
    Columbia SK v.
    common cold v's
    coryza v.
    cowpox v.
    Coxsackie v.
    Crimean hemorrhagic fe-
      ver v.
    Crimean-Congo hemor-
      rhagic fever v.
    croup-associated v.
    cytomegalic inclusion
      disease v.
    defective v.
    dengue v.
    DNA v.
    DNA oncogenic v.
    Dobrava v.
    Dobrava-Belgrade v.
    Duvenhage v.
    double-stranded v.
    eastern equine encephalo-
      myelitis v.
    EB v.
    Ebola v.
    echovirus
    ectromelia v.
    EEE v.
    encephalomyocarditis v.
      (EMC virus)

virus *(continued)*
    enteric v's
    enteric orphan v's
    enveloped v.
    epidemic keratoconjunctiv-
      itis v.
    Epstein-Barr v. (EBV)
    equine encephalomyeli-
      tis v.
    Everglades v.
    exanthematous disease v.
    v. fixé
    fixed v.
    foamy v's
    fowlpox v.
    Germisten v.
    Guama v.
    Guama group v's
    Guanarito v.
    Guaroa v.
    Hantaan v.
    Hanzalova v.
    helper v.
    hemadsorption v. *(types 1
      and 2)*
    hepatitis v.
    hepatitis A v.
    hepatitis B v.
    hepatitis C v.
    hepatitis C–like v's
    hepatitis D v.
    hepatitis delta v.
    hepatitis E v.
    hepatitis G v.
    hepatitis GB v.
    herpangina v.
    herpesvirus
    herpes simplex v.
    human immunodeficien-
      cy v.
    human parainfluenza v. (1–
      4)
    human respiratory syncy-
      tial v.
    human T-cell leukemia v.
    human T-cell lymphotro-
      pic v. *(types I, II, III)*
    human T-lymphotropic v.
      (1, 2)

virus *(continued)*
 hybrid v.
 Hypr v.
 igbo-ora v.
 Ilheus v.
 v.-induced leukemia
 v.-induced lymphoma
 influenza v.
 influenza A v.
 influenza B v.
 influenza C v.
 Jamestown Canyon v.
 Japanese encephalitis v.
 JC v.
 Junin v.
 Kemerovo v.
 Kirsten murine sarcoma v.
 Koongol v.
 Korean hemorrhagic fever v.
 Kumba v.
 Kumlinge v.
 Kunjin v.
 Kyasanur Forest disease v.
 La Crosse v.
 Lansing v.
 Lassa v.
 latent v.
 LCM (lymphocytic cho-
  riomeningitis) v.
 Leon v.
 leukemia v.
 louping ill v.
 lymphadenopathy v. (LAV)
 lymphadenopathy-associa-
  ted v.
 lymphocystis v's
 lymphocyte-associated v.
 lymphocytic choriomenin-
  gitis v. (LCMV)
 lytic v.
 M-25 v.
 Machupo v.
 maedi/visna v.
 Makonde v.
 Marburg v.
 masked v.
 Mayaro v.

virus *(continued)*
 measles v.
 measles-like v's
 v.-mediated transformation
 Mengo v.
 milker's node v.
 Modoc v.
 molluscum contagiosum v.
 monkeypox v.
 Montana myotic leukoen-
  cephalitis v.
 mouse mammary tumor v.
  (MMTV)
 Mucambo v.
 mucosal disease v.
 mumps v.
 murine mammary tumor v.
  (MMTV)
 Murray Valley encephali-
  tis v.
 naked v.
 Nakiwogo v.
 Negishi v.
 Neudoerfl v.
 neurotropic v.
 v. neutralizing capacity
 newborn pneumonitis v.
 Newcastle disease v.
 Nipah v.
 non-A, non-B hepatitis v.
 nonenveloped v.
 non-oncogenic v.
 Norwalk v.
 Nyando v.
 Omsk hemorrhagic fever v.
 oncogenic v's
 o'nyong-nyong v.
 orf v.
 Oropouche v.
 orphan v's
 Orungo v.
 papilloma v.
 pappataci fever v.
 parainfluenza v.
 paravaccinia v.
 v. particle
 pharyngoconjunctival fe-
  ver v.

virus *(continued)*
  phlebotomus fever v.
  Pichinde v.
  Piry v.
  polio v.
  poliomyelitis v.
  polyomavirus
  Pongola v.
  Powassan v.
  pox v.
  pseudocowpox v.
  pseudorabies v.
  Puumala v.
  Quaranfil v.
  rabbit myxoma v.
  rabies v.
  rabies-like v's
  v. replication
  respiratory v's
  respiratory syncytial v's
  Rift Valley fever v.
  Rio Bravo v.
  RNA v.
  RNA oncogenic v.
  Rocio v.
  Ross River v.
  Rous sarcoma v.
  RS v.
  rubella v.
  Russian spring-summer en-
    cephalitis v.
  Sabia v.
  St. Louis encephalitis v.
  salivary gland v.
  sandfly fever v's
  sandfly fever-Naples v.
  sandfly fever-Sicilian v.
  satellite v.
  Semliki Forest v.
  Semunya v.
  Sendai v.
  Seoul v.
  Sepik v.
  Simbu v.
  Simbu group v.
  simian v. 40 (SV40)
  simian immunodeficien-
    cy v. (SIV)

virus *(continued)*
  Sindbis v.
  Sin Nombre v.
  slow v.
  smallpox v.
  v.-specific RNA
  Spondweni v.
  street v.
  v. suspension
  swine influenza v.
  Tacaribe v.
  Tahyna v.
  Tamiami v.
  tanapox v.
  temperate v.
  Thogoto v.
  Thogoto-like v's
  tick-borne v's
  tick-borne encephalitis v's
  v. titration
  tobacco mosaic v.
  Toscana v.
  tumor v.
  Turlock v.
  U v.
  Uganda S v.
  Uppsala v.
  Uukuniemi v.
  v. vaccine
  vaccinia v.
  varicella v.
  varicella-zoster v.
  variola v.
  Venezuelan equine en-
    cephalomyelitis v. (VEE
    virus)
  vesicular stomatitis v.
  vesicular stomatitis–like
    v's
  v. virulence
  Wesselsbron v.
  western equine encephalo-
    myelitis v. (WEE virus)
  West Nile v.
  Whataroa v.
  Wyeomyia v.
  Yaba monkey tumor v.
  Yale SK v.

virus *(continued)*
 yellow fever v.
 Zika v.

virusemia

virustatic

visceral
 v. larva migrans
 v. schistosomiasis

vision

vitamin
 v. A
 v. B$_{12}$
 v. B$_{12}$ deficiency
 v. D$_2$
 v. D$_3$
 v. D intoxication
 v. D resistance

vitiligo

vitrectomy

vitronectin (S protein)
 v. receptor

VLA
 very late activation
  VLA antigen
 very late antigen
  VLA-1
  VLA-2
  VLA-3
  VLA-4
  VLA-5
  VLA-6

VLDL
 very-low-density lipoprotein

VMA
 vanillylmandelic acid

Volkmann's membrane

Vollmer
 V's patch skin test
 V's patch test

volume
 blood v.
 cell v.
 v. contraction
 v. hypertension
 v. receptors
 v. regulation
 v.-regulatory decrease
  (VRD)
 urine v.

volume-mediated
 v.-m. hypertension
 v.-m. thirst

volvulosis

vomiting in allergies

von Behring antitoxin

von Gierke disease

von Graefe's sign

von Hippel-Lindau disease

von Krogh transformation

von Pirquet
 von P. hypothesis
 von P. reaction
 von P. test

von Recklinghausen disease

von Willebrand
 von W's disease
 von W's factor

vox cholerica

VpreB

vpr gene (*of HIV*)

vpu gene (*of HIV*)

vpx gene (*of HIV-2*)

VRD
 volume-regulatory decrease

V (variable) region

VSG
    variable surface glycopro-
      tein

vulvovaginal candidiasis

vulvovaginitis
    atrophic v.

vulvovaginitis *(continued)*
    Candida v.
    candidal v.

VZIG
    varicella-zoster immune
      globulin

W
  W box

Waaler-Rose test

WAIHA
  warm autoimmune hemo-
    lytic anemia

waist/hip ratio

Waldenström's macroglobulinemia

Waldeyer's ring

wandering
  w. goiter
  w. histiocyte

war fever

warm
  w. agglutinin
  w. antibody
  w. autoimmune hemolytic
    anemia (WAIHA)
  w. hemagglutinin
  w. nodule
  w.-reactive antibody

wart
  Peruvian w.

Warthin-Finkeldey cells

wasserhelle
  w. cell

Wassermann
  W. antibody
  W. antigen
  W. test

waste
  infectious w.
  w. management

wasting
  w. disease
  w. syndrome

water
  w.-borne infection

water (continued)
  w. deprivation
  w. deprivation test
  w. intake
  w. intoxication
  w. metabolism
  w. permeability
  w. repletion reaction
  total body w.

water balance derangement
  hypertonic w. b. d.
  hypotonic w. b. d.

water-clear cell
  w.-c. c. hyperplasia

water drinking
  compulsive w. d.
  psychogenic w. d.

Waterhouse-Friderichsen syndrome

watery diarrhea syndrome

wax
  tubercle bacillus w.

WB
  Western blot

W box

WDHA
  watery diarrhea, hypokale-
    mia, achlorhydria
      WDHA syndrome

WDHH
  watery diarrhea, hypokale-
    mia, hypochlorhydria
      WDHH syndrome

WEE
  western equine encephalo-
    myelitis
      WEE virus

Wegener's granulomatosis

Weibel-Palade bodies

weight
> body w.
> molecular w.

weight/height
> w./h. ratio
> w./h. tables

Weil
> W's disease
> W.-Felix reaction
> W.-Felix test
> W's syndrome

Weiner theory

Wermer's syndrome

Werner-His disease

Wernicke-Korsakoff syndrome

Wesselsbron
> W. disease
> W. virus

West African trypanosomiasis

Western
> W. blot (WB)
> W. blot analysis
> W. blot assay
> W. blot hybridization
> W. blot immunoassay
> W. blot technique
> W. blot test
> W. blotting

western
> w. equine encephalitis (WEE)
> w. equine encephalomyelitis (WEE)
> w. equine encephalomyelitis virus

West Nile virus

Whataroa virus

Whatman paper

wheal
> w. and erythema reaction

wheal (continued)
> w. and flare reaction
> w. and flare response

Whipple's triad

white
> w. adipose tissue
> w. adrenal line
> w. blood cells
> w.-graft reaction
> w. head
> w. piedra
> w. pulp

whitepox

Whitmore
> W's disease
> W's fever

Whitten effect

WHO
> World Health Organization
> WHO classification

whole
> w. complement assay
> w. complement titer
> w. organism vaccine

whoop

whooping cough
> w. c. toxin

Widal
> W. reaction
> W. test

Widowitz's sign

Wilder's sign

Willis' pancreas

Wilson's disease

window
> anticore w.
> aortopulmonary w.
> skin w.

Winkler's bodies

Winslow's pancreas

Wiskott-Aldrich syndrome

Witebsky
    W's criteria
    W's postulates

withdrawal bleeding

witkop

Wohlbach's n's

Wolff-Chaikoff effect

Wölfler's gland

Wolfram syndrome

Wolhynia fever

Wolman's disease

woody thyroiditis

woolsorter
    w's disease
    w's pneumonia

workup
    diagnostic w.

World Health Organization
    (WHO)

worm
    w. abscess
    parasitic w.

wound
    w. healing

woven bone

wrestler's herpes

Wright's stain

Wuchereria bancrofti

wuchereriasis

Wu and Kabat plots

Wyeomyia virus

X
X autosome translocation
X body
X box
X chromatin
X chromosome
X zone

xanthoma diabeticorum

X autosome translocation

X body

X box

X chromatin

X chromosome

xenoantigen

xenocytophilic

xenogeneic
x. antibodies
x. antigen
x. graft
x. transplantation

xenograft
concordant x.
discordant x.

xenoimmunization

Xenopus
X. complement
X. cytokines
X. cytotoxic cells
X. immunoglobulins
X. lymphomyelocyte tissues
X. MHC (major histocompatibility complex)
X. models for studying immunity
X. oocytes

xenoreactive
x. antibody

xenotropic

xerostomia

xid (X-linked immunodeficiency)

x-irradiation

XLA
X-linked agammaglobulinemia

X-linked
X-l. agammaglobulinemia (XLA)
X-l. familial hypophosphatemia
X-l. hyper IgM syndrome
X-l. hypogammaglobulinemia
X-l. hypophosphatemia
X-l. immune deficiency
X-l. immunodeficiency
X-l. infantile agammaglobulinemia
X-l. infantile hypogammaglobulinemia
X-l. lymphoproliferative disease
X-l. lymphoproliferative syndrome
X-l. severe combined immunodeficiency (X-linked SCID)

XO gonadal dysgenesis (*same as* Turner syndrome)

XO karyotype

XO/XX mosaicism

x-ray
skull x-r.

XX
XX disorder
XX gonadal dysgenesis
XX male syndrome
XX true hemaphroditism

X–X translocation

XXY syndrome

Y
- Y body
- Y box
- Y chromatin
- Y chromosome
- Y chromosome genes

Yaba monkey tumor virus

yabapox

YAG-type laser

Yale SK virus

Yangtze Valley fever

Yatapoxvirus

Yates' correction

yaws

Y body

Y box

Y chromatin

Y chromosome

Y chromosome genes

yeast
- y. cell test

yellow
- y. fever
- y. fever vaccine
- y. fever virus

Yersinia
- *Y.* arthritis
- *Y. enterocolitica*
- *Y. frederiksenii*
- *Y. intermedia*
- *Y. kristensenii*
- *Y. pestis*
- *Y. pseudotuberculosis*

yersiniosis

yohimbe

yolk sac

Yssel's medium

YY disorder

Zahorsky's syndrome

Zamboni fixation

ZAP
  zeta-associated protein
    ZAP-70
    ZAP kinase

zeitgebers (*Ger. "time-givers"*)

zeta (ζ)
  z.-associated protein-70
  z. chain
  z. potential

Ziagen

zidovudine

ZIFT
  zygote intrafallopian trans-
    fer

Zika virus

zinc deficiency

zirconium sensitivity

Zollinger-Ellison syndrome

zona *pl.* zonae
  z. fasciculata
  z. glomerulosa
  z. pellucida
  z. reticularis

zone
  active z's
  androgenic z.
  z. of antibody excess
  z. of antigen excess
  cortical z.
  definitive z. of adrenal cor-
    tex
  z. of equivalence
  fascicular z.
  fetal z. of adrenal cortex
  glomerular z.
  mantle z.

zone *(continued)*
  marginal z.
  z. of optimal proportions
  reticular z.
  sudanophobic z.
  thymus-dependent z.
  thymus-independent z.
  X z.

zoning

zoodermic

zoografting

zoohormone

zoonosis *pl.* zoonoses

zoonotic
  z. risk

zoophilic

zoophilous

zooplasty

zooprecipitin

zooprophylaxis

zoosis

zoster
  z. immune globulin (ZIG)
  z. sine eruptione
  z. sine herpete

zosteriform

zosteroid

Zygomycetes

zygomycosis
  rhinocerebral z.
  rhinofacial z.
  subcutaneous z.

zygote
  z. intrafallopian transfer
    (ZIFT)

zymogen

zymosan

Drugs Used in Immunology and Endocrinology

Below are the names of generic and ℞ brand name drugs used in immunology and endocrinology, as shown in the *Saunders Pharmaceutical Xref Book*. The drugs are categorized by their "indications"—also called "designated use," "approved use," or "therapeutic action"—which group together drugs used for a similar purpose. The indications shown below are broad categories of therapeutic action. Individual drugs may be placed in subcategories or have specifically targeted diseases beyond the scope of this listing. For complete information about the drugs listed below, including each drug's availability, specific indications, forms of administration, and dosages, please consult the current edition of *Saunders Pharmaceutical Word Book*.

AIDS [*see: HIV Infections*]

Antibiotics
[*see also: Antidiarrheal Agents, Intestinal Antibacterials; Antiprotozoals; Antituberculosis Agents*]

Antibiotics, Aminoglycosides
amikacin
amikacin sulfate
Amikin
Garamycin
Garamycin Pediatric
gentamicin sulfate
Humatin
Jenamicin
kanamycin sulfate
Kantrex
MiKasome
Mycifradin Sulfate
Nebcin
Neo-fradin
Neo-Tabs
neomycin sulfate
netilmicin sulfate
Netromycin
paromomycin sulfate
Scheinpharm Tobramycin ⊛
Septopal

Antibiotics, Aminoglycosides (continued)
streptomycin sulfate
TOBI
tobramycin
tobramycin sulfate

Antibiotics, Carbapenems
imipenem
Lorabid
loracarbef
meropenem
Merrem
Primaxin I.M.
Primaxin I.V.

Antibiotics, Cephalosporins
Ancef
Apo-Cefaclor ⊛
Biocef
Ceclor
Ceclor CD
Ceclor CDpak
Cedax
cefaclor
cefadroxil
Cefadyl
cefamandole nafate
cefazolin sodium
cefdinir
cefditoren pivoxil

Antibiotics, Cephalosporins (continued)

cefepime HCl
cefixime
Cefizox
cefmetazole sodium
Cefobid
cefodizime
cefonicid sodium
cefoperazone sodium
Cefotan
cefotaxime sodium
cefotetan disodium
cefoxitin sodium
cefpodoxime proxetil
cefprozil
ceftazidime
ceftibuten
Ceftin
ceftizoxime sodium
ceftriaxone sodium
cefuroxime axetil
cefuroxime sodium
Cefzil
cephalexin
cephalexin HCl
cephalothin sodium
cephapirin sodium
cephradine
Ceptaz
Claforan
Duricef
Fortaz
Keflex
Keflin, Neutral
Keftab
Kefurox
Kefzol
Mandol
Maxipime
Mefoxin
Modivid
Monocid
Novo-Cefaclor ⑭
Omnicef
Rocephin
Spectracef
Suprax
Tazicef
Tazidime

Antibiotics, Cephalosporins (continued)

Vantin
Velosef
Zefazone
Zinacef
Zolicef

Antibiotics, Fluoroquinolones

alatrofloxacin mesylate
Apo-Norflox ⑭
Apo-Oflox ⑭
Avelox
Cipro
ciprofloxacin
enoxacin
Floxin
gatifloxacin
grepafloxacin HCl
Levaquin
levofloxacin
lomefloxacin HCl
Maxaquin; Maxaquin-3
moxifloxacin HCl
norfloxacin
Noroxin
Novo-Norfloxacin ⑭
ofloxacin
Penetrex
Raxar
sparfloxacin
Tequin
trovafloxacin mesylate
Trovan
Trovan/Zithromax Compliance Pak
Zagam

Antibiotics, Glycopeptides

Lyphocin
Targocid
teicoplanin
Vancocin
Vancoled
vancomycin HCl

Antibiotics, Lincosamides

Cleocin
Cleocin Pediatric
Cleocin Phosphate
clindamycin
clindamycin HCl
clindamycin palmitate HCl
clindamycin phosphate

Antibiotics, Lincosamides (continued)
Dalacin C (CAN)
Dalacin C Phosphate (CAN)
HyClinda
Lincocin
lincomycin HCl
Lincorex
Antibiotics, Macrolides
azithromycin
Biaxin
Biaxin XL
clarithromycin
dirithromycin
Dynabac
E.E.S.
E.E.S. 200
E.E.S. 400
Eramycin
Ery-Tab
EryPed
EryPed 200; EryPed 400
Erythrocin
Erythrocin Stearate
erythromycin
erythromycin estolate
erythromycin ethylsuccinate (EES)
erythromycin gluceptate
erythromycin lactobionate
erythromycin stearate
Eryzole
Ilosone
Ilotycin Gluceptate
PCE
Pediazole
Prevpac
Robimycin
Tao
troleandomycin
Trovan/Zithromax Compliance Pak
Zithromax
Zithromax (CAN)
Antibiotics, Penicillins
amoxicillin
amoxicillin sodium
Amoxil
ampicillin
ampicillin sodium
Augmentin
bacampicillin HCl

Antibiotics, Penicillins (continued)
Bactocill
Beepen-VK
Betapen-VK
Bicillin C-R; Bicillin C-R 900/300
Bicillin L-A
Biomox
carbenicillin indanyl sodium
cloxacillin sodium
Cloxapen
Crysticillin 300 A.S.; Crysticillin 600 A.S.
D-Amp
dicloxacillin sodium
Dycill
Dynapen
Gen-Amoxicillin (CAN)
Geocillin
Ledercillin VK
Marcillin
methicillin sodium
Mezlin
mezlocillin
Nafcil
nafcillin sodium
Nallpen
Omnipen
Omnipen-N
oxacillin sodium
Pathocil
Pen-V
Pen-Vee K
penicillin G benzathine
penicillin G potassium
penicillin G procaine
penicillin G sodium
penicillin V potassium
Penicillin VK
Permapen
Pfizerpen
Pfizerpen-AS
piperacillin sodium
Pipracil
Polycillin
Polycillin-N
Polycillin-PRB
Polymox
Principen
Probampacin
Prostaphlin

Antibiotics, Penicillins (continued)
Robicillin VK
Spectrobid
Staphcillin
Tegopen
Ticar
ticarcillin disodium
Timentin
Totacillin
Totacillin-N
Trimox
Unasyn
Unipen
V-Cillin K
Veetids
Veetids '125'; Veetids '250'
Wycillin
Wymox
Zosyn

Antibiotics, Sulfonamides
Bactrim IV
Bactrim Pediatric
Bactrim; Bactrim DS
Cotrim Pediatric
Cotrim; Cotrim D.S.
Eryzole
Gantanol
Gantrisin
Pediazole
Septra
Septra DS
Septra IV
sulfacytine
sulfadoxine
sulfamethizole
sulfamethoxazole (SMX; SMZ)
Sulfatrim
sulfisoxazole
sulfisoxazole acetyl
Thiosulfil Forte
trisulfapyrimidines

Antibiotics, Tetracyclines
Achromycin V
Bio-Tab
Declomycin
demeclocycline HCl
Doryx
Doxy 100; Doxy 200
Doxy Caps
Doxychel Hyclate

Antibiotics, Tetracyclines (continued)
doxycycline
doxycycline calcium
doxycycline hyclate
Dynacin
Helidac
Minocin
minocycline HCl
Monodox
Nor-Tet
oxytetracycline
oxytetracycline HCl
Panmycin
Periostat
Robitet
Sumycin
Sumycin '250'; Sumycin '500'
Teline; Teline-500
Terramycin
Terramycin IM
Tetracap
tetracycline HCl
Tetralan
Tetralan "250"; Tetralan-500
Tetram
Uri-Tet
Vectrin
Vibra-Tabs
Vibramycin

Antibiotics, Other (including Synergists)
Aerosporin
Albamycin
Altracin
Azactam
aztreonam
Baci-IM
bacitracin
bactericidal and permeability-increasing (BPI) protein, recombinant
Bactrim IV
Bactrim Pediatric
Bactrim; Bactrim DS
Centoxin
chloramphenicol
chloramphenicol sodium succinate
Chloromycetin
Chloromycetin Sodium Succinate
Cidecin

Antibiotics, Other (including Synergists) (continued)
clavulanate potassium
clofazimine
colistimethate sodium
colistin sulfate
Coly-Mycin M
Coly-Mycin S
Cotrim Pediatric
Cotrim; Cotrim D.S.
dalfopristin
daptomycin
evernimicin
Factive
Flagyl
Flagyl ER
Flagyl IV
Flagyl IV RTU
furazolidone
Furoxone
gemifloxacin mesylate
Helidac
Ketek
Lamprene
linezolid
Metaret
Metro I.V.
metronidazole
metronidazole HCl
Mycobutin
nebacumab
Neuprex
Normix
novobiocin calcium
polymyxin B sulfate
Primsol
Proloprim
Protostat
quinupristin
Renoquid
rifabutin
rifaximin
Rifaximin
ritamycin
Rituxan
rituximab
Septra
Septra DS
Septra IV
spectinomycin HCl

Antibiotics, Other (including Synergists) (continued)
Spexil
sulbactam sodium
Sulfatrim
suramin hexasodium
Synercid
telithromycin
trimethoprim (TMP)
Trimpex
Trobicin
trospectomycin sulfate
Unasyn
Ziracin
Zovant
Zyvox

Antiemetics and Antinauseants
alosetron HCl
Anergan 50
Antivert; Antivert/25; Antivert/50
Antrizine
Anzemet
Apo-Domperidone Ⓒᴬᴺ
Apo-Perphenazine Ⓒᴬᴺ
Apo-Trifluoperazine Ⓒᴬᴺ
Arrestin
chlorpromazine
chlorpromazine HCl
Clopra
Compazine
dimenhydrinate
Dimetabs
Dinate
diphenidol HCl
dolasetron mesylate
domperidone
Dramamine
Dramanate
Dramilin
Dramoject
dronabinol
droperidol
Dymenate
E-Vista
Emitasol
granisetron HCl
Hydrate
hydroxyzine HCl

Antiemetics and Antinauseants (continued)
Hyzine-50
Inapsine
K-Phen-50
Kytril
Marinol
Marmine
Maxolon
meclizine HCl
Meni-D
metoclopramide HCl
metoclopramide monohydrochloride monohydrate
MK-869
Motilium ⓒⒶⓃ
Norzine
Novo-Domperidone ⓒⒶⓃ
Nu-Prochlor ⓒⒶⓃ
Octamide PFS
ondansetron HCl
Ormazine
Pentazine
perphenazine
Phenameth
Phenazine 25
Phenazine 50
Phenergan
Phenergan Fortis
Phenergan Plain
Phenoject-50
phosphorated carbohydrate solution (hyperosmolar solution with phosphoric acid)
Pramidin
Pro-50
prochlorperazine
prochlorperazine bimaleate
prochlorperazine edisylate
prochlorperazine maleate
prochlorperazine mesylate
Prometh
Prometh-50
promethazine HCl
Prorex-25; Prorex-50
Prothazine
Prothazine Plain
Quiess
Reclomide
Reglan

Antiemetics and Antinauseants (continued)
Ru-Vert-M
Scopace
scopolamine hydrobromide
Stelazine
Stemetil ⓒⒶⓃ
T-Gen
Tebamide
thiethylperazine
thiethylperazine malate
Thorazine
Ticon
Tigan
Torecan
Transderm Scōp
Triban; Pediatric Triban
trifluoperazine HCl
Trilafon
Trimazide
trimethobenzamide HCl
V-Gan 25; V-Gan 50
Vistacon
Vistaject-25; Vistaject-50
Vistaril
Vistazine 50
Vontrol
Zofran
Zofran ODT

Antineoplastics, Therapeutic Vaccines (Theraccines)
AdjuVax-100a
Avicine
BrevaRex
Gastrimmune
GVAX
M-Vax
Melacine
melanoma vaccine
monoclonal antibody B43.13
NovoVac
O-Vax
OncoVax-CL
OncoVax-Pr
OvaRex
TA-HPV
Theratope-STn
vaccinia virus vaccine for human papillomavirus (HPV), recombinant

Antituberculosis Agents
[see also: Antibiotics]
aminosalicylate sodium (p-aminosalicylate sodium)
aminosalicylic acid (4-aminosalicylic acid)
aminosidine
BCG vaccine (bacillus Calmette-Guérin)
Capastat Sulfate
capreomycin sulfate
clofazimine
cycloserine (L-cycloserine)
ethambutol HCl
ethionamide
Gabbromicina
isoniazid
Lamprene
Laniazid
Laniazid C.T.
Myambutol
Nydrazid
Paromomycin
Paser
Priftin
pyrazinamide (PZA)
Rifadin
Rifamate
rifampin
rifapentine
Rifater
Rimactane
Rimactane/INH
Seromycin
Sodium P.A.S.
streptomycin sulfate
Tice BCG
Trecator-SC

Antivenin [see: Immunizing Agents, Immune Extracts]

Antivirals
[see also: HIV Infections, Viral]
Antivirals, Systemic
abacavir succinate
acyclovir
acyclovir sodium
adefovir dipivoxil
amantadine HCl

Antivirals, Systemic (continued)
Apo-Acyclovir Ⓒᴬᴺ
atevirdine mesylate
Aztec
Combivir
Crixivan
Cytovene
didanosine
Doxovir
emtricitabine
Epivir
Epivir-HBV
famciclovir
Famvir
Flumadine
Fortovase
ganciclovir
ganciclovir sodium
Genvir
Heptovir Ⓒᴬᴺ
Hivid
indinavir sulfate
interferon alfa-2b (IFN-α2)
interferon alfa-n1
Intron A
Invirase
lamivudine
lysine (L-lysine)
Norvir
oseltamivir phosphate
Ostavir
Papirine
pleconaril
Preveon
Rebetol
Rebetron
Relenza
Retrovir
ribavirin
rimantadine HCl
ritonavir
saquinavir
saquinavir mesylate
stavudine
Symadine
Symmetrel
Tamiflu
tuvirumab
valacyclovir HCl
valganciclovir HCl

Antivirals, Systemic (continued)
Valtrex
vidarabine
Videx
Virazole
Wellferon
zalcitabine
zanamivir
Zeffix
Zerit
Ziagen
zidovudine
Zovirax

Diabetes Agents
Diabetes Agents, Insulin
AERx
Humalog
Humalog Mix 75/25
insulin
insulin aspart
insulin glargine
insulin lispro
insulin lispro protamine
Lantus
NovoLog
NovoPen 1.5
NovoRapid
Oralgen; Oralin ⓒⒶⓃ
Regular Iletin II U-500 (concentrated)
Diabetes Agents, Oral Agents
acetohexamide
Actos
Amaryl
Avandia
Basen
bromocriptine mesylate
chlorpropamide
Diaβeta (or DiaBeta)
Diab II
Diabinese
Diapid
Dymelor
Ergoset
Euglucon ⓒⒶⓃ
Gen-Gliclazide ⓒⒶⓃ
gliclazide
glimepiride

Diabetes Agents, Oral Agents (continued)
glipizide
GlucoNorm ⓒⒶⓃ
Glucophage
Glucotrol
Glucotrol XL
Glucovance
Glustat
glyburide
Glynase
Glyset
IGF-1/BP3 complex
INS-1
lypressin
metformin HCl
Micronase
Micronized Glyburide
miglitol
moxonidine
nateglinide
Oralgen; Oralin ⓒⒶⓃ
Orinase
Physiotens
pioglitazone HCl
pramlintide
pramlintide acetate
Prandase ⓒⒶⓃ
Prandin
Precose
repaglinide
Rezulin
rosiglitazone maleate
Starlix
Symlin
tolazamide
tolbutamide
Tolinase
troglitazone
voglibose
Diabetes Agents, Related Disorders
alprostadil, liposomal
Alredase
Apligraf
Apo-Domperidone ⓒⒶⓃ
Axokine
becaplermin
Cytolex
Dermagraft; Dermagraft-TC
domperidone

Diabetes Agents, Related Disorders (continued
epalrestat
graftskin
Locilex
memantine
Motilium ⓒⓐⓝ
Novo-Domperidone ⓒⓐⓝ
pexiganan acetate
pimagedine HCl
Regranex
tolrestat

HIV Infections
[see also: Antibiotics; Antiemetics and Antinauseants; Antituberculosis Agents; Antivirals; Immunizing Agents; Immunostimulants]
HIV Infections, Bacterial
aminosidine
azithromycin
Biaxin
Biaxin XL
clarithromycin
diethylhomospermine (DEHOP; DEHSPM)
ethambutol HCl
gentamicin sulfate
isoniazid
Laniazid
Laniazid C.T.
letrazuril
Maitec
Myambutol
Mycobutin
Nydrazid
Paromomycin
Priftin
rifabutin
Rifadin
Rifamate
rifampin
rifapentine
Rifater
Rimactane
Rimactane/INH
Synsorb Cd
Zithromax
Zithromax ⓒⓐⓝ

HIV Infections, Fungal
Abelcet
AmBisome
Amphotec
amphotericin B cholesteryl sulfate
amphotericin B deoxycholate
amphotericin B lipid complex (ABLC)
Apo-Ketoconazole ⓒⓐⓝ
Diflucan
fluconazole
Fungizone
itraconazole
ketoconazole
Nizoral
Sporanox
HIV Infections, Parasitic
albendazole
atovaquone
azithromycin
Bactrim IV
Bactrim Pediatric
Bactrim; Bactrim DS
Biaxin
Biaxin XL
clarithromycin
Cotrim Pediatric
Cotrim; Cotrim D.S.
Daraprim
Mepron
NeuTrexin
NebuPent
Pentacarinat
Pentam 300
pentamidine isethionate
Pneumopent
pyrimethamine
Septra
Septra DS
Septra IV
sulfadiazine
sulfamethoxazole (SMX; SMZ)
Sulfatrim
trimethoprim (TMP)
trimetrexate glucuronate
Zithromax
Zithromax ⓒⓐⓝ
HIV Infections, Viral
abacavir succinate
abacavir sulfate

HIV Infections, Viral (continued)

acemannan
activated cellular therapy (ACT)
adefovir dipivoxil
Agenerase
AIDS vaccine
AIDSVax
Alferon LDO
Ampligen
amprenavir
amprenavir & indinavir sulfate
amprenavir & lamivudine & zidovudine
amprenavir & nelfinavir mesylate
amprenavir & saquinavir
Anticort
AR-177
atevirdine mesylate
Aztec
benzimidavir
Bravavir
Bucast
calanolide A
Carrisyn
CD4, human truncated 369 AA
  polypeptide
CD4, recombinant soluble human
  (rCD4)
celgosivir HCl
cidofovir
Combivir
Coviracil
Crixivan
crofelemer
Cymeval
cytolin
Cytovene
delavirdine mesylate
dextran sulfate
didanosine
didanosine & nevirapine & zidovudine
didanosine & zidovudine
docosanol (n-docosanol)
efavirenz
efavirenz & lamivudine & zidovudine
emtricitabine
Epivir
filgrastim
fomivirsen sodium

HIV Infections, Viral (continued)

Fortovase
Forvade
foscarnet sodium
Foscavir
ganciclovir
ganciclovir sodium
Genevax-HIV
gp120 (glycoprotein 120) antigens
gp160 (glycoprotein 160) antigens
HIV immunotherapeutic (HIV-IT);
  HIV therapeutic
HIV-1 peptide vaccine
Hivid
hypericin
Inactivin
indinavir sulfate
indinavir sulfate & amprenavir
inosine pranobex
interferon alfa-n3
interleukin-10 (IL-10)
Invirase
Isoprinosine
lamivudine
lamivudine & saquinavir mesylate &
  ritonavir
lamivudine & zidovudine & amprenavir
lamivudine & zidovudine & efavirenz
Lidakol
lodenosine
lopinavir
MultiKine
nelfinavir mesylate
nelfinavir mesylate & amprenavir
nevirapine
nevirapine & zidovudine & didanosine
Norvir
Novapren
Panavir
pentafuside
poly I: poly C12U
Preveon
probucol
procaine HCl
Protovir
Receptin
Remune
Rescriptor

HIV Infections, Viral (continued)
Retrovir
ritonavir
ritonavir & lamivudine & saquinavir mesylate
ritonavir & zidovudine & saquinavir
mesylate
saquinavir
saquinavir & amprenavir
saquinavir mesylate
saquinavir mesylate & ritonavir &
lamivudine
saquinavir mesylate & ritonavir &
zidovudine
Savvy
Scriptene
sevirumab
Soluble T4
sorivudine
stavudine
Sustiva
T-cell gene therapy
TAT antagonist
tenofovir disoproxil fumarate (tenofovir DF)
Tenovil
tetrachlorodecaoxide
thymopentin
Timunox
tipranavir disodium
tirilazad mesylate
trichosanthin
tucaresol
tumor necrosis factor (TNF)
Uendex
valganciclovir HCl
VaxSyn HIV-1
vidarabine
Videx
VIMRxyn
Vira-A
Viracept
Viramune
Virend
Vistide
Vitrasert
Vitravene
zalcitabine
Zerit
Ziagen

HIV Infections, Viral (continued)
zidovudine
zidovudine & amprenavir & lamivudine
zidovudine & didanosine
zidovudine & didanosine & nevirapine
zidovudine & efavirenz & lamivudine
zidovudine & saquinavir mesylate &
ritonavir
Zintevir
**HIV Infections, Other Related Dis-
orders**
Alferon N
alitretinoin
alitretinoin & interferon
amikacin
9-aminocamptothecin (9-AC)
Androderm
AndroGel
Androgel-DHT
Atragen
Avonex
Betaseron
bexarotene
Cachexon
Caelyx ⒢
Coactinon
crofelemer
Cryptaz
Cryptosporidium parvum bovine
colostrum IgG concentrate
DaunoXome
daunorubicin citrate, liposomal
diethylhomospermine (DEHOP;
DEHSPM)
dihydrotestosterone (DHT)
docosanol (n-docosanol)
doxorubicin HCl, liposome-encapsu-
lated (LED)
dronabinol
edodekin alfa
emivirine
epoetin alfa (EPO)
Epogen
gallium nitrate
Geref
L-glutathione, reduced
Hepandrin
Immuno-C

HIV Infections, Other Related Disorders (continued)

interferon & alitretinoin
interferon alfa
interferon alfa-2a (IFN-αA; rIFN-A)
interferon alfa-2b (IFN-α2)
interferon beta (IFN-B)
interferon beta-1a
interferon beta-1b
Intron A
Lidakol
LymphoCide
Marinol
Megace
megestrol acetate
memantine
MiKasome
monoclonal antibody LL2, humanized
monoclonal antibody to CD22 antigen on B-cells, radiolabeled
Nipent
nitazoxanide (NTZ)
Omniferon
Oxandrin
oxandrolone
Panretin
PEG-Intron A
pentostatin
phenylhydrazone
poloxamer 331
Procrit
Proleukin
Protox
Provir
r-IFN-beta
R-Frone
rifalazil
Roferon-A
sermorelin acetate
Sporidin-G
SU-5416
Targretin
testosterone
thalidomide
Thalomid
TheraDerm
topotecan HCl
Veldona
Virulizin

Hormones
Hormones, Anterior Pituitary

Cortrosyn
cosyntropin
Genotropin
Geref
Humatrope
Norditropin
Norditropin SimpleXx
Nutropin
Nutropin AQ
Nutropin Depot
pegvisomant
Protropin
Protropin II
Saizen
sermorelin acetate
Serostim
somatrem
somatropin
Somavert
Umatrope

Hormones, Hypothalamic

buserelin acetate
deslorelin
Factrel
gonadorelin acetate
gonadorelin HCl
goserelin acetate
histrelin
histrelin acetate
Lupron Depot; Lupron Depot-Ped
Lupron Depot–3 month; Lupron Depot–4 month
Lupron; Lupron Pediatric
Lutrepulse
nafarelin acetate
octreotide acetate
ProMaxx-100
Reducin
Sandostatin
Sandostatin LAR Depot
Somagard
somatostatin (SS)
Supprelin
Suprefact ⒸⒶⓃ
Suprefact; Suprefact Depot ⒸⒶⓃ
Synarel
Zecnil
Zoladex

Hormones, Pancreatic
  GlucaGen Emergency Kit
  glucagon
  Glucagon Emergency Kit
Hormones, Posterior Pituitary
  DDAVP
  desmopressin acetate
  Diapid
  lypressin
  oxytocin
  Pitocin
  Pitressin Synthetic
  Stimate
  Syntocinon
  vasopressin (VP)
Hypoglycemics [see: Diabetes Agents]

Immunizing Agents
  [see also: Immunostimulants]
Immunizing Agents, Bacterial Vaccines
  Acel-Imune
  Acel-P ⓒⒶ
  ActHIB
  ActHIB/Tripedia
  BCG vaccine (bacillus Calmette-Guérin)
  Certiva
  cholera vaccine
  Comvax
  diphtheria & tetanus toxoids & acellular pertussis vaccine (DTaP)
  diphtheria & tetanus toxoids & whole-cell pertussis vaccine (DTwP)
  diphtheria & tetanus toxoids, adsorbed (DT; Td)
  diphtheria toxoid, adsorbed
  Hemophilus b conjugate vaccine
  HibTITER
  ImmuCyst ⓒⒶ
  Infanrix
  lipoprotein OspA, recombinant
  LYMErix
  meningococcal polysaccharide vaccine, group A
  meningococcal polysaccharide vaccine, group C

Immunizing Agents, Bacterial Vaccines (continued)
  meningococcal polysaccharide vaccine, group W-135
  meningococcal polysaccharide vaccine, group Y
  Menomune-A/C/Y/W-135
  mixed respiratory vaccine (MRV)
  MRV
  OmniHIB
  OncoTICE ⓒⒶ
  Pacis ⓒⒶ
  PedvaxHIB
  pertussis vaccine adsorbed
  plague vaccine
  Pneumo 23 ⓒⒶ
  pneumococcal polysaccharide vaccine
  pneumococcal vaccine, 7-valent
  pneumococcal vaccine, polyvalent
  Pneumovax 23
  Pnu-Imune 23
  Prevnar
  ProHIBiT
  Quilimmune-P
  SPL-Serologic types I and III
  StaphVAX
  staphage lysate (SPL)
  tetanus toxoid
  Tetramune
  TheraCys
  Tice BCG
  Tri-Immunol
  TriHIBit
  Tripedia
  Typherex
  Typhim Vi
  typhoid vaccine
  typhoid Vi capsular polysaccharide vaccine
  Typhoid Vaccine (AKD)
  Typhoid Vaccine (H-P)
  Vivotif Berna
Immunizing Agents, Immune Extracts
  antivenin (Crotalidae) polyvalent (ovine) Fab
  antivenin (Latrodectus mactans)
  CroTab
  diphtheria antitoxin

Immunizing Agents, Immunoglobulins

Atgam
CytoGam
cytomegalovirus immune globulin, human
Gamastan
Gamimune N
Gammagard S/D
Gammar
Gammar-IV
Gammar-P IV
Gamulin Rh
globulin, immune
H-BIG
Hep-B-Gammagee
hepatitis B immune globulin (HBIG)
HIV immune globulin (HIVIG)
HIV-IG
Hyper-Tet
Hyperab
HyperHep
Hypermune RSV
HypRho-D; HypRho-D Mini-Dose
Imogam
Iveegam
lymphocyte immune globulin, antithymocyte
MICRhoGAM
Mini-Gamulin Rh
Nabi-HB
Nashville Rabbit Antithymocyte Serum
Polygam
Polygam S/D
rabies immune globulin (RIG)
RespiGam
respiratory syncytial virus immune globulin (RSV-IG)
$Rh_0(D)$ immune globulin
RhoGAM
Sandoglobulin
tetanus immune globulin (TIG)
varicella-zoster immune globulin (VZIG)
Venoglobulin-I
Venoglobulin-S
WinRho SD; WinRho SDF

Immunizing Agents, Viral Vaccines

[see also: HIV Infections, Viral]

Immunizing Agents, Viral Vaccines (continued)

AIDS vaccine
AIDSVax
Arilvax
Attenuvax
Biavax II
ChimeriVax
Comvax
Engerix-B
FluMist
Fluogen
FluShield
Fluvirin
Fluzone
Genevax-HIV
gp120 (glycoprotein 120) antigens
Havrix
Hepagene
hepatitis A vaccine, inactivated
hepatitis B virus vaccine, inactivated
HIV-1 peptide vaccine
Imovax
influenza virus vaccine
IPOL
Japanese encephalitis (JE) virus vaccine
JE-VAX
M-M-R II
M-R-Vax II
measles & rubella virus vaccine, live
measles, mumps & rubella virus vaccine, live
measles virus vaccine, live
Meruvax II
mumps virus vaccine, live
Mumpsvax
Orimune
poliovirus vaccine, inactivated (IPV)
poliovirus vaccine, live oral (OPV)
Priorix ⓐ
RabAvert
rabies vaccine
Recombivax HB
Remune
Rotamune
RotaShield
rotavirus vaccine
rubella & mumps virus vaccine, live
rubella virus vaccine, live

Immunizing Agents, Viral Vaccines (continued)
thymalfasin
Vaqta
varicella virus vaccine
Varivax
Vaxigrip ⒸⒶ
yellow fever vaccine
YF-Vax
Zadaxin

Immunizing Agents, Immunostim-ulating Adjuncts
aldesleukin
Alferon LDO
Alferon N
ancestim
Avonex
Betaseron
diethyldithiocarbamate
filgrastim
Infergen
interferon alfa
Intron A
levamisole HCl
Maxamine
Neupogen
Omniferon
PEG-Intron A
Proleukin
r-IFN-beta
R-Frone
Rebetron
Rebif ⒸⒶ
Roferon-A
Stemgen
tetrachlorodecaoxide
Veldona
Wellferon
Wellferon ⒸⒶ

Immunostimulants
[*see also: HIV Infections; Immunizing Agents*]
acetylcysteine (*N*-acetylcysteine)
Actimmune
Aldara
Aliminase
Ampligen
beta alethine

Immunostimulants (continued)
Beta LT
Betafectin
cilmostim
coenzyme Q10
Copaxone
disaccharide tripeptide glycerol dipalmitoyl
Ergamisol
Fluimucil
glatiramer acetate
Iamin
ImmTher
imiquimod
Imreg-1
Imuthiol
interferon alfa
interferon alfa-2a (IFN-αA; rIFN-A)
interferon alfa-2b (IFN-α2)
interferon alfa-n1
interferon alfa-n3
interferon alfacon-1
interferon beta (IFN-B)
interferon beta-1a
interferon beta-1b
interferon gamma-1b
interleukin-4 receptor (IL-4R)
Leucomax
Leucotropin
Leukine
Linomide
lisofylline (LSF)
Macstim
Megagen
megakaryocyte growth and develop-ment factor, pegylated, recombi-nant human
milodistim
molgramostim
Neumega
Nuvance
oprelvekin
oxothiazolidine carboxylate (L-2-oxothiazolidine-4-carboxylic acid)
PGG glucan
Pixykine
poly I: poly C12U
prezatide copper acetate
Procysteine
regramostim

Immunostimulants (continued)
Remune
roquinimex
sargramostim
Stimulon
T-cell gene therapy
thalidomide
Thalomid
thymopentin
Timunox
tucaresol
Vendona

Immunosuppressants
abetimus sodium
anti-human thymocyte immuno-
    globulin, rabbit
Atgam
azathioprine
azathioprine sodium
basiliximab
Campath 1H
CellCept
Centara
cyclosporine
dacliximab
daclizumab

Immunosuppressants (continued)
Imuran
lymphocyte immune globulin, anti-
    thymocyte
muromonab-CD3
mycophenolate mofetil
mycophenolate mofetil HCl
Nashville Rabbit Antithymocyte
    Serum
Neoral
Orthoclone OKT3
priliximab
Prograf
Rapamune
Sandimmune
Sandimmune Neoral ⒸⒶⓃ
SangCya
Simulect
sirolimus
tacrolimus
Thymoglobulin
triptolide
Zenapax
Nausea [see: *Antiemetics and Antinau-
seants*]
Tuberculosis [see: *Antituberculosis
Agents*]
Vaccines [see: *Immunizing Agents*]

9577